250 best
beans, lentils
& tofu recipes

Healthy, Wholesome Foods

Robert
ROSE

250 Best Beans, Lentils & Tofu Recipes
Text copyright © 2012 Robert Rose Inc.
Photographs copyright © 2012 Robert Rose Inc.
Cover and text design copyright © 2012 Robert Rose Inc.

Part of this book was previously published by Robert Rose Inc. in 2000 under the title *The Beans, Lentils & Tofu Gourmet*.

For a complete list of contributing authors, see page 278.
For complete cataloguing information, see page 288.

Disclaimer
The recipes in this book have been carefully tested by our kitchen and our tasters. To the best of our knowledge, they are safe and nutritious for ordinary use and users. For those people with food or other allergies, or who have special food requirements or health issues, please read the suggested contents of each recipe carefully and determine whether or not they may create a problem for you. All recipes are used at the risk of the consumer.

We cannot be responsible for any hazards, loss or damage that may occur as a result of any recipe use.

For those with special needs, allergies, requirements or health problems, in the event of any doubt, please contact your medical adviser prior to the use of any recipe.

Design and Production: PageWave Graphics Inc.
Editor: Judith Finlayson
Copyeditor: Gillian Watts
Proofreader: Gillian Watts
Indexer: Gillian Watts

Photography: Colin Erricson and Mark T. Shapiro
Cover image: Teriyaki Rice Noodles with Veggies and Beans (page 217)

We acknowledge the financial support of the Government of Canada through the Book Publishing Industry Development Program (BPIDP) for our publishing activities.

Published by Robert Rose Inc.
120 Eglinton Avenue East, Suite 800, Toronto, Ontario, Canada M4P 1E2
Tel: (416) 322-6552 Fax: (416) 322-6936
www.robertrose.ca

Printed and bound in Canada

1 2 3 4 5 6 7 8 9 FP 20 19 18 17 16 15 14 13 12

Contents

Foreword 4

Introduction 5

Appetizers 15

Soups 39

Salads and Dressings 73

Wraps, Rolls, Sandwiches and Burgers 99

Chilies 123

Curry and Dal 149

Mains with Meat, Poultry, Fish and Seafood 173

Meatless Mains 215

Sides and Small Plates 263

Contributors 278

Index 279

Foreword

Great discoveries are often accidental. If Archimedes hadn't been taking a bath, he wouldn't have devised the basic principle of hydrostatics. And if Isaac Newton had not been in the path of a falling apple, he might never have given us the theory of gravity. Christopher Columbus, too, was no stranger to chance. He set sail for Cathay in search of valuable spices such as cinnamon and cloves; instead, he landed in the New World, where he discovered allspice, cocoa, chile peppers — and the haricot bean.

Not that beans, as such, were new to European cooks. Beans (and their botanical relation, lentils) had been cultivated by the ancient Egyptians, as well as the Greeks and the Romans, among others. Both beans and lentils made their way across Europe as civilization moved north and west. By the time Columbus set sail for America, Europe's favorite bean was the broad (or fava) bean. The haricot bean, small, white and oval in shape, was something quite new. Its discovery further enriched Europeans' knowledge of that category of food we know today as legumes, which includes chickpeas, beans, soybeans and lentils.

Today legumes remain one of the world's most widely consumed and versatile foods. But the fact is that, in North America at least, beans and lentils (and their soybean-derived relative tofu) have something of an image problem. They are often perceived as difficult to cook. In addition, they have acquired a reputation for being bland and unexciting. However, as the recipes in this book demonstrate, nothing could be farther from the truth.

Over the centuries, tofu and legumes have earned their stripes as key ingredients in many signature dishes of countries around the world. What would Italy be without pasta e fagioli, the Middle East without hummus, India without dal, Greece without fassolada, Mexico without frijoles refritos or France without cassoulet? Who could imagine East Asian cuisine without the ubiquitous tofu, sliced, diced, stuffed and stir-fried, to be eaten with equal gusto in both street bazaars and the most elegant restaurants? And how many North Americans would enjoy life without the occasional feast of chili or old-fashioned baked beans?

At Robert Rose we've published many cookbooks over the years that contain some absolutely outstanding recipes for these very versatile ingredients. So it seemed natural that we collect many of these dishes in a single volume. And here it is: *250 Best Beans, Lentils and Tofu Recipes*. Quite simply, we think it's the best collection of its kind.

These recipes offer a spectacular variety of tastes, textures and cooking styles. Yet they are also relatively quick and easy to prepare and use ingredients that can be found in most supermarkets. We've also included 32 pages of beautiful color photographs to provide additional inspiration, as well as an introduction to the essentials of storing, cooking and enjoying beans, lentils and tofu.

We invite you to discover the rich variety of dishes that await you in this book. Like Columbus, you may be surprised by what you find.

— *The Editors at Robert Rose*

Introduction

Legumes (dried beans, peas and lentils) have played a significant role in many cuisines, from South Asia and the Middle East to Europe, the Americas and beyond. These crops were among the first foods our ancestors farmed, likely because, during the hunter-gatherer stage of our evolution, we ate them fresh from the wild, splitting the pods open and consuming the tender seeds. At some point we discovered how to preserve this agricultural bounty by drying the seeds in the sun. In fact, if it weren't for legumes, many of our ancestors wouldn't have survived. Because they were easy to store, these dried seeds were a crucial source of nutrition in an age that lacked refrigeration, when seasonal supplies of fresh produce were unavailable.

As history and culinary expertise evolved, in various parts of the world the cooking of legumes developed into something approaching an art form. Consider Italy, for instance, where humble *fagioli* form the backbone of traditional rustic cooking, starring in soups, stews and sauces — the kind of classic comfort food that Italians have excelled at for generations. The French lay claim to *lentilles du Puy*, small but flavorful green lentils, and flageolets, which many consider the ne plus ultra of dried beans. Their way with lesser varieties is defined by that iconic French country dish cassoulet, a richly flavored mélange of white beans, lamb, pork and duck, traditionally simmered in an earthenware pot. In the Middle East, hummus — a cumin-spiked purée of chickpeas, olive oil and lemon juice, often finished with tahini — is perhaps the best-known export. And then, of course, there is Indian dal, with its complex blend of seasonings, perhaps one of the most creative methods for elevating the simple pulse.

While other cultures were devising ways to cook the humble legume, farther east, Asians were busy refining the art of tofu, a curd made from soybeans, which are native to that region. Tofu was first used in China around 200 BCE. Today it is a dietary staple throughout Asia, where, in addition to being a significant component of a vegetarian diet, it is often combined with meat or fish and served stuffed or as part of a stir-fry.

Bean Cuisine

It's not surprising that legumes are so popular. In addition to being extremely economical and nutritious, they are delicious hot or cold, are visually appealing and come in many different shapes, sizes and colors — including yellow chickpeas, red or white kidney beans and multicolored lentils. They are highly adaptable, too. Legumes combine well with a wide variety of flavors and foods, running the gamut from graceful and elegant (Lentil and Pancetta Antipasto, page 37) to rib-sticking and hearty (Wagon Boss Chili, page 129). Whatever your dietary preferences, you can expect to enjoy delicious main courses featuring legumes, from vegan-friendly Roasted Vegetable Lasagna (page 230) to rich meat dishes such as Lamb with Flageolet Gratin (page 200).

Buying and Storing Legumes

Dried beans and lentils can be purchased packaged at supermarkets or from bulk and natural foods stores. They should be stored in a dry, airtight container at room temperature. Since they lose their moisture over time, they are best used within a year of purchase. Beans that have been on hand for a while take longer to soak and to cook and are likely to be tougher than those that have been stored for only a few months.

Once cooked, legumes should be covered and stored in the refrigerator, where they will keep for up to five days. Cooked legumes can also be frozen in an airtight, freezer-friendly container. They will keep in the freezer for up to six months.

Preparing Legumes

Dried beans and lentils more than double in size after cooking. Because their sizes and shapes vary, it's difficult to give exact ratios between uncooked and cooked quantities, but you're fairly safe using 1 cup (250 mL) uncooked legumes in a recipe that requires 2 cups (500 mL) of any cooked lentil or bean.

If you have purchased your legumes in bulk and aren't sure about the source, before using them check for contaminants. Spread them out on a rimmed baking sheet and sort through to remove any that are damaged or discolored, along with any bits of dirt or stones.

Soaking Dried Beans

Unlike dried beans, lentils do not need to be soaked before they are cooked. However, some chefs also feel that dried beans do not require presoaking. Although they may be correct from a culinary perspective, there is sound scientific evidence that soaking dried beans before cooking draws out gas-producing substances. Moreover, the process makes some of the nutrients in beans more biologically available. The research also indicates that the soaking water should be discarded, not maintained. When you throw away the soaking water, you are getting rid of significant amounts of gas-creating substances and only a smattering of nutrients.

To Salt or Not to Salt

Conventional wisdom suggests that salting beans during the soaking or cooking process will make them tough. However, various people — including food scientists Shirley Corriher and Harold McGee — have tested this hypothesis and concluded that it has no validity. The experts differ about whether it is preferable to salt during the soaking or the cooking stage, but they agree that adding salt during at least one of these stages will produce beans that are more tender and flavorful.

There are two basic approaches to soaking beans: the long-soak and quick-soak methods.

Long-Soak Method

With the long-soak method, your beans will take less time to cook and will hold their shape better. Place the beans in a large bowl and cover with water. Add salt to taste, if desired. You'll need 3 parts water to 1 part beans, by volume. Set aside at room temperature overnight or for up to 12 hours. If the weather is hot and humid, you may want to change the water once to ensure that the beans don't begin to ferment. Drain and rinse thoroughly under cold running water.

Quick-Soak Method

Combine 1 part dried beans and 3 parts water in a large saucepan. Add salt to taste, if desired. Bring to a boil and boil rapidly for 3 minutes. Turn off the heat, cover and set aside for 1 hour. Drain and rinse thoroughly under cold running water.

Presoaking in the Microwave

This method works only for smaller quantities (up to 1 cup/250 mL) of beans. In a 12-cup (3 L) microwavable bowl, combine 3 cups (750 mL) hot water with 1 cup (250 mL) dried beans. Add salt to taste, if desired. Cover tightly with plastic wrap and microwave on High for 10 to 15 minutes. Set aside for an hour. Drain and rinse under cold water. Use in recipes or cook as described on page 8.

Presoaking in the Pressure Cooker

If you have a pressure cooker, you can presoak your beans using the following method. Place beans and water in the pressure cooker, using 3 cups (750 mL) water for every 1 cup (250 mL) beans, plus 1 tbsp (15 mL) vegetable oil if you have a "jiggle-top" cooker. Lock the lid in place and bring up to full pressure over high heat. What you do next depends on the size and type of beans you are preparing.

- For small beans, remove the cooker from the heat immediately and let the pressure come down naturally for 10 minutes before releasing remaining steam using the quick-release valve.
- For larger beans, cook under pressure for 1 minute, then allow the pressure to come down naturally for 10 minutes.
- For chickpeas and very large beans, cook for 2 to 3 minutes at high pressure before allowing the

pressure to come down naturally for 10 minutes; then release any pressure with the quick-release valve.

Checking whether pressure-soaked beans are fully soaked

The goal of soaking is to have water penetrate to the center of the bean. You can check for this by cutting one open to make sure the color is even. An opaque spot in the center indicates that the bean needs further soaking or that you will have to add a few minutes of cooking time while pressure-cooking the beans.

The "Gas Problem"

Although soaking beans before cooking them helps to alleviate the gas problem, flatulence may still be an undesirable side effect of consuming legumes — a result of their high fiber content. Fortunately there are techniques for mitigating this problem. One way to reduce abdominal discomfort is to introduce legumes into your diet gradually, eating more easily digested varieties such as split peas and lentils and increasing the quantities slowly so your body can adapt over time. You should also avoid eating legumes along with other gas-producing vegetables such as cabbage, cauliflower, broccoli and Brussels sprouts.

Indian cooks, who have been making dal for centuries, know a thing or two about limiting this problem. They often season their lentils with spices that aid digestion, such as gingerroot or asafetida. In Mexico, where beans are a dietary staple, epazote, a pungent and bitter-tasting herb, is thought to do the trick. Another technique is to add a pinch of baking soda to the water in which the dried legumes are soaked. Finally, a digestive enzyme such as Beano can help to break down the fiber, making it easier to digest.

Cooking Dried Beans

There are a number of methods for cooking beans after they have been soaked: on the stovetop or in a microwave oven, slow cooker or pressure cooker. (For the slow cooker method, see Basic Beans in the Slow Cooker, page 277.)

Once the beans are in the cooking pot, you can start the seasoning process. Add salt if you wish (see To Salt or Not to Salt, page 6) and, if desired, add flavor enhancements such as a clove-studded onion, garlic, bay leaves or a bouquet garni made of parsley, celery, thyme and bay leaf, tied together in a piece of cheesecloth.

Stovetop Method

Place the beans in a large saucepan and add 3 parts water to 1 part beans. Cover and bring to a boil over medium heat. Reduce heat and simmer as gently as possible until the beans are tender and the skin just begins to break easily. This usually takes about 1 hour, depending upon the variety.

Microwave Method

This method works only for smaller quantities (up to 1 cup/250 mL). In a microwavable bowl, combine 1 cup (250 mL) soaked, drained beans with 4 cups (1 L) hot water. Add salt to taste, if desired. Cover tightly with plastic wrap and microwave on High for 35 minutes. Allow to rest, covered, for an additional 20 minutes.

Cooking Legumes in the Pressure Cooker

If you enjoy legumes or cook a lot of vegetarian dishes, the pressure cooker is a like a miracle. It allows you to cook inexpensive and healthy dried beans in minutes. Still, some precautions are necessary when you're cooking beans and lentils under pressure.

- Leave room for the beans to cook. Make sure you never overload the pressure cooker when cooking beans. Because beans and lentils froth up and expand substantially while cooking (up to four times their dry size and weight), never fill the pressure cooker more than one-third full.
- Use enough water. Always use at least 2 cups (500 mL) water or other liquid for every 1 cup (250 mL) dry beans in a recipe. If you have an old-fashioned jiggle-top pressure cooker, always watch it carefully while cooking beans, since the vent can easily become clogged. If it does, you will hear a loud hissing noise. Immediately remove the cooker from the heat and release the pressure.

Using Canned Legumes

When time is of the essence, canned beans are a great option: the time-consuming work of soaking and cooking has been done for you. Canned legumes are almost as nutritious as home-cooked versions. However, there are two cautions. Because the sodium content may be high, look for brands with reduced sodium or no salt added. Also, check to make sure the cans are not lined with bisphenol A (BPA), which has been identified as a potential toxin.

You can substitute canned legumes for cooked dried ones in equal quantities in any recipe. Where a recipe calls for 2 cups (500 mL) cooked beans, you can use a standard 14 to 19 oz (398 to 540 mL) can in most recipes. Unless otherwise specified, be sure to drain and rinse canned beans well under cold running water before adding to your recipe.

Pressure-Cooking Legumes

Legumes	Cooking time (approx.)	Water per 1 cup (250 mL) beans soaked overnight or pressure soaked (unless otherwise indicated) plus time for natural pressure release
Adzuki (Japanese brown) beans	5 to 6 minutes	3 cups (750 mL)
Anasazi beans	5 to 6 minutes	3 cups (750 mL)
Appaloosa beans	8 to 10 minutes	3 cups (750 mL)
Black beans	8 to 9 minutes	3 cups (750 mL)
Black-eyed peas (no soaking)	10 minutes	3 cups (750 mL)
Butter beans, unsalted	5 to 6 minutes	3 cups (750 mL)
Cannellini (white) beans	8 to 10 minutes	3 cups (750 mL)
Chickpeas (garbanzo beans)	10 to 15 minutes	3 cups (750 mL)
Cranberry (borlotti) beans	6 to 8 minutes	3 cups (750 mL)
Fava beans	12 to 15 minutes	3 cups (750 mL)
Flageolets	8 to 10 minutes	3 cups (750 mL)
Great Northern beans	8 to 10 minutes	3 cups (750 mL)
Lentils, brown (no soaking)	10 minutes	cover by 2 inches (5 cm)
Lentils, French (no soaking)	12 minutes	cover by 2 inches (5 cm)
Lentils, red (no soaking)	5 minutes	cover by 2 inches (5 cm)
Lima beans, baby	5 to 6 minutes	3 cups (750 mL)
Lima beans, Christmas	6 to 8 minutes	3 cups (750 mL)
Lima beans, large	4 to 6 minutes	3 cups (750 mL)
Navy beans	4 to 5 minutes	3 cups (750 mL)
Peas, split (no soaking)	8 to 10 minutes	3 cups (750 mL)
Peas, whole	5 to 8 minutes	3 cups (750 mL)
Pigeon peas	5 to 8 minutes	3 cups (750 mL)
Pinto beans	4 to 6 minutes	3 cups (750 mL)
Rattlesnake beans	4 to 6 minutes	3 cups (750 mL)
Scarlet runner beans	8 to 10 minutes	3 cups (750 mL)
Soybeans, white	10 to 14 minutes	3 cups (750 mL)
Soybeans, black	16 to 18 minutes	3 cups (750 mL)
Tongues of fire beans	8 to 10 minutes	3 cups (750 mL)

As noted above in Presoaking in the Pressure Cooker, jiggle-top pressure cooker users should add 1 tbsp (15 mL) oil to the water before cooking, to help reduce foaming and potential clogging.

- Watch your cooking time. Cooking times for beans can vary substantially, depending on a variety of factors such as the age and dryness of the beans. Even local humidity can affect cooking times. Where a recipe offers a range of cooking times, it's always best to start with the shorter one. You can always finish the beans conventionally or add another minute or two of pressure cooking if they're not quite done. To check for doneness, cut a bean in half with a sharp knife and look at the center. If the beans are done, they will be tender and one color throughout.
- Let the pressure drop naturally. When the cooking time is complete, remove the cooker from the heat and allow it to stand until the pressure indicator drops. This helps to avoid clogging the center pipe and safety valve with pulpy cooking liquid. It also prevents the beans from splitting.
- Keep your cooker clean. Always clean the pressure regulator and lid carefully after cooking beans, to make sure there are no obstructions.

Cooking Lentils and Split Peas

Unlike dried beans and chickpeas, lentils and split peas usually do not need to be presoaked. In a colander or sieve, rinse under cold water until the water runs clear and the legumes are thoroughly washed. Depending on the type, their cooking time varies from 10 minutes for red, pink and French lentils to 45 minutes for split peas. To ensure proper cooking times, follow the recipes in this book.

Cooking with Tofu

Although tofu is quite bland, it has a remarkable ability to soak up flavors and makes an excellent background for robust sauces. It is fabulous in soups and, paired with other ingredients, makes a flavorful main course. It can even be used in sandwiches and salad dressings. Because it is a prepared food, tofu is very convenient. It is also quite delicious once you learn to think of it as an ingredient rather than a meal in itself.

There are three main types of tofu. Firm tofu is dense and solid, holding its shape in stir-fries and soups or under the broiler and on the grill; it is higher in protein, fat and calcium than other varieties. Soft tofu works best when blended or mashed with other ingredients, and silken tofu is a creamy, custard-like product that works well in purées. Silken tofu is particularly good for dips and sauces.

Whatever recipes you choose to make from this book, introducing more tofu into your diet will add variety and nutrition to your meal planning.

Buying and Storing Tofu

Tofu is sold in water-filled tubs or vacuum packs and can be found in the produce or dairy section of supermarkets. Since it has a limited shelf life, check the "best before" date on the package. After the package has been opened, drain the liquid, place any unused portions in a bowl and cover with fresh cold water. Store, covered, in the refrigerator. Tofu will keep for one week if the water is changed daily. If it develops a sour smell, throw it out.

The Health Benefits of Legumes

Legumes Are Very Good for You

Many major health organizations agree that legumes can play a key role in our efforts to prevent chronic diseases. Research has shown that people with a healthy lifestyle who regularly consume legumes as part of a nutritious diet are less likely to develop cardiovascular disease, certain types of cancer and Type 2 diabetes. Eating more legumes may also help you to lose weight and keep it off. While the exact recommendations vary, health organizations recommend that people eat more legumes — up to 3 cups (750 mL) per week. Eating this quantity may reduce the possibility that you will develop metabolic syndrome: a cluster of risk factors such as increased belly fat and high blood pressure, as well as elevated cholesterol, triglycerides, insulin and blood sugar, all of which have been linked to heart disease, stroke, Type 2 diabetes and cancer.

Additionally, legumes contain various nutrients such as vitamins and minerals, protein and fiber. These include a type of non-digestible fiber called oligosaccharides, which act as a prebiotic, or a food source for the healthy bacteria that live in your digestive system. By consuming more prebiotic fiber, you can help to ensure that you have enough healthy bacteria to keep your digestive system on track.

Nutrients in Legumes

Although the nutrient content varies among the different types of lentils, dried beans, chickpeas and peas, all these foodstuffs share some common nutritional characteristics. A typical serving of legumes is high in dietary fiber, a good source of low-fat vegetable protein, and low in both sugar and sodium. All provide valuable micronutrients in varying degrees.

These include
- the B vitamins thiamin (B_1) and folate;
- minerals such as potassium, magnesium, manganese, copper, iron, zinc and phosphorus; and
- phytonutrients such as antioxidants.

Legumes Provide an Abundance of Fiber

Health organizations recommend at least 25 grams of fiber a day for women and at least 38 grams for men. The problem is, on average, most North Americans consume only about 11 grams of this important nutrient each day. Although their fiber content varies among the different types, you can expect $1/2$ cup (125 mL) of any cooked legume to provide, on average, about 7 grams of fiber.

The benefits of a diet that provides plentiful amounts of fiber have been well documented. It reduces your risk of developing heart disease, diabetes and cancer, among other conditions. And, because they fill you up, eating foods that are high in fiber may encourage you to eat less overall. In other words, consumption of fiber may be an ally in helping you to lose weight and to keep it off.

Legumes Provide Two Types of Fiber
There are two main types of fiber — soluble and insoluble — and legumes provide both. Insoluble fiber is the kind your mother probably told you about. Commonly called roughage, it helps to keep you regular and is an important component of a healthy diet.

The other kind of fiber, soluble fiber, is in some ways even more beneficial than so-called roughage. Once again depending on the variety, expect legumes to provide about 1 to 2 grams of soluble fiber per ½-cup (125 mL) serving. Soluble fiber has been linked with a variety of health benefits. Because it helps to blunt, or slow down, the digestion and absorption of carbohydrate in food, it helps to keep your blood sugar and insulin levels on an even keel, reducing the possibility that you will develop Type 2 diabetes. A higher intake of foods that are rich in soluble fiber may help people who do have diabetes to better control their blood sugar. Consumption of soluble fiber has also been shown to lower the levels of LDL ("bad") cholesterol in your blood.

day to obtain the complete range of amino acids.

Contrary to traditional wisdom, foods such as beans and rice do not need to be consumed at the same meal. In the past it was thought that the amino acids in one food would complement those lacking in the other food, and together the meal would provide a "complete" protein. We now know that all amino acids, regardless of their food source, go into a general "amino acid pool fund," not unlike when you deposit money into a bank account. Your body will simply use (make a withdrawal of) the particular amino acid it needs when it is carrying on important work such as making immune cells, maintaining muscle or rebuilding and maintaining bones, skin and more!

Legumes Are Anti-inflammatory

Studies show that as part of a healthy diet that includes many anti-inflammatory foods, legumes can help to lower markers of inflammation such as CRP and complement C3. High levels of these markers have been linked with chronic illnesses, including several cancers, arthritis, cardiovascular disease, obesity and diabetes.

Legumes Are a Good Source of Protein

Dried beans, peas, chickpeas and lentils provide low-fat vegetable protein, and as such are an ideal staple for vegan and vegetarian diets. However, they do not contain the entire range of essential amino acids that would allow them to be classified as a "complete" protein. Vegans and vegetarians should ensure that they also eat adequate amounts of grains and cereals, seeds and nuts every

Legumes Are Synergistic

Legumes provide a variety of phytonutrients, such as antioxidants, which are beneficial compounds in plant foods. Unlike vitamins and minerals, phytonutrients are not considered essential for health, but they help to make the difference between simply surviving and thriving. Phytonutrients promote health and reduce the risk for chronic disease. For example, in one 2011 study that investigated the antioxidant capacity of specific fruits, vegetables and legumes, researchers found not only that legumes are antioxidant-rich but also that by combining a legume with a fruit, for instance, the total antioxidant capacity of both foods was increased. In other words, pairing the foods created synergy. This emphasizes the importance of eating a variety of plant foods, throughout the day, to ensure that you get the most out of this teamwork.

Legumes Are Rich in Minerals

Legumes provide valuable minerals, such as potassium, magnesium, phosphorus, manganese, iron and zinc. Both potassium and magnesium help to keep your blood pressure under control and have, in various studies, been linked with reduced risk of ischemic stroke (80 percent of strokes are ischemic, which means caused by a blood clot). Both minerals also play a role in keeping your bones and teeth strong, with some assistance from manganese and phosphorus. In addition, magnesium helps to regulate blood sugar, and higher intakes have been shown to reduce the risk for insulin resistance and Type 2 diabetes. A diet high in magnesium may also reduce your risk of developing colon cancer. Zinc has many functions, not the least of which is helping to keep your immune system strong and maintaining taste acuity, which means that it supports the way your taste buds help you enjoy the foods you eat.

The Benefits of Eating Tofu

Among its many benefits, tofu is an excellent source of high-quality vegetable protein: a 1/2-cup (125 mL) serving of tofu provides between 5 to 10 grams of soy protein. It is also low on the glycemic index, which means that it is beneficial if you are watching your blood sugar levels.

When calcium is used as the curdling agent, tofu is an excellent source of that mineral. For example, a 1/2-cup (125 mL) serving of regular tofu made with calcium sulfate contains 430 milligrams of calcium — that's over 40 percent of the recommended daily intake for adults.

Because tofu is made from soybeans, it's trans fat–free and a source of the essential polyunsaturated fatty acids alpha-linolenic acid (the plant form of omega-3 fat) and linoleic acid (omega-6). Essential fats are those that cannot be made by the body and must be obtained from our diet.

Isoflavones and Health

Phytoestrogens are compounds that are found in nearly 300 plants in the human diet. These compounds were termed "phytoestrogens" because they have modest estrogen-like properties when consumed. While there are several different types, the three more important ones are lignans, coumestans and isoflavones; the isoflavones of most interest are glyciten, daidzein and genistein. Soybeans contain the highest amount of isoflavones, and thus tofu is a major source as well. A 1/2-cup (125 mL) serving of tofu contains about 40 milligrams of isoflavones, which means it is considered an excellent source of these compounds.

Research suggests that isoflavones offer many health benefits in the form of whole-soy foods, prepared and consumed in amounts consistent with the traditional diets of people who regularly consume soy foods. Eaten this way, isoflavones reduce the risk for breast and prostate cancer, heart disease and osteoporosis. Recent research has found that consuming as little as 25 to 30 milligrams of isoflavones per day, on average, can confer these benefits.

Isoflavones from soy, including tofu, help to keep estrogen levels in balance by increasing the level of sex-hormone-binding globulin, a protein that binds to estrogen in the blood and inhibits the enzyme aromatase, which is needed to convert pre-estrogen into active estrogen. Isoflavones also help to temper estrogen's activity in the body by binding to estrogen receptors on cells, as well as by reducing inflammation, a risk factor for both cardiovascular disease and cancer.

Food Sources Are Best

Isoflavone supplements should not be confused with the isoflavones found in whole foods. Not only have studies using isoflavone supplements not found benefits similar to those using soy foods, many have produced detrimental results. As a result, most health organizations advise against the use of isoflavone supplements. This is another example that shows how whole foods often work better than isolated nutrients. It may be that the compounds found in whole soybeans work together in concert to confer a health benefit, or that soybeans may contain another compound, as yet unidentified, that is responsible for these benefits.

Buy Organic

Most of the soybeans grown in North America are grown from genetically modified seeds. If you are concerned about GMOs (genetically modified organisms), look for tofu that is certified organic in origin. Buying organic tofu also ensures that you are reducing your exposure to chemical fertilizers, herbicides and pesticides, which may, over the long term, have negative effects.

Appetizers

White Bean Salsa. 16

Crostini 17

Pita Chips 17

White Bean with Mint. 18

Basil and White Bean Spread 18

Lemon-Laced Butterbean Dip 19

Black Bean Nachos 20

Refried Nachos 21

Grande Beef Nachos 22

Beyond Bean Dip 23

Warm Mexican Layered Dip 24

Spicy Bean Dip 25

Slow Cooker Black Bean and
    Salsa Dip 26

Wild West Bean Caviar with
    Roasted Tomatoes. 27

Black Bean and Corn Salsa Mini
    Tostadas with Chipotle Sour Cream . . . 28

Pico de Gallo 29

Black Bean and Roasted Corn Salsa 29

Black Bean Chipotle Dip 30

Smoked Oyster Hummus 31

Red Pepper Hummus. 31

Hummus from Scratch 32

Red Hot Hummus. 33

Roasted Vegetable Hummus 34

Roasted Eggplant and Artichoke Dip 35

Santorini-Style Fava Spread 36

Lentil and Pancetta Antipasto 37

Lentils with Spicy Sausage 38

White Bean Salsa

This brilliant, out of the pantry appetizer is the equivalent of that extra pair of sheer black stockings you have tucked in the back of your lingerie drawer — a kind of insurance policy, if you will. Guests will lap up this lemony, garlicky salsa, so be sure to keep a few extra cans of white beans in the pantry at all times.

Makes about 24 crostini

Vegan Friendly

Hands-on time:
20 minutes

Start to finish:
20 minutes

Make Ahead

The salsa can be made and kept at room temperature for up to 3 hours or refrigerated for up to 8 hours. Let come to room temperature before continuing with the recipe.

1	can (14 to 19 oz/398 to 540 mL) cannellini or navy beans, drained and rinsed	1
1	green onion, white and green parts, minced	1
1/4 cup	extra virgin olive oil, divided	60 mL
1 tsp	grated lemon zest	5 mL
1 1/2 tbsp	freshly squeezed lemon juice	22 mL
1	clove garlic, minced	1
1/4 tsp	salt	1 mL
1/8 tsp	cayenne pepper	0.5 mL
	Freshly ground black pepper	
3 tbsp	minced flat-leaf parsley, divided	45 mL
	Crostini (page 17) or Pita Chips (page 17)	
1/4 cup	goat cheese, softened, optional	60 mL

1. In a large bowl, combine beans, green onion, 2 tbsp (30 mL) of the olive oil, lemon zest, lemon juice, garlic, salt, cayenne, black pepper and 2 tbsp (30 mL) of the parsley. Taste for seasoning and add more salt, pepper or lemon juice, if necessary.

2. Just before serving, spread toasted bread with goat cheese, if using, and top with a heaping tbsp (15 mL) of the salsa. Sprinkle over remaining parsley.

Variation

Transfer the salsa to a decorative bowl, sprinkle on the remaining parsley and serve with pita chips. Or add a finely chopped tomato or avocado for even more visual and textural interest.

> **Canned White Beans.** The darlings of our pantry, canned beans wait patiently in the wings to come to our rescue whenever we need delicious food fast. Canned white beans provide a blank palette on which to paint your favorite tastes and textures. Explore other spicy add-ins such as cumin or coriander and fresh herbs such as thyme, basil or cilantro.

Crostini

These small, crispy bread slices make a great foundation for an infinite number of toppings.

Hands-on time:
10 minutes

Start to finish:
20 minutes

Tip

It's best to use an Italian or French loaf that is about 3 inches (7.5 cm) in diameter for this recipe.

• **Preheat broiler**

1	loaf Italian or French bread, cut into ½-inch (1 cm) thick slices (see Tip, left)	1
¼ cup	olive oil	60 mL

1. Brush bread slices lightly on both sides with olive oil. Arrange on a baking sheet. Broil on highest rack, turning once, for 3 to 4 minutes total or until lightly browned. Let cool. The bread slices can be toasted several hours in advance and kept at room temperature in an airtight container.

Pita Chips

Pita chips are tasty, homemade crispy breads that taste so much better than anything you can buy readymade.

Hands-on time:
30 minutes

Start to finish:
30 minutes

Make Ahead

Pita chips can be made 1 day ahead and kept at room temperature.

• **Preheat oven to 400°F (200°C)**

8	6-inch (15 cm) or small pita rounds, cut into 6 wedges and separated	8
⅓ cup	olive oil or unsalted butter, melted	75 mL
	Kosher salt	

1. Brush inside of each pita wedge with olive oil and arrange on a baking sheet. Sprinkle with salt and bake in preheated oven for about 8 minutes or until chips are crisp. Let cool on pan. Store in an airtight container at room temperature for up to 1 day.

Fagioli bianchi alla menta

White Bean with Mint

This spread is wonderful served on crostini.

Tip

Blanch mint and
parsley leaves
in boiling water
for 10 seconds;
remove immediately
and drain.

• **Food processor**

1 cup	whole mint leaves, blanched and drained (see Tip, left)	250 mL
1 cup	whole flat-leaf parsley leaves, blanched and drained	250 mL
4	cloves garlic, peeled	4
1½ cups	cooked cannellini beans (white kidney beans)	375 mL
2 tbsp	extra virgin olive oil	30 mL
	Salt and freshly ground black pepper	

1. In a food processor, combine mint, parsley and garlic; process until finely chopped. Add beans; process for 1 minute or until well-combined, scraping down sides of bowl at halfway point. Add oil; process until smooth. Season to taste with salt and pepper.

Basil and White Bean Spread

Don't tell and no one will ever guess how easy it is to make this delicious and sophisticated spread. Serve this with Crostini (page 17) brushed with Garlic-Infused Olive Oil (page 19). Sliced baguette and crackers work well, too.

Start to finish:
10 minutes

Tip

It is easy to make your
own garlic-infused
olive oil — just be sure
to use it immediately
as infused oils are a
favored medium for
bacteria growth.

• **Food processor**

1	can (19 oz/540 mL) white kidney beans, drained and rinsed	1
2 cups	packed flat-leaf parsley leaves (see Tips, page 19)	500 mL
2 tbsp	prepared basil pesto sauce	30 mL
1 tbsp	minced garlic	15 mL
1 tbsp	lemon juice	15 mL
	Salt and freshly ground black pepper	

1. In a food processor fitted with metal blade, combine beans, parsley, basil pesto, garlic and lemon juice. Process until smooth. Season with salt and black pepper to taste.

Lemon-Laced Butterbean Dip

Delicious and healthful, this Mediterranean-inspired dip is very easy to make. Serve it with toasted pita, sliced baguette, Crostini (page 17) brushed with Garlic-Infused Olive Oil (see below) or vegetable dippers.

Makes about 1 cup (250 mL)

Vegan Friendly

Tips

To quick soak lima beans, bring to a boil in 6 cups (1.5 L) water over medium heat. Boil rapidly for 3 minutes. Cover, turn off element and let stand for 1 hour. Drain.

Make sure you have thoroughly dried the parsley (patting between layers of paper towel) before adding to the food processor; otherwise the spread may be watery.

- **Food processor**

1 cup	dried lima beans, soaked (see Tips, left)	250 mL
¼ cup	freshly squeezed lemon juice	60 mL
¼ cup	extra virgin olive oil	60 mL
1 tsp	salt	5 mL
	Freshly ground black pepper	
½ cup	loosely packed Italian flat-leaf parsley leaves	125 mL
4	green onions, white part only, cut into chunks	4

1. In a large pot of water, cook soaked beans until tender, about 30 minutes. Scoop out about 1 cup (250 mL) of the cooking liquid and set aside. Drain beans and pop out of their skins.

2. In a food processor fitted with metal blade, pulse cooked beans, lemon juice, olive oil, salt, and pepper to taste, to blend, about 5 times. Gradually add just enough bean cooking water through the feed tube to make a smooth emulsion, pulsing to blend, about 10 times. Add parsley and green onions and pulse until chopped and integrated, about 5 times. Cover and refrigerate for up to 2 days until ready to use.

> **Garlic-Infused Olive Oil:** In a clean jar or cruet, combine ¼ cup (60 mL) olive oil and 1 tbsp (15 mL) minced garlic. Cover and let steep at room temperature for several hours. Strain through a fine sieve or funnel lined with a paper coffee filter. Discard garlic.

Black Bean Nachos

Cowboys may not have eaten nachos at the turn of the century but we certainly consume a lot of corn chips today, a testament to the spread of Tex-Mex cooking throughout the West. Today, nachos have become the national snack in cowboy country. In small-town cafés, rural bars or casual city restaurants, you'll always find nachos to start a meal.

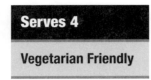

Serves 4

Vegetarian Friendly

Tip

Use canned beans, rinsed and drained, or cook your own. Start with 1 cup (250 mL) dried black beans.

Salsa

2	plum tomatoes, seeded and chopped	2
¼ cup	chopped onions	60 mL
1 tbsp	freshly squeezed lime juice	15 mL
1	jalapeño pepper, seeded and minced	1
2 tbsp	minced cilantro	30 mL
1 tbsp	chopped parsley	15 mL
1 tsp	chopped fresh thyme	5 mL
1 tsp	chopped fresh oregano	5 mL
1	green onion, chopped	1

Refried Beans

1 cup	cooked black beans	250 mL
1 tbsp	olive oil	15 mL
1 tbsp	minced garlic	15 mL
2	hot chile peppers, minced	2
¼ cup	chopped cilantro	60 mL
	Salt to taste	

Guacamole

2	ripe avocados	2
3 tbsp	freshly squeezed lime juice	45 mL
1 tsp	minced garlic	5 mL
¼ tsp	dried thyme leaves	1 mL
¼ tsp	dried oregano	1 mL
1	jalapeño pepper, chopped	1
12 cups	combination of yellow and blue tortilla chips	3 L
8 oz	Monterey Jack cheese, shredded	250 g

1. *Salsa:* In a bowl, stir together tomatoes, onions, lime juice, jalapeño, cilantro, parsley, thyme, oregano and green onion. Marinate for 1 hour in the refrigerator.

2. *Refried Beans:* Mash beans with a fork or purée in food processor. In a frying pan, heat olive oil over medium heat. Add mashed beans, garlic, chile peppers, and cilantro; cook, stirring, for 3 minutes or until soft and fragrant. Season with salt to taste. Set aside.

3. *Guacamole:* In a bowl and using a fork, mash avocado with lime juice. Stir in garlic, thyme, oregano and jalapeño. Set aside.

4. *Assembly:* Preheat oven to 400°F (200°C). Put tortilla chips in a large ovenproof dish. Distribute refried beans and salsa evenly over chips. Sprinkle with cheese. Bake for 5 minutes or until cheese is melted and dish is hot. Serve with guacamole on the side.

Refried Nachos

A favorite of teenagers, nachos are also a great comfort food dish. In this recipe, the degree of spice depends upon the heat of the salsa. If you are heat averse, use a mild salsa. If you are a heat seeker, use a spicy one.

Makes about 4 cups (1 L)

Tips

To microwave, place beans, salsa and chiles in a microwave-safe dish. Microwave on High until bubbling, about 4 minutes. Stir in cheese and microwave until melted, about $1\frac{1}{2}$ minutes.

To jack up the heat, add a finely chopped jalapeño pepper along with the beans.

If you like a hint of smoke as well as heat, add a finely chopped chipotle pepper in adobo sauce.

1	can (14 oz/398 mL) refried beans	1
1 cup	prepared tomato salsa	250 mL
1	can (4.5 oz/127 mL) chopped green chiles, drained	1
2 cups	shredded Cheddar or Monterey Jack cheese	500 mL
	Tortilla chips or tostadas	

1. In a saucepan over medium heat, bring beans, salsa and chiles to a boil. (You can also do this in the microwave; see Tips, left.) Stir in cheese until melted. Serve with tortilla chips or tostadas for dipping.

Variations

Mexican Pita Pizzas: Place pita breads in a large baking dish and spread with nacho mixture. Bake in 400°F (200°C) oven until the mixture is hot and bubbling, about 10 minutes. Serve with a knife and fork.

Bean Tacos: Warm 4 to 6 taco shells according to package directions. Fill with bean mixture and garnish with any combination of lettuce, tomato, green or red onion, avocado and/or sour cream.

Grande Beef Nachos

When you get a crowd over you need to serve something fast and hearty. This dish can be put together in just a few minutes.

Serves 6

Tips

For this quantity of beans, use 1 can (14 to 19 oz/398 to 540 mL), drained and rinsed, or cook 1 cup (250 mL) dried beans.

Do not place the hot meat mixture over the corn chips until you are ready to microwave. It will make your chips soggy.

You can also make this in the oven. Place under preheated broiler until cheese melts, 2 to 5 minutes.

- **Food processor**

1	bag (12 oz/375 g) tortilla chips	1
8 oz	Cheddar cheese, cut into chunks	250 g
8 oz	Monterey Jack cheese, cut into chunks	250 g
1	onion, cut into quarters	1
2 cups	drained cooked pinto or black beans (see Tips, left)	500 mL
1 tsp	chili powder	5 mL
1 tsp	paprika	5 mL
³⁄₄ tsp	salt	3 mL
³⁄₄ tsp	dried onion flakes	3 mL
¹⁄₄ tsp	cayenne pepper	1 mL
¹⁄₄ tsp	onion powder	1 mL
¹⁄₈ tsp	ground oregano	0.5 mL
8 oz	lean ground beef	250 g
¹⁄₄ cup	sour cream	60 mL

1. On a microwave-safe platter, place chips in a single layer. Set aside.
2. In a food processor fitted with shredding blade, shred Cheddar and Monterey Jack cheeses. Transfer to a bowl and set aside.
3. Replace shredding blade with metal blade. With motor running, drop onion though feed tube and process until finely chopped. Into the work bowl, add beans, chili powder, paprika, salt, onion flakes, cayenne pepper, onion powder and oregano and process until smooth, 2 to 3 minutes, stopping and scraping down sides of the bowl once or twice.
4. In a large skillet over medium heat, cook ground beef until no longer pink, 10 to 15 minutes. Drain off fat. Add bean mixture and cook, stirring, until hot.
5. Spoon beef mixture over chips. Sprinkle cheese mixture over top. Microwave for 20 seconds or until cheese is bubbling. Garnish with sour cream.

Variation

Use ground sausage (casings removed) in place of the ground beef to add a little zip.

Beyond Bean Dip

Although the texture of canned beans is inferior for dishes that call for whole beans, they are simple and fast to use — especially for dips or refried bean dishes. Rinse and drain canned beans before using.

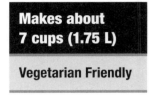

Makes about 7 cups (1.75 L)

Vegetarian Friendly

• **Food processor**

Bean Layer

1	can (14 oz/398 mL) refried beans or 1 can (19 oz/540 mL) pinto beans	1
¼ cup	sour cream	60 mL
1	jalapeño pepper, seeded and minced	1
1	clove garlic, minced	1
1 tsp	chili powder	5 mL
½ tsp	ground cumin	2 mL

Guacamole Layer

2	ripe avocados	2
3 tbsp	lemon juice or lime juice	45 mL
3	green onions, minced	3
1 tsp	minced jalapeño pepper	5 mL

Garnish

1 cup	sour cream	250 mL
1 cup	shredded Cheddar cheese	250 mL
2	green onions, chopped	2
½ cup	sliced black olives	125 mL
1	tomato, seeded and chopped	1
	Regular and blue corn tortilla chips as accompaniments	

1. If using pinto beans, rinse and drain. Purée beans in food processor; transfer to a bowl. Stir in sour cream, jalapeño, garlic, chili powder and cumin. Set aside.

2. In another bowl, mash avocados with lemon juice. Stir in green onions and jalapeño pepper. Set aside.

3. Spread bean dip in a thin layer over a deep 12-inch (30 cm) platter. Carefully spread guacamole over bean layer. Spread with sour cream, making sure to cover guacamole completely to keep it from darkening. Starting at the outside edge of the plate, make a 2-inch (5 cm) ring of shredded cheese. Inside that ring, sprinkle green onions in a ring. Follow with black olives and finish with a pile of chopped tomato in the center of the plate. Serve with lots of regular and blue corn tortilla chips for scooping.

Warm Mexican Layered Dip

This layered dip is easy to assemble and is always popular with a crowd. It makes a hearty buffet dish served with tortilla chips or small steamed tortillas.

Makes 6 to 8 servings

Tips

Use a nonstick skillet when browning ground turkey, chicken or beef, as it eliminates the need for oil or butter.

If you prefer to use pre-shredded cheese or don't have a kitchen scale, you'll need 1 cup (250 mL) each Cheddar and Monterey Jack.

- **Preheat oven to 400°F (200°C)**
- **9-inch (23 cm) square glass or ceramic baking dish, greased**

1 lb	ground turkey or beef	500 g
1	jar (15 oz/426 mL) salsa	1
1	envelope (1¼ oz/37 g) taco seasoning mix	1
1	can (16 oz/454 mL) refried beans	1
1 cup	sour cream	250 mL
4 oz	Cheddar cheese, shredded	125 g
4 oz	Monterey Jack cheese, shredded	125 g

1. Heat a large nonstick skillet over medium-high heat. Cook turkey, breaking it up with the back of a spoon and stirring occasionally, for 8 to 10 minutes or until no longer pink. Stir in salsa and taco seasoning.

2. Spread turkey mixture in prepared baking dish. Layer refried beans, sour cream, Cheddar and Monterey Jack on top.

3. Bake in preheated oven for 25 to 30 minutes or until bubbling.

Spicy Bean Dip

Made with red kidney beans, black beans or pinto beans, this bean purée is a popular addition to south-of-the-border-style snacks.

Makes 2 cups (500 mL)

Tip

Use ½ cup (125 mL) dried beans, soaked and cooked (see pages 6 to 10) instead of canned beans. Reserve about ½ cup (125 mL) of the bean cooking liquid to add to the puréed beans as required.

- **Food processor**

1 tbsp	vegetable oil	15 mL
1	onion, finely chopped	1
1	clove garlic, minced	1
1 tsp	chili powder	5 mL
1	jalapeño pepper, seeded and finely chopped	1
1	can (14 to 19 oz/398 to 540 mL) red kidney beans (see Tip, left)	1
	Salt and freshly ground black pepper	
¼ to ½ cup	water	60 to 125 mL

1. In a large skillet, heat oil over medium heat. Add onion and sauté until softened and nicely browned, 8 to 10 minutes. Add garlic, chili powder and jalapeño and sauté for 1 to 2 minutes. Set aside.

2. In a food processor, purée beans until almost smooth. Add beans to onion mixture and season lightly with salt and pepper. Add ¼ cup (60 mL) water and cook, stirring diligently, for 5 minutes. Add more water, if needed, until beans are heated through and of good spreading consistency — not too runny and not too stiff. Transfer to a serving bowl and serve hot or cover and keep in the refrigerator for up to 1 week. Reheat gently, as required.

Variation

Hot Spicy Bean Dip: Add 1 cup (250 mL) shredded Monterey Jack or mild Cheddar cheese to bean purée. Transfer mixture to a small ovenproof bowl and cover with foil. Before serving, bake in a preheated 350°F (180°C) oven until beans are bubbling, 5 to 10 minutes. Brown top lightly under the broiler. Serve hot with corn chips or crisp breads for dipping.

Slow Cooker Black Bean and Salsa Dip

This tasty Cuban-inspired dip, which can be made from ingredients you're likely to have on hand, is nutritious and flavorful.

Makes about 3 cups (750 mL)

Vegetarian Friendly

Tips

For this quantity of beans, soak, cook and drain 1 cup (250 mL) dried black beans (see pages 6 to 10) or drain and rinse 1 can (14 to 19 oz/398 to 540 mL) black beans.

For the best flavor, toast and grind cumin seeds yourself. Place in a dry skillet over medium heat, and cook, stirring, until fragrant, about 3 minutes. Immediately transfer to a spice grinder or mortar and grind finely.

For a smoother dip, purée the beans in a food processor or mash with a potato masher before adding to stoneware.

If you use a five-alarm salsa in this dip, you may want to omit the jalapeño pepper.

Roast your own pepper or use a bottled roasted red pepper.

- **Small to medium (1½ to 3½ quart) slow cooker**

2 cups	cooked black beans (see Tips, left)	500 mL
8 oz	cream cheese, cubed	250 g
½ cup	tomato salsa	125 mL
¼ cup	sour cream	60 mL
1 tsp	chili powder	5 mL
1 tsp	ground cumin (see Tips, left)	5 mL
1 tsp	cracked black peppercorns	5 mL
1	jalapeño pepper, finely chopped, optional (see Tips, left)	1
1	roasted red bell pepper, finely chopped, optional (see below)	1
	Finely chopped green onion, optional	
	Finely chopped cilantro, optional	

1. In slow cooker stoneware, combine beans, cream cheese, salsa, sour cream, chili powder, cumin, peppercorns, and jalapeño pepper and bell pepper, if using. Cover and cook on High for 1 hour. Stir again and cook on High for an additional 30 minutes, until mixture is hot and bubbly.

2. Serve immediately or set temperature at Warm until ready to serve. Garnish with green onion and/or cilantro, if desired.

> **To roast peppers:** Preheat oven to 400°F (200°C). Place pepper(s) on a baking sheet and roast, turning two or three times, until the skin on all sides is blackened. (This will take about 25 minutes.) Transfer pepper(s) to a heatproof bowl. Cover with a plate and let stand until cool. Remove and, using a sharp knife, lift off skins. Discard skins and slice according to recipe instructions.

Wild West Bean Caviar with Roasted Tomatoes

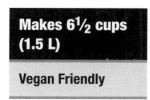

Makes 6½ cups (1.5 L)

Vegan Friendly

● **Preheat broiler or barbecue**

3	ripe tomatoes	3
2 tbsp	olive oil	30 mL
¼ cup	red wine vinegar, plus a pinch of granulated sugar or balsamic vinegar	60 mL
1 tbsp	lime juice	15 mL
3	cloves garlic, minced	3
½ tsp	salt	2 mL
6 cups	cooked black beans or black-eyed peas	1.5 L
½ cup	chopped red onions	125 mL
½ cup	chopped cilantro	125 mL
1	jalapeño pepper, seeded and minced	1
	Corn chips or pita chips	

1. Under the broiler or on the barbecue, cook tomatoes for 10 minutes, turning occasionally, or until charred on all sides. Cool; peel, seed and core. In a food processor, combine tomato flesh, olive oil, vinegar, lime juice, garlic and salt; process until smooth.

2. In a bowl, stir together roasted tomato sauce, beans, red onions, cilantro and jalapeño pepper. Let stand at room temperature for 30 minutes to allow flavors to develop.

3. Serve with corn chips and pita chips for scooping, or serve as a starter salad or side dish.

Black Bean and Corn Salsa Mini Tostadas with Chipotle Sour Cream

Once you've made Pico de Gallo, these lovely little smoky tostadas are just a hop, skip and a margarita away. We simply add corn, black beans and avocado to our basic salsa, spoon it onto a tortilla chip (we especially like to use the ones shaped like little scoops) and drizzle with a chipotle- and lime-flavored sour cream. Any leftover salsa makes a great filling for a veggie burrito.

Makes about 50 tiny tostadas

Vegetarian Friendly

Hands-on time:
35 minutes

Start to finish:
1 hour 25 minutes

Tip

We love canned beans. They're easy and convenient, and let's face it, it's not always in the cards to stand over a simmering pot for 2 hours. But it is important to find good-quality canned beans. It's frustrating to open a can of beans and have them come out in a solid mass of mush.

Make Ahead

The corn and black bean salsa can be made 2 hours ahead. The chipotle sour cream can be made up to 1 day ahead. The tostadas should be assembled just before serving.

1	recipe Pico de Gallo (page 29)	1
1	can (14 to 19 oz/398 to 540 mL) black beans, drained and rinsed	1
1½ cups	frozen corn kernels, thawed	375 mL
1	avocado, cut into small dice	1
1 cup	sour cream	250 mL
1 tbsp	finely minced chipotle chile pepper in adobo sauce	15 mL
1 tbsp	freshly squeezed lime juice	15 mL
2 tbsp	milk, plus more if necessary	30 mL
¼ tsp	salt	1 mL
	Tortilla chips (preferably scoop-style)	

1. In a large bowl, combine Pico de Gallo, black beans, corn and avocado. Taste and season with more salt, if necessary. Set aside.

2. In a medium bowl, combine sour cream, chipotle with sauce, lime juice, milk and salt. The mixture should be the consistency of whipping cream. Add more milk if too thick.

3. Place several tortilla chips on a serving plate. Place a spoonful of black bean and corn salsa on each tortilla chip. Drizzle chipotle cream over top of each tostada. Serve.

A Sharp Knife

There are two types of pico de gallo. One is the colorful, salad-like salsa where the ingredients have all been finely diced by hand with a sharp knife and then gently combined. The other is a uniformly pinkish mixture where all the ingredients have been tossed into a food processor and pulsed into an indiscernible mass. Hmm. Which one sounds more appetizing?

Pico de Gallo

Just the name puts us in the mood for Mexican food. Pico de Gallo is a delightfully simple, uncooked salsa made of ripe tomatoes, onion, cilantro and chiles. Its bright flavor comes from a liberal splash of freshly squeezed lime juice. Tortilla chips are the obvious accompaniment to this zesty condiment, but there are a million different uses. We love it on scrambled eggs or on a salad with tortilla chip croutons or as a topping to a south-of-the-border bruschetta. It's great on tacos, too!

**Makes about
2 cups (500 mL)**

Vegan Friendly

Hands-on time:
20 minutes

Start to finish:
50 minutes

Make Ahead
Make this up to
4 hours ahead. Cover
and refrigerate.

1 lb	ripe tomatoes, seeded and chopped	500 g
½ cup	finely chopped red onion	125 mL
¼ cup	finely chopped fresh cilantro	60 mL
2 tbsp	freshly squeezed lime juice	30 mL
1	small clove garlic, minced	1
1 to 2 tbsp	minced jalapeño or serrano chiles	15 to 30 mL
	Salt	

1. In a medium bowl, combine tomatoes, red onion, cilantro, lime juice, garlic and jalapeño, adding minced chiles to taste. Toss to blend well. Season with salt to taste. Let stand at room temperature for at least 30 minutes to allow the flavors to develop.

Black Bean and Roasted Corn Salsa

This dip is very easy; everything is mixed in the food processor.

**Makes 2 cups
(500 mL)**

Vegan Friendly

Tip
If you can't find
roasted corn, you can
roast 2 cups (500 mL)
fresh or thawed
frozen corn kernels
in a single layer in
a dry skillet over
medium heat, stirring
constantly, until lightly
browned.

• **Food processor**

2 cups	drained cooked black beans	500 mL
12 oz	cream cheese, cubed and softened, or vegan alternative	375 g
⅓ cup	roasted red pepper (about 1 small)	75 mL
2	chipotle peppers in adobo sauce, drained	2
2 tbsp	chopped fresh cilantro leaves	30 mL
1 tbsp	taco seasoning	15 mL
2 tsp	freshly squeezed lime juice	10 mL
1	bag (12 oz/375 g) roasted corn (see Tip, left)	1

1. In a food processor fitted with metal blade, process black beans, cream cheese, red pepper, chipotle peppers, cilantro, taco seasoning and lime juice until smooth, about 3 minutes, stopping and scraping down sides of the bowl once or twice. Transfer to a bowl and fold in roasted corn.

Black Bean Chipotle Dip

This dip has a south-of-the-border kick. It gets even hotter the next day. Serve with crackers, chips or toast points.

Makes 2 to 3 cups (500 to 750 mL)

Vegan Friendly

Tips

For this quantity of beans, use 1 can (14 to 19 oz/398 to 540 mL), drained and rinsed, or cook 1 cup (250 mL) dried beans.

Dip will keep, covered and refrigerated, for up to 1 week. The flavors get stronger after a day or two.

- **Food processor**

2 cups	drained cooked black beans (see Tips, left)	500 mL
12 oz	cream cheese, cubed and softened, or vegan alternative	375 g
$\frac{1}{3}$ cup	roasted red peppers (about 1 small)	75 mL
$\frac{1}{2}$ to 1	chipotle pepper in adobo sauce, drained	$\frac{1}{2}$ to 1
1 tbsp	fresh cilantro leaves	15 mL
1 tbsp	taco seasoning	15 mL
1 tsp	freshly squeezed lime juice	5 mL

1. In a food processor fitted with metal blade, process black beans, cream cheese, red peppers, chipotle pepper to taste, cilantro, taco seasoning and lime juice until smooth, about 2 minutes, stopping and scraping down sides of the bowl once or twice. Transfer to a serving dish.

Variation

Substitute pinto beans for the black beans for a lighter-looking dip.

Smoked Oyster Hummus

This intriguing spread is a variation on traditional Middle Eastern hummus. It always gets rave reviews. Serve with pita bread, pita toasts or crudités.

Makes about 3 cups (750 mL)

Tips

Taste the oysters before using to ensure their flavor meets your approval, as it can vary from brand to brand, affecting the result.

Use a bottled pepper or roast your own (see page 26).

2 cups	cooked chickpeas, drained and rinsed	500 mL
1/4 cup	freshly squeezed lemon juice	60 mL
1/4 cup	extra virgin olive oil	60 mL
1	large roasted red pepper (see Tips, left)	1
4	cloves garlic	4
1/2 tsp	salt	2 mL
1	can (3 oz/90 g) smoked oysters, drained	1
	Freshly ground black pepper	

1. In a food processor fitted with the metal blade, process chickpeas, lemon juice, olive oil, roasted pepper, garlic and salt until smooth, stopping and scraping down sides of the bowl as necessary.
2. Add oysters and pulse just to chop and combine, about 5 times. Season with pepper to taste.

Red Pepper Hummus

This hummus is a twist on regular hummus that gives all sandwiches a wonderful kick. It also works great as an appetizer served with pita triangles and crudités.

Makes 1 1/2 cups (375 mL)

Vegan Friendly

Tips

Tahini is made of ground sesame seeds. Look for it in the international section of grocery stores.

If you can't find tahini, try smooth peanut butter instead.

Substitute cannellini or white beans for the chickpeas.

- **Food processor**

1	can (14 to 19 oz/398 to 540 mL) chickpeas, drained and rinsed	1
1/3 cup	roasted red peppers from a jar, drained	75 mL
2	cloves garlic, coarsely chopped	2
1/4 cup	tahini (see Tips, left)	60 mL
2 tbsp	minced Italian flat-leaf parsley	30 mL
2 tbsp	freshly squeezed lemon juice	30 mL
1 1/2 tsp	ground cumin	7 mL
1/4 tsp	kosher salt	1 mL
1/4 tsp	cayenne pepper	1 mL

1. In a food processor, purée chickpeas, roasted peppers, garlic, tahini, parsley, lemon juice, cumin, salt and cayenne until smooth. Use immediately or cover and refrigerate for up to 2 days.

Hummus from Scratch

Although it's more work, cooking dried chickpeas rather than using canned chickpeas produces the tastiest hummus. Try this and see if you agree. Serve with warm pita. Although it's a bit unconventional, hummus makes a great sauce for grilled kabobs, particularly lamb. It is also great as a topping for roasted eggplant (see Variation, opposite).

Makes about 3 cups (750 mL)

Vegan Friendly

Tips

If you're in a hurry, instead of setting the chickpeas aside to soak, cover the pot and bring to a boil. Boil for 3 minutes. Turn off heat and soak for 1 hour. Drain and rinse thoroughly with cold water. Then proceed with cooking as in Step 2.

For the best flavor, toast and grind cumin seeds yourself. Place in a dry skillet over medium heat, and cook, stirring, until fragrant, about 3 minutes. Immediately transfer to a spice grinder or mortar and grind finely.

• Food processor

1 cup	dried chickpeas (see Tips, left)	250 mL
	Garlic, bay leaves or bouquet garni, optional	
1/3 cup	tahini paste	75 mL
1/3 cup	extra virgin olive oil	75 mL
1/4 cup	freshly squeezed lemon juice	60 mL
1/4 cup	Italian flat-leaf parsley leaves	60 mL
2	cloves garlic (approx.)	2
1 tsp	ground cumin (see Tips, left)	5 mL
1 tsp	salt (approx.)	5 mL
1/2 tsp	freshly ground black pepper	2 mL
1/4 tsp	cayenne pepper, optional	1 mL
	Sweet paprika, optional	

1. In a large saucepan, combine chickpeas and 3 cups (750 mL) cold water. Set aside to soak for at least 6 hours or overnight. Drain and rinse thoroughly with cold water.

2. Return drained chickpeas to saucepan and add 3 cups (750 mL) cold fresh water. If desired, season with garlic, bay leaves or a bouquet garni made from your favorite herbs tied together in a cheesecloth bag. Cover and bring to a boil over medium-high heat. Reduce heat and simmer until chickpeas are tender, about 1 hour. Scoop out about 1 cup (250 mL) of the cooking water and set aside. Drain and rinse chickpeas.

3. In a food processor fitted with the metal blade, process cooked chickpeas, tahini, olive oil, 1/4 cup (60 mL) of the cooking water, and lemon juice until smooth, about 30 seconds, stopping and scraping down sides of the bowl as necessary. If necessary, add additional cooking water and pulse to blend. (You want the mixture to be quite creamy.) Add parsley, garlic, cumin, salt, pepper, and cayenne, if using, and process until smooth, about 15 seconds. Taste and adjust garlic, lemon juice and/or salt to suit your taste. Process again, if necessary. Spoon into a serving bowl and dust with paprika, if using.

Variation

Roasted Eggplant with Hummus: Cut 1 eggplant into
1/2-inch (1 cm) thick slices. Brush with olive oil and
bake in a 400°F (200°C) oven for about 25 minutes.
Top with hummus.

Red Hot Hummus

Go easy on the chili paste until you get the heat just the way you like it. Substitute 1 to 2 tsp (5 to 10 mL) powdered chili pepper or hot pepper flakes for the paste.

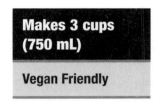

**Makes 3 cups
(750 mL)**

Vegan Friendly

Tip

You can use 2 cups
(500 mL) cooked
chickpeas, drained
and rinsed, instead
of canned.

● **Food processor**

	Juice of 1 lime or lemon	
2 tbsp	whole chia seeds	30 mL
1/2 cup	coarsely chopped sun-dried tomatoes	125 mL
1 cup	hot water	250 mL
1	can (14 to 19 oz/398 to 540 mL) chickpeas, drained and rinsed (see Tip, left)	1
2	cloves garlic	2
1 tbsp	toasted sesame oil	15 mL
1/4 cup	olive oil	60 mL
1 to 2 tbsp	chili paste	15 to 30 mL
	Sea salt and freshly ground pepper	

1. In a bowl, combine lemon juice and chia seeds. In
   a separate bowl, combine sun-dried tomatoes and
   hot water. Set both aside for at least 20 minutes or
   until seeds are gelatinous.

2. In a food processor, combine chickpeas, garlic and
   sesame oil. Process for 20 seconds. With the motor
   running, add lemon juice and chia seed mixture and
   sun-dried tomato mixture through the feed tube. Keep
   the motor running and slowly add olive oil through the
   opening. Process until well blended, about 20 seconds.
   Add chili paste, salt and pepper to taste and process
   for 5 seconds to blend into the hummus.

3. Transfer mixture to a clean container with lid. Store
   hummus in the refrigerator for up to 3 days.

Roasted Vegetable Hummus

Cinnamon gives a spicy nudge to this Middle Eastern staple. This is a fairly thick dip that is best made in a food processor (see Tips, below).

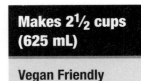

Makes 2½ cups (625 mL)

Vegan Friendly

Tips

To use a blender, add ¼ cup (60 mL) apple juice before processing in Step 2.

You can use 2 cups (500 mL) cooked chickpeas, drained and rinsed, instead of canned.

- **Preheat oven to 400°F (200°C)**
- **Rimmed baking sheet**
- **Food processor**

6	cloves garlic	6
2	onions, quartered	2
2	carrots, cut into 1-inch (2.5 cm) pieces	2
1	red bell pepper, quartered	1
5 tbsp	olive oil, divided	75 mL
1	can (14 to 19 oz/398 to 540 mL) chickpeas, drained and rinsed (see Tips, left)	1
2 tbsp	freshly squeezed lemon juice	30 mL
2 tbsp	tahini	30 mL
½ tsp	ground cinnamon	2 mL
½ tsp	sea salt	2 mL

1. On baking sheet, combine garlic, onions, carrots and red pepper. Drizzle 2 tbsp (30 mL) of the oil over and toss well to coat. Roast in preheated oven for 40 minutes or until soft and browned. Edges of vegetables may be slightly burnt and crisp. Let cool.

2. In a food processor, combine roasted vegetables, remaining olive oil, chickpeas, lemon juice, tahini, cinnamon and salt. Blend until smooth.

3. Transfer mixture to a clean container with lid. Store hummus tightly covered in the refrigerator for up to 3 days.

Roasted Eggplant and Artichoke Dip

Without the cream cheese and fat-laden sauces typically used in dips, this vegan version is tasty and much healthier.

Makes about 3 cups (750 mL)

Vegan Friendly

Tip

You can use 2 cups (500 mL) cooked black beans, drained and rinsed, instead of canned.

- **Preheat oven to 400°F (200°C)**
- **Rimmed baking sheet**
- **Food processor**

6	cloves garlic	6
2	onions, quartered	2
1	eggplant, peeled and cut into eighths	1
4 tbsp	olive oil, divided	60 mL
2 tbsp	freshly squeezed lemon juice	30 mL
1	can (14 oz/398 mL) artichokes, drained	1
1	can (14 to 19 oz/398 to 540 mL) black beans, drained and rinsed (see Tip, left)	1
½ tsp	ground cumin	2 mL
½ tsp	sea salt	2 mL
¼ cup	unsweetened apple juice (approx.)	60 mL

1. On baking sheet, combine garlic, onions and eggplant. Drizzle 2 tbsp (30 mL) of the oil over and toss well to coat. Roast in preheated oven for 40 minutes or until soft and browned. Let cool.

2. In a food processor, combine roasted vegetables, remaining olive oil, lemon juice, artichokes, black beans, cumin and salt. Blend until smooth. With the motor running, add apple juice though the feed tube until desired consistency is reached.

3. Transfer mixture to a clean container with lid. Store dip tightly covered in the refrigerator for up to 3 days.

Santorini-Style Fava Spread

This spread, which is Greek in origin, is unusual and particularly delicious. Although fava beans do figure in Greek cuisine, for most Greek people fava *is synonymous with yellow split peas, one of the major indigenous foods of the island of Santorini, from which they make many dishes, including this spread. Serve this with warm toasted pita and wait for the compliments.*

**Makes about
2 cups (500 mL)**

Vegan Friendly

Make Ahead

Complete Step 1. Cover and refrigerate for up to 2 days. When you're ready to serve, heat peas on the stovetop until bubbles form about the edges. Complete the recipe.

- **Small (1$\frac{1}{2}$ to 2 quart) slow cooker**
- **Food processor**

$\frac{1}{2}$ cup	extra virgin olive oil, divided	125 mL
$\frac{1}{2}$ cup	diced shallots (about 2 large)	125 mL
2 tsp	dried oregano	10 mL
1 tsp	salt	5 mL
$\frac{1}{2}$ tsp	cracked black peppercorns	2 mL
1 cup	yellow split peas	250 mL
4 cups	water	1 L
6	oil-packed sun-dried tomato halves, drained and coarsely chopped	6
4	cloves garlic, chopped	4
$\frac{1}{4}$ cup	coarsely chopped Italian flat-leaf parsley	60 mL
4	fresh basil leaves, hand-torn	4
3 tbsp	red wine vinegar	45 mL
	Salt and freshly ground black pepper	
	Toasted pita bread	

1. In a skillet, heat 1 tbsp (15 mL) of the oil over medium heat. Add shallots and cook, stirring, until softened, about 3 minutes. Add oregano, salt and peppercorns and cook, stirring, for 1 minute. Add split peas and cook, stirring, until coated. Add water and bring to a boil. Boil for 2 minutes.

2. Transfer to slow cooker stoneware. Cover and cook on Low for 8 hours or on High for 4 hours, until peas have virtually disintegrated. Drain off excess water, if necessary. Transfer solids to a food processor. Add sun-dried tomatoes, garlic, parsley, basil and red wine vinegar. Pulse 7 or 8 times to chop and blend ingredients. With motor running, add remaining olive oil in a steady stream through the feed tube. Season to taste with additional salt and pepper and drizzle with additional olive oil, if desired. Serve warm with toasted pita.

Lentil and Pancetta Antipasto

Pancetta is Italian bacon cured with nutmeg, cinnamon or cloves to give it a distinctive flavor. If pancetta is unavailable, regular bacon can be substituted, but the flavor won't be as authentically Italian. For a colorful antipasti platter to serve as a sit-down appetizer, spoon this salad onto a platter, along with antipasto, a couple of tomatoes cut into wedges, a selection of olives and some sliced mozzarella or bocconcini cheese.

Serves 6

Make Ahead

Antipasto can be refrigerated, covered, for up to 24 hours. Let stand at room temperature for 30 minutes before serving.

1 cup	green lentils	250 mL
4	sprigs fresh oregano or marjoram	4
2 oz	pancetta, chopped	60 g
2	stalks celery, finely chopped	2
½	medium red onion, finely chopped	½
¼ cup	chopped fresh Italian flat-leafed parsley	60 mL
1	clove garlic, minced	1
2 tbsp	olive oil	30 mL
1 tbsp	chopped fresh oregano or marjoram	15 mL
1 tbsp	red wine vinegar	15 mL
½ tsp	black pepper	2 mL
¼ tsp	salt	1 mL

1. Rinse lentils under running water, picking them over and discarding any grit. Drain well. Bring a medium saucepan of water to a boil over high heat. Add lentils and oregano sprigs; cook, uncovered, for 15 to 20 minutes or until lentils are tender but still firm. Drain well, discarding oregano; transfer lentils to a large serving bowl.

2. In a small heavy skillet, cook pancetta over medium-high heat for 2 to 3 minutes or until just starting to crisp. With a slotted spoon, remove pancetta from skillet; drain on a paper-towel-lined plate.

3. Add pancetta, celery, onion, parsley and garlic to lentils; toss well. Sprinkle with oil, oregano, vinegar, pepper and salt; toss well. If desired, season to taste with additional salt and pepper. Serve at room temperature.

Lentils with Spicy Sausage

North Americans are finally acknowledging the lowly lentil for the miracle food that it is. Not only total protein nutrition, but also delicious and endlessly adaptable, with a slew of tasty recipes to choose from. Here's a winter-type lentil that can make for either a good entrée on its own, or a hearty main course served with boiled potato and green salad. The butter enhancement is optional if it offends the calorie-wise, but it will obviously add a welcome richness to the proceedings.

Serves 4 to 6 as an appetizer or 3 to 4 as a main course

• **Preheat oven to 400°F (200°C)**

1 cup	green lentils	250 mL
4 cups	boiling water	1 L
4 or 5	cloves garlic, sliced	4 or 5
1	bay leaf	1
½ tsp	dried thyme	2 mL
¼ tsp	freshly ground black pepper	1 mL
8 oz	spicy sausage (merguez, chorizo or spicy Italian)	250 g
½ cup	sliced onions	125 mL
1 tbsp	butter (optional)	15 mL
1 tsp	white wine vinegar	5 mL
	Salt to taste	
	Several sprigs fresh parsley, chopped	

1. In a pot, soak lentils in 2 cups (500 mL) of the boiling water for 20 minutes. (Lentils will swell up and absorb most of the water.) Add remaining 2 cups (500 mL) boiling water; stir in the garlic, bay leaf, thyme and pepper. Cook, uncovered, over medium heat for 30 minutes, stirring very occasionally. At the end of this period the lentils should be tender but still holding their shape; if too much water has boiled off (there should be enough moisture to give a saucy appearance to the lentils), add ½ to 1 cup (125 to 250 mL) more water as needed.

2. Meanwhile, broil sausage and onions for 3 to 4 minutes on each side. (They should not cook through; neither should the onions burn.) Remove and slice sausage into ½-inch (1 cm) pieces. Set aside sausage and onions together.

3. When the lentils are done, transfer to an ovenproof dish. Add butter (if using), vinegar and salt. Stir to mix. Add sausage and onions; stir until well distributed. Bake uncovered in preheated oven for 30 minutes. Serve immediately, garnished with chopped fresh parsley.

Soups

Bok Choy, Noodle and Tofu Chicken
Soup 40

Curry-Fried Tofu Soup with
Vegetables and Udon Noodles 41

Pasta e Fagioli 42

Mixed Vegetable Herb Broth
with Soft Tofu 43

White Bean Soup with Swiss Chard 44

Corn and Rice Chowder
with Parsley Persillade 45

Ribollita 46

Minestrone Genovese 48

Wild Mushroom and Navy Bean Soup . . . 49

Wheat Berry Minestrone 50

Navy Bean and Ham Soup 51

Cabbage, Bean and Bacon Chowder 52

Firehouse Chili Soup 53

Lamb Soup with Red Wine
Romano Beans and Chèvre 54

Spicy Black Bean Gazpacho 55

Succotash Sausage Soup 56

Black Bean and Sausage Gumbo 57

Caribbean Black Bean Soup 58

Black Bean, Butternut Squash
and Poblano Chile Soup 59

Chicken, Pinto Beans and
Green Chile Soup 60

Pappardelle and Chickpea Soup 61

Quick Chickpea and Pasta Soup 62

Chickpea Soup with Chorizo
and Garlic 63

Harira 64

Hearty Potato and Leek Soup 65

Coconut Curried Chickpea Soup 66

Lentil Soup with Rice 67

Curried Squash and Red Lentil Soup
with Coconut 68

Savory Red Lentil Soup 69

Green Lentil Soup 70

Roasted Garlic and Lentil Soup 71

Moroccan Spiced Lentil Soup 72

Bok Choy, Noodle and Tofu Chicken Soup

Tips

Napa cabbage, found in the produce section of grocery stores, can replace bok choy.

Spaghettini or capellini can also be used.

Try adding 3 oz (75 g) shrimp or cubed boneless chicken with the pasta.

Make Ahead

This soup is best prepared just before serving so the pasta and vegetables do not get overcooked and lose their color.

2 tsp	sesame oil	10 mL
1½ tsp	minced gingerroot	7 mL
1 tsp	crushed garlic	5 mL
2½ cups	chopped bok choy	625 mL
⅔ cup	chopped green onions	150 mL
⅓ cup	chicken stock	75 mL
6 cups	chicken stock	1.5 L
2 tbsp	soy sauce	30 mL
¾ cup	broken rice vermicelli	175 mL
½ cup	chopped snow peas	125 mL
½ cup	diced red bell peppers	125 mL
1 cup	firm tofu, cut into small cubes	250 mL

1. In a large nonstick saucepan, heat oil over medium-high heat; add ginger, garlic, bok choy, green onions and ⅓ cup (75 mL) stock. Sauté, covered, for approximately 5 minutes.

2. Add 6 cups (1.5 L) stock; bring to boil and add soy sauce, vermicelli, snow peas, red peppers and tofu. Reduce heat to medium and cook for 3 minutes or until pasta is cooked.

Curry-Fried Tofu Soup with Vegetables and Udon Noodles

We recommend that you make the effort to find Madras curry powder for this recipe. (Look for it in Asian markets.) Rusty in color and usually containing bay leaves, it is fuller and more complex than regular curry powder, which contains more turmeric and tends to be bitter.

Serves 4

Vegetarian Friendly

Tip

To make the bouquet garni for this recipe, place 3 slices of gingerroot, 1 clove garlic, 1 stalk lemon grass, smashed and sliced (or 1 tbsp/15 mL) lemon zest), 2 star anise, and 2 thumb-sized pieces of dried tangerine peel, rinsed (or 2 tsp/10 mL orange zest), in a piece of cheesecloth and tie securely with kitchen twine.

	Bouquet garni (see Tip, left)	
6 cups	vegetable or chicken stock	1.5 L
1	package (1 lb/500 g) medium-firm tofu	1
2 tbsp	Madras curry powder	30 mL
1/4 tsp	salt	1 mL
4	packages (7 oz/200 g) udon noodles or 1 lb (500 g) fresh spaghetti	4
2 cups	bean sprouts	500 mL
2 tbsp	vegetable oil	30 mL
1 cup	carrots, cut into matchsticks	250 mL
2 cups	broccoli florets	500 mL
1/2 tsp	salt	2 mL
4	sprigs cilantro	4

1. In a large saucepan or stockpot over high heat, bring bouquet garni and stock to a boil. Lower heat to medium and cook for 3 minutes. Cover and allow to steep for 15 minutes. Remove bouquet garni.

2. Cut tofu into 2-inch (5 cm) squares, about 1/2 inch (1 cm) thick. Pat dry with paper towels. In a mixing bowl, combine curry powder and salt; dredge tofu in mixture until lightly but evenly coated.

3. In a large pot of boiling salted water, cook noodles until al dente, about 2 minutes. Drain and divide between 4 serving bowls. Top with equally divided portions of bean sprouts.

4. In a nonstick wok or skillet, heat oil over medium-high heat for 30 seconds. Add tofu and fry until golden brown and slightly crisp on the outside, about 1 minute per side.

5. Meanwhile, bring broth to a boil. Add carrots and broccoli and cook for 3 minutes or until vegetables are just tender. Season with salt. Pour boiling broth and vegetables over noodle mixture. Top with tofu. Garnish with cilantro and serve immediately.

Pasta e Fagioli

This delicious Italian soup is great winter fare. For a stick-to-your ribs meal, serve with hot whole-grain rolls.

Serves 8

Tips

For this quantity of beans, soak and cook 1 cup (250 mL) dried beans or use 1 can (14 to 19 oz/398 to 540 mL) white kidney (cannellini) beans, drained and rinsed.

If you have a leftover boot (the tough outer rind) of Parmesan in the fridge add it to the soup along with the stock. It will add pleasant creaminess.

Three chiles add a pleasant hint of heat to the soup. Use more if you are a heat seeker.

If you don't have fresh rosemary, use ½ tsp (2 mL) dried.

• Food processor

2 cups	drained cooked white kidney (cannellini) beans, divided	500 mL
4 oz	chunk pancetta, coarsely chopped	125 g
2	onions, quartered	2
2	each carrots and celery stalks, peeled and cut into 3-inch (7.5 cm) lengths	2
2	cloves garlic, coarsely chopped	2
1 tbsp	olive oil	15 mL
1	sprig fresh rosemary	1
1 tsp	dried oregano	5 mL
½ tsp	cracked black peppercorns	2 mL
3	dried red chile peppers (approx.)	3
2	bay leaves	2
6 cups	chicken broth	1.5 L
1	can (28 oz/796 mL) diced tomatoes	1
1 cup	tiny pasta, such as ditalini or orzo	250 mL
1 tbsp	butter, optional	15 mL
½ cup	finely chopped parsley leaves	125 mL
	Freshly grated Parmesan cheese	
	Extra virgin olive oil	

1. In a food processor fitted with the metal blade, pulse 1 cup (250 mL) of the beans until mashed, about 5 times. Transfer to a bowl and set aside. In same work bowl, pulse pancetta, onions, carrots, celery and garlic until finely chopped, about 15 times.

2. In a stockpot or large saucepan, heat oil over medium heat. Add pancetta mixture and stir well. Cover, reduce heat to low and cook until vegetables are soft and pancetta has rendered most of its fat, about 10 minutes. Add rosemary, oregano, peppercorns, chile peppers and bay leaves and cook, stirring, for 1 minute. Add broth, tomatoes with juice, remaining 1 cup (250 mL) whole beans and mashed beans and bring to a boil. Cover, reduce heat to low and simmer until vegetables are tender and flavors meld, about 20 minutes.

3. Meanwhile, in a large pot of boiling salted water, cook pasta until al dente. Drain well, toss with butter, if using, and stir into soup. Remove and discard bay leaves and chile peppers. To serve, ladle into warm bowls and garnish with parsley, Parmesan and a drizzle of olive oil.

Mixed Vegetable Herb Broth with Soft Tofu

The Asian flavor of miso, combined with traditional Western herbs, enhances this savory vegetable soup.

Serves 4 to 6

Vegetarian Friendly

1 tbsp	butter	15 mL
½ cup	diced onions	125 mL
1 cup	diced carrots	250 mL
5 cups	chicken or vegetable stock	1.25 L
3 tbsp	white or red miso paste	45 mL
1 cup	frozen peas	250 mL
1 cup	frozen corn kernels	250 mL
1 lb	soft tofu, cut into ½-inch (1 cm) cubes	500 g
2 tbsp	chopped basil	30 mL
2 tbsp	chopped parsley, preferably flat-leaf Italian variety	30 mL
1 tbsp	chopped chives	15 mL
	Seasoned salt and freshly ground black pepper to taste	

1. In a large saucepan or soup pot, melt butter over medium heat. Add onions and carrots; sauté for 1 minute. Add stock and miso and bring to a boil. Add peas and corn; cook for 2 minutes. Skim off any impurities that float to the top.

2. Gently stir tofu, basil, parsley and chives into the soup and return to a boil. Season to taste with seasoned salt and pepper. Remove from heat and serve immediately.

Zuppa di fagioli con biete

White Bean Soup with Swiss Chard

This may be the best bean soup ever. The cooking time will depend on the freshness of the soaked beans. Health food stores are a good source for high-quality organic beans and pulses. Don't add salt to the beans' cooking water; this toughens them and encourages them to split open.

Serves 4 to 6

2 cups	dried cannellini beans (white kidney beans) or navy beans, soaked overnight in water to cover	500 mL
1 tbsp	olive oil	15 mL
8 oz	mushrooms, finely chopped (about 3 cups/ 750 mL)	250 g
3	cloves garlic, minced	3
1	onion, chopped	1
½ tsp	freshly grated nutmeg	2 mL
6 cups	chicken stock	1.5 L
1 lb	Swiss chard, washed, stemmed and chopped (about 6 cups/1.5 L)	500 g
	Salt and freshly ground black pepper to taste	
3 cups	ricotta cheese	750 mL
8	slices rustic country-style bread	8
¾ cup	grated Pecorino Romano	175 mL
¼ cup	chopped flat-leaf parsley	60 mL

1. Drain beans and place in a large saucepan. Add water to cover by 2 inches (5 cm); bring to a boil. Reduce heat to simmer and cook for 1½ hours or until beans are tender, skimming any foam that rises to the surface. Drain beans, discarding cooking liquid.

2. Wipe saucepan clean. Heat olive oil in saucepan over medium heat. Add mushrooms, garlic, onion and nutmeg; cook, stirring often, for 5 minutes or until vegetables are softened. Stir in cooked beans and chicken stock; bring to a boil. Reduce heat to medium-low and cook for 20 minutes. Stir in Swiss chard; cook for 2 minutes or until wilted. Season to taste with salt and pepper.

3. Preheat broiler. Spread ricotta cheese on bread slices. Top with Pecorino Romano. Broil for 2 minutes or until cheese is golden.

4. Ladle soup into soup plates. Place a piece of cheese toast in the center of each serving. Sprinkle with parsley. Serve with extra toasts on the side.

Corn and Rice Chowder with Parsley Persillade

Here we have the perfect balance of incomplete proteins together in one dish — corn, rice and beans. Persillade is the term given to a fine mince of garlic and parsley that is usually added at the end to sautéed dishes, vegetables stews and soups. Use it as a substitute for salt or butter on vegetables.

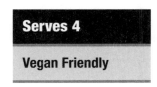

Serves 4

Vegan Friendly

Tips

Store persillade, tightly covered, in the refrigerator up to 4 days.

Use fresh corn kernels sliced off the cob when available; at all other times frozen corn is best.

Parsley Persillade

1/4 cup	finely chopped fresh parsley	60 mL
1	clove garlic, finely chopped	1
2 tbsp	finely ground almonds	30 mL

Chowder

3 cups	rice or soy milk	750 mL
1 cup	chopped onion	250 mL
1	leek, white and light green parts, chopped	1
1 1/3 cups	sweet corn kernels (see Tips, left)	325 mL
1	can (14 oz/398 mL) lima beans, drained and rinsed, or 1 2/3 cups (400 mL) cooked lima beans	1
1 cup	cooked wild rice	250 mL
1/2 tsp	salt	2 mL

1. *Parsley Persillade:* In a small bowl, combine parsley, garlic and almonds.

2. *Chowder:* In a large saucepan, heat milk to just under a boil over medium heat. Add onion and leek. Cover, reduce heat to low and simmer gently for 10 minutes. Add corn. Cover and simmer for 5 minutes.

3. Stir in lima beans, wild rice and salt and heat through. Taste and add more salt, if required. Ladle into soup bowls. Garnish with about 1 tbsp (15 mL) Parsley Persillade.

Ribollita

Hearty bean soups are almost a way of life in Italy — especially in Tuscany, where the residents have long been known as mangia fagioli *or "bean eaters." Sustaining, filling and satisfying, these soups (which also include minestrone and pasta e fagioli) form the basis of the next day's supper. This is the inspiration for sturdy ribollita, which means "reboiled."*

Serves 6 to 8

Vegetarian Friendly

- **12-cup (3 L) soup tureen or casserole dish**
- **Food processor or blender**

3 tbsp	olive oil	45 mL
3	cloves garlic, finely chopped	3
2	medium leeks, green part only, trimmed, washed and finely chopped	2
1	onion, finely chopped	1
1	carrot, finely chopped	1
1	stalk celery, finely chopped	1
2 tsp	finely chopped rosemary	10 mL
1	small dried chile pepper	1
1 1/4 cups	dried cannellini beans (white kidney beans) or navy beans, soaked overnight in water to cover	300 mL
	Salt and freshly ground black pepper to taste	
1/2 cup	extra virgin olive oil	125 mL
2	cloves garlic, crushed	2
2	whole sprigs thyme	2
8	slices oven-toasted or grilled bread, brushed with olive oil and rubbed with garlic	8
1 cup	grated Parmigiano-Reggiano	250 mL

1. In a large saucepan, heat olive oil over medium heat. Add garlic, leeks, onion, carrot, celery, rosemary and chile; cook, stirring frequently, for 10 minutes or until vegetables are softened and starting to brown. Stir in drained beans and 10 cups (2.5 L) water. Bring to a boil; reduce heat to simmer and cook 1 1/2 hours or until beans are tender, skimming any foam that rises to the surface.

2. With a slotted spoon, transfer half of the cooked beans and vegetables to a food processor or blender; purée. Return bean purée to saucepan; stir to blend. Season to taste with salt and pepper. Keep soup at a low simmer.

3. Preheat oven to 375°F (190°C). In a small skillet, heat olive oil over medium heat. Add garlic and thyme; cook for 2 minutes or until garlic is golden. Strain oil into a heatproof bowl; discard solids.

4. Put toasts in bottom of soup tureen or casserole dish; sprinkle with half of the cheese. Pour bean soup over toasts. Drizzle garlic-thyme oil over the surface. Sprinkle with remaining cheese. Bake, uncovered, for 30 minutes or until cheese is golden. Serve from tureen at the table.

Minestrone Genovese

A specialty of Genoa, Italy, this robust soup is distinguished by the addition of basil pesto. The porcini mushrooms add earthiness and the brown rice, along with the traditional puréed beans, helps to thicken the soup. Served with whole-grain bread and a tossed salad, this makes a substantial and satisfying meal.

Makes 6 main-course servings

Vegetarian Friendly

Tips

If you prefer, use 1 cup (250 mL) dried white kidney beans, soaked and cooked (see pages 6 to 10).

Unless you have a stove with a true simmer, after reducing the heat to low place a heat diffuser under the pot to prevent the mixture from boiling. This device also helps to ensure the grains will cook evenly and prevents hot spots, which might cause scorching, from forming. Heat diffusers are available at kitchen supply and hardware stores and are made to work on gas or electric stoves.

- **Food processor**

1	package ($\frac{1}{2}$ oz/14 g) dried porcini mushrooms	1
2 cups	hot water	500 mL
1	can (14 to 19 oz/398 to 540 mL) white kidney beans, drained and rinsed (see Tips, left), divided	1
6 cups	vegetable or chicken stock, divided	1.5 L
2 tbsp	tomato paste	30 mL
1 tbsp	olive oil	15 mL
2	onions, finely chopped	2
2	carrots, peeled and diced	2
2	stalks celery, diced	2
4	cloves garlic, minced	4
1	dried red chile pepper, optional	1
	Salt and freshly ground black pepper	
1 cup	short-grain brown rice, rinsed and drained	250 mL
4 cups	shredded cabbage	1 L
1 cup	sliced green beans	250 mL
$\frac{1}{4}$ cup	basil pesto	60 mL
	Freshly grated Parmesan cheese	

1. In a bowl, soak dried mushrooms in hot water for 30 minutes. Strain through a coffee filter or a sieve lined with a damp paper towel, reserving liquid. Pat mushrooms dry and chop finely. Set aside.

2. In a food processor fitted with the metal blade, combine 1 cup (250 mL) of the beans, 1 cup (250 mL) of the stock and tomato paste and purée until smooth. Set aside.

3. In a large saucepan or stockpot, heat oil over medium heat for 30 seconds. Add onions, carrots and celery and cook, stirring, until carrots are softened, about 7 minutes. Add garlic, reserved chopped mushrooms, chile pepper, if using, and salt and pepper to taste. Cook, stirring, for 1 minute. Add rice and toss until well coated with mixture. Add whole and puréed beans, remaining stock and mushroom soaking liquid and bring to a boil.

4. Reduce heat to low. Cover and simmer for 45 minutes. Return to a boil. Stir in cabbage and green beans and cook until beans and rice are tender, about 8 minutes. Remove from heat and stir in pesto. Ladle into bowls and top with Parmesan.

Wild Mushroom and Navy Bean Soup

Wild mushrooms are so easy to find in grocery stores nowadays that it is a crime not to use them. They add big flavor to soups, and we love the colors and shapes for the visual interest they add.

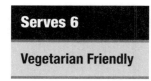

Serves 6

Vegetarian Friendly

Tip

To clean mushrooms, you can either rinse them quickly in water or wipe them with a damp paper towel. Mushrooms will be much happier in your refrigerator if you store them in a paper bag.

¼ cup	unsalted butter	60 mL
1½ lbs	wild (exotic) mushrooms, sliced	750 g
3	cloves garlic, minced	3
1 cup	thinly sliced green onions	250 mL
½ tsp	salt	2 mL
2 tbsp	all-purpose flour	30 mL
6 cups	beef or mushroom stock	1.5 L
½ cup	dry white wine	125 mL
2	cans (each 14 to 19 oz/398 to 540 mL) navy beans, drained and rinsed	2
1 cup	whipping (35%) cream	250 mL
Pinch	cayenne pepper	Pinch
	Freshly ground black pepper	
¼ cup	minced fresh chives	60 mL

1. In a large pot, melt butter over medium heat. Add mushrooms, garlic, green onions and salt; sauté until mushrooms have released their liquid and are browned, about 10 minutes. Sprinkle with flour and sauté for 2 minutes.

2. Gradually whisk in stock and wine. Add beans and bring to a boil, stirring often. Reduce heat and simmer for about 20 minutes to blend the flavors. Stir in cream, cayenne and salt and black pepper to taste; reheat over medium heat until steaming, stirring often.

3. Ladle into heated bowls and garnish with chives.

Wheat Berry Minestrone

Here's a hearty meal-in-a-bowl that makes a delicious lunch or light supper any time of the year. Serve this soup for supper, accompanied by whole-grain bread and a simple green salad.

Serves 6

Vegan Friendly

Tips

For this quantity of beans, use 1 can (14 to 19 oz/398 to 540 mL), drained and rinsed, or cook 1 cup (250 mL) dried beans.

For enhanced flavor, if you have a boot of Parmesan, the tough rind that is left over from a whole piece, add it to the soup along with the tomatoes.

When using leafy greens, such as kale or Swiss chard, be sure to remove the tough stems before chopping. Also, since they can be quite gritty pay extra attention when washing.

To make crostini: Brush 8 to 10 baguette slices with olive oil on both sides. Toast under preheated broiler, turning once, until golden, about 2 minutes per side.

- **Food processor**

2	onions, quartered	2
4	stalks celery, cut into 3-inch (7.5 cm) lengths	4
4	cloves garlic, chopped	4
1 tbsp	oil	15 mL
2 tsp	dried Italian seasoning	10 mL
1 tsp	salt	5 mL
1/4 tsp	cayenne pepper	1 mL
2 cups	drained cooked white kidney beans (see Tips, left)	500 mL
4 cups	chicken or vegetable broth, divided	1 L
1 cup	wheat, spelt or Kamut berries, rinsed and drained	250 mL
1	can (14 oz/398 mL) diced tomatoes with juice	1
8 cups	coarsely chopped trimmed kale or Swiss chard (see Tips, left)	2 L
	Salt and freshly ground black pepper	
	Crostini, optional (see Tips, left)	
	Freshly grated Parmesan cheese or vegan alternative, optional	
	Extra virgin olive oil	

1. In a food processor fitted with metal blade, pulse onions, celery and garlic until finely chopped, about 15 times. In a large saucepan or stockpot, heat oil over medium heat. Add onion mixture and cook, stirring, until vegetables are softened, about 5 minutes. Add Italian seasoning, salt and cayenne and cook, stirring, for 1 minute.

2. Meanwhile, in same work bowl, purée beans with 1 cup (250 mL) of the broth until smooth. Add to saucepan along with wheat berries, tomatoes with juice, 2 cups (500 mL) water and remaining 3 cups (750 mL) of the broth and bring to a boil.

Tip

Puréeing the beans with some of the broth gives this soup a creamy texture without the addition of cream.

3. Cover, reduce heat to low and simmer until wheat berries are almost tender, about 1 hour. Stir in kale. Cover and cook until kale and wheat berries are tender, about 15 minutes. Season with salt and pepper to taste.

4. When ready to serve, ladle soup into warm bowls. Float 1 or 2 crostini in each bowl, if using. Sprinkle liberally with Parmesan, if using, and drizzle with olive oil.

Navy Bean and Ham Soup

We return to this soup time and time again when we're looking for the simple flavors of ham and beans.

Serves 6 to 8

Tip

Here's how to quick-soak dried beans: In a colander, rinse beans under cold water and discard any discolored ones. In a saucepan, combine beans with enough cold water to cover them by 2 inches (5 cm). Bring to a boil over medium heat and boil for 2 minutes. Remove from heat and let soak, covered, for 1 hour.

8 cups	cold water	2 L
2 cups	dried navy beans, soaked overnight or quick-soaked (see Tip, left) and drained	500 mL
2	large smoked ham hocks (about 1¾ lbs/875 g total)	2
1	onion, coarsely chopped	1
1	carrot, coarsely chopped	1
1	clove garlic, coarsely chopped	1
2	sprigs fresh thyme	2
1	bay leaf	1
	Salt and freshly ground black pepper	
2 tbsp	chopped fresh parsley	30 mL

1. In a large pot, bring water, beans, ham hocks, onion, carrot, garlic, thyme and bay leaf to a boil over medium heat. Reduce heat and simmer until beans are tender, about 1½ hours. Discard thyme sprigs and bay leaf.

2. Remove ham hocks from the soup and let cool slightly. Pick the meat from the bones and shred into bite-size pieces. Discard bones, fat and skin. Return meat to the soup and simmer until heated through. Season with salt and pepper to taste.

3. Ladle into heated bowls and garnish with parsley.

Cabbage, Bean and Bacon Chowder

The Great Northern bean is large and white, and is the North American version of the haricot bean or Italian cannellini bean. Substitute white kidney beans if Great Northern beans are unavailable.

Serves 6

2 tbsp	canola oil	30 mL
8 oz	lean Canadian back bacon, chopped	250 g
1	large onion, chopped	1
2	cloves garlic, minced	2
1	jalapeño pepper, seeded and chopped	1
2	carrots, chopped	2
1	potato, chopped	1
1	small white turnip, chopped	1
8 cups	beef stock	2 L
1 lb	green cabbage, finely shredded	500 g
1	can (19 oz/540 mL) Great Northern beans, rinsed and drained	1
	Salt and pepper to taste	

1. In a large saucepan, heat oil over medium-high heat. Add back bacon, onion, garlic and jalapeño pepper; cook 4 minutes or until softened.

2. Stir in the carrots, potato, turnip and stock; bring to a boil. Reduce heat to medium-low and cook, covered, for 15 to 25 minutes or until vegetables are tender.

3. Stir in cabbage and cook for 15 minutes or until cabbage is tender. Stir in beans and heat through. Season to taste with salt and pepper.

Firehouse Chili Soup

Quick to throw together, this beefy soup is sure to fire up hearty appetites.

Serves 6 to 8

Tip

If you can't find Southwest-style tomatoes, regular canned diced tomatoes will also work.

1/4 cup	olive oil	60 mL
1 cup	chopped onion	250 mL
1 lb	lean ground beef	500 g
4	cloves garlic, minced	4
2	cans (each 14 to 19 oz/398 to 540 mL) red kidney beans, drained and rinsed	2
1	can (14 oz/398 mL) Southwest-style diced tomatoes, with juice	1
4 cups	beef stock	1 L
2 tbsp	chili powder (or to taste)	30 mL
1 tsp	dried oregano	5 mL
1 tsp	salt	5 mL
1/2 tsp	freshly ground black pepper	2 mL
1 tbsp	Worcestershire sauce	15 mL
2 tsp	balsamic vinegar	10 mL
1 cup	shredded Cheddar cheese (optional)	250 mL
1	avocado, diced (optional)	1

1. In a large pot, heat oil over medium heat. Add onion and sauté until softened, about 6 minutes. Add ground beef and garlic; sauté, breaking beef up with the back of a wooden spoon, until no longer pink, about 5 minutes. Drain any excess fat.

2. Add beans, tomatoes with juice, stock, chili powder, oregano, salt, black pepper, Worcestershire sauce and vinegar; bring to a boil. Cover, reduce heat to low and simmer gently for 30 minutes to blend the flavors. Taste and adjust seasoning with salt and black pepper, if necessary.

3. Ladle into heated bowls and garnish with cheese and avocado, if desired.

Variations

Try using your favorite bulk sausage (or sausage meat removed from casings) instead of ground beef.

Substitute canned white kidney beans for the red kidney beans and ground turkey for the beef.

Lamb Soup with Red Wine, Romano Beans and Chèvre

This soup is really a meal in itself — and the smell of it simmering in the oven is mouthwatering. If you want to scale down this recipe, you can use a smaller cut of lamb, such as a center leg roast.

Serves 10

Tip

Unlike beef, where there are many cuts of meat, lamb offers a more limited selection. A leg of lamb, which comes from the rear leg of the animal, can be bought in a number of ways. The heavier the leg, the older and fattier the lamb. (Generally, to be called a lamb, the animal must be under 1 year old.) Look for pink meat with creamy white fat.

Romano beans are also known as cranberry or borlotti beans.

● **Preheat oven to 375°F (190°C)**

1	leg of lamb (about 5 to 6 lbs/2.5 to 3 kg)	1
	Salt and pepper	
2 tbsp	olive oil	30 mL
2 tbsp	butter	30 mL
2	onions, chopped	2
2	carrots, chopped	2
2	parsnips, chopped	2
1	fennel bulb, cored and chopped	1
2	cloves garlic, pressed	2
½ cup	red currant jelly	125 mL
½ cup	balsamic vinegar	125 mL
3 cups	red wine	750 mL
4 cups	water	1 L
1 lb	plum tomatoes, chopped	500 g
1 cup	romano beans, soaked overnight and drained	250 mL
1	bay leaf	1
	Fresh thyme, to taste	
	Fresh tarragon, to taste	
	Freshly grated Parmesan cheese	
	Fresh chèvre (goat cheese), crumbled	
	Zest of 1 orange	

1. Season the lamb with salt and pepper. In a large, heavy ovenproof casserole dish with a lid, heat olive oil and butter over medium-high heat until bubbling. Add lamb and sear on all sides until browned. Place casserole in preheated oven and roast for 45 minutes. Remove from oven and, with a slotted spoon, transfer lamb to a bowl.

2. To the casserole dish, add onions, carrots, parsnips and fennel; cook over medium heat until browned. Add pressed garlic and cook for 2 minutes or until slightly browned.

3. Stir in red currant jelly, balsamic vinegar, wine, water, tomatoes and Romano beans. Add the lamb along with the bay leaf, thyme and tarragon. Cover and simmer in the oven for another hour.

4. Remove casserole from oven. Cut lamb into pieces and return to stock. Adjust seasoning and serve in warm bowls, garnished with Parmesan, crumbled chèvre and orange zest.

Spicy Black Bean Gazpacho

A generous bowlful of this nourishing soup makes an ideal lunch or light supper. Just add some pita bread or whole-grain crackers.

Serves 6

Vegetarian Friendly

Tips

Tabasco is a preferred brand of hot pepper sauce, especially for tomato-based dishes.

Cold soups taste best when refrigerated overnight, giving the flavors a chance to blend. Always check the seasoning of a cold soup, however. Often you will need to add extra salt, pepper or hot pepper sauce.

• **Food processor**

1	red bell pepper, coarsely chopped	1
3	green onions, coarsely chopped	3
3	ripe tomatoes, coarsely chopped	3
1	large clove garlic, minced	1
1	can (19 oz/540 mL) black beans, rinsed and drained	1
1	can (19 oz/540 mL) tomato juice	1
2 tbsp	balsamic vinegar	30 mL
1 tbsp	red wine vinegar	15 mL
	Salt and pepper	
1/2 to 1 tsp	hot pepper sauce	2 to 5 mL
1/3 cup	chopped fresh cilantro or parsley	75 mL
	Light sour cream or plain yogurt	

1. In a food processor, finely chop red pepper and green onions, using on-off turns; transfer to a large bowl. Add tomatoes to food processor; finely chop, using on-off turns. Add to pepper-onion mixture along with black beans and tomato juice. Add balsamic and red wine vinegars; season with salt, pepper and hot pepper sauce to taste. Cover and refrigerate for 4 hours, preferably overnight.

2. Add about 1/3 cup (75 mL) cold water to thin soup, if desired. Adjust seasoning with vinegars, salt, pepper and hot pepper sauce. Ladle into chilled bowls; sprinkle with cilantro and top with a spoonful of sour cream.

Succotash Sausage Soup

Succotash is a favorite late-summer side dish. In this creamy soup, we've made it a meal by adding hearty kielbasa sausage.

Serves 6 to 8

Tip

To trim leeks, cut off and discard the root end and the dark green tops (or save the tops for stock). Cut leeks lengthwise and wash under running water to remove any grit or dirt. Then cut as directed in the recipe.

1/4 cup	unsalted butter	60 mL
1 lb	kielbasa sausage, cut into thin half-moons	500 g
2 cups	chopped leeks, white and light green parts only	500 mL
3	garlic cloves, chopped	3
1	large red bell pepper, finely chopped	1
3 tbsp	all-purpose flour	45 mL
1 tbsp	chopped fresh thyme	15 mL
6 cups	chicken stock	1.5 L
2 cups	frozen baby lima beans, thawed	500 mL
1/2 tsp	salt	2 mL
1/4 tsp	freshly ground black pepper	1 mL
1	can (14 oz/398 mL) cream-style corn	1
1 1/2 cups	fresh or frozen white corn kernels, thawed if frozen	375 mL
1/2 cup	whipping (35%) cream Fresh thyme leaves	125 mL

1. In a large, heavy pot, melt butter over medium heat. Add sausage, leeks, garlic and red pepper; sauté until vegetables are softened and sausage is browned, about 6 minutes. Sprinkle with flour and thyme; sauté for 2 minutes.

2. Gradually whisk in stock. Add lima beans, salt and pepper; bring to a boil, stirring often. Reduce heat and simmer, stirring occasionally, until lima beans are tender, about 10 minutes. Add cream-style corn and corn kernels; simmer for 10 minutes. Stir in cream. Taste and adjust seasoning with salt and pepper, if necessary. Reheat until steaming, stirring often. Do not let boil.

3. Ladle into heated bowls and garnish each with a few thyme leaves.

Black Bean and Sausage Gumbo

This hearty soup is really almost a stew. Serve it as a main course with cornbread and beer or ladle it over hot cooked rice in deep soup plates.

Serves 8 to 10

Tip

Use canned black beans, rinsed and drained, or start with 2 cups (500 mL) dried black beans.

$\frac{1}{2}$ cup	canola oil	125 mL
$\frac{1}{2}$ cup	all-purpose flour	125 mL
4	onions, chopped	4
4	stalks celery, chopped	4
1	red bell pepper, chopped	1
6	cloves garlic, pressed	6
8 cups	chicken stock	2 L
5 cups	cooked black beans (see Tip, left)	1.25 L
$\frac{1}{4}$ cup	Worcestershire sauce	60 mL
2 lbs	spicy Italian sausages, cooked and sliced	1 kg
$\frac{1}{2}$ tsp	chopped fresh thyme	2 mL
	Salt and pepper to taste	
$\frac{1}{2}$ cup	minced fresh parsley	125 mL
$\frac{1}{2}$ cup	chopped green onions	125 mL
$\frac{1}{2}$ cup	seeded and chopped tomatoes	125 mL
	Cornbread or hot cooked rice as accompaniment	

1. In a stockpot, cook oil and flour over medium heat, stirring constantly, for 10 minutes or until you have a brown roux the color of peanut butter. Be careful, this gets very hot and burns easily.

2. Stir in onions, celery, red pepper and garlic; cook, covered and stirring occasionally, for 8 minutes or until vegetables are tender. Stir in stock, beans, Worcestershire sauce, sausage and thyme; bring to a boil. Reduce heat to medium-low and cook, covered, for 30 minutes. Season to taste with salt and pepper. Stir in parsley and green onions. Place a mound of hot cooked rice in each serving bowl and spoon gumbo over top. Serve garnished with tomatoes.

Caribbean Black Bean Soup

Natives of the Caribbean love to combine sweet and savory elements in a dish. We love it as well. That's why, for this soup, we paired the smoky flavors of black beans and bacon with the bright notes of a tropical fruit salsa.

Serves 6 to 8

Tip

For a thicker consistency, after Step 2, mash some of the beans with a potato masher or process 2 cups (500 mL) of the soup in a blender or food processor.

2 tbsp	unsalted butter	30 mL
8	slices bacon, chopped	8
1	onion, chopped	1
3	cloves garlic, minced	3
1	carrot, chopped	1
1	stalk celery, chopped	1
1 tsp	dried thyme	5 mL
1 tsp	ground cumin	5 mL
6 cups	beef stock	1.5 L
2 cups	water	500 mL
2 cups	dried black beans, soaked overnight or quick-soaked (see pages 6 and 7) and drained	500 mL
1	bay leaf	1
1 tsp	salt	5 mL
1/2 tsp	freshly ground black pepper	2 mL
1	lime, cut into 6 to 8 wedges	1

Fruit Salsa

2	oranges, sectioned	2
1	banana, diced	1
1/2 cup	finely chopped red onion	125 mL
1/4 cup	chopped fresh cilantro	60 mL
2 tbsp	freshly squeezed lime juice	30 mL

1. In a large pot, melt butter over medium heat. Add bacon and sauté until it renders its fat but is still soft, about 2 minutes. Add onion and sauté until softened, about 6 minutes. Add garlic, carrot, celery, thyme and cumin; sauté until vegetables are softened, about 5 minutes.

2. Add stock, water, beans and bay leaf; bring to a boil. Reduce heat and simmer for 1 hour. Add salt and pepper; simmer until beans are tender, about 30 minutes. Taste and adjust seasoning with salt and pepper, if necessary. Discard bay leaf.

3. *Prepare the fruit salsa:* In a small bowl, combine oranges, banana, red onion, cilantro and lime juice.

4. Ladle soup into heated bowls and garnish each with a heaping tablespoon (15 mL) of fruit salsa and a lime wedge. Diners may squeeze the lime over their soup, if they desire.

Black Bean, Butternut Squash and Poblano Chile Soup

The savory combination of earthy black beans, smoky chipotle chiles and sweet butternut squash is absolutely irresistible.

Serves 6 to 8

Vegetarian Friendly

Tip

You can often find butternut squash already peeled and diced in your grocer's produce aisles, which makes this already easy soup even easier.

1 tbsp	olive oil	15 mL
2	cloves garlic, minced	2
2	large poblano chile peppers, seeded and chopped	2
1	onion, chopped	1
1 tbsp	cumin seeds	15 mL
2	cans (each 14 to 19 oz/398 to 540 mL) black beans, drained and rinsed	2
1	butternut squash (about 1$\frac{1}{2}$ lbs/750 g), peeled and cut into $\frac{1}{2}$-inch (1 cm) dice	1
1	can (14 oz/398 mL) diced tomatoes, with juice	1
6 cups	chicken or vegetable stock	1.5 L
1 tbsp	minced drained chipotle chile peppers in adobo sauce	15 mL
1 tsp	salt	5 mL
	Sour cream	

1. In a large, heavy pot, heat oil over medium heat. Add garlic, poblano chiles, onion and cumin seeds; sauté until onion is softened, about 6 minutes.

2. Add beans, squash, tomatoes with juice, stock, chipotle chiles and salt; bring to a boil. Reduce heat and simmer, stirring occasionally, until squash is tender, about 30 minutes.

3. Ladle into heated bowls and garnish each with a dollop of sour cream.

Chicken, Pinto Beans and Green Chile Soup

Who doesn't love a 30-minute meal? We know we do, especially on a hectic weeknight when we want something good but don't have time to put together anything too involved. This is the perfect soup on those busy nights.

Serves 8

Tip

San Marzano tomatoes, imported from Italy, are thought by many to be the best canned tomatoes in the world. They hail from a small town of the same name near Naples, whose volcanic soil is thought to filter impurities from the water and render tomatoes with a thick flesh, fewer seeds and a stronger taste. Look for the words "San Marzano" on the label to be sure you're getting the best.

1 tbsp	olive oil	15 mL
2	poblano chile peppers, seeded and chopped	2
1	onion, chopped	1
3	cloves garlic, minced	3
2 tsp	ground cumin	10 mL
1 tsp	dried oregano	5 mL
1 tsp	ground coriander	5 mL
1/4 tsp	cayenne pepper	1 mL
1	can (14 oz/398 mL) diced tomatoes, with juice	1
5 cups	chicken stock	1.25 L
1 tsp	salt	5 mL
1/4 tsp	freshly ground black pepper	1 mL
2	cans (each 14 to 19 oz/398 to 540 mL) pinto beans, drained and rinsed	2
3 cups	shredded cooked chicken	750 mL
1/2 cup	shredded Monterey Jack or Cheddar cheese	125 mL
1/2 cup	sour cream	125 mL

1. In a large pot, heat oil over medium heat. Add poblano chiles and onion; sauté until softened, about 6 minutes. Add garlic, cumin, oregano, coriander and cayenne; sauté for 2 minutes.

2. Stir in tomatoes with juice, stock, salt and black pepper; bring to a boil. Reduce heat and simmer for 20 minutes to blend the flavors. Add beans and chicken; heat until steaming, about 5 minutes. Taste and adjust seasoning with salt, if necessary.

3. Ladle into heated bowls and garnish with cheese and sour cream.

Pasta e Ceci

Pappardelle and Chickpea Soup

Pappardelle are long, ribbon-like strips of pasta, about ³/₄ inch (2 cm) in width. They are often used with rich, creamy sauces, with porcini and, famously, with rabbit. This ancient version pairs the pasta with chickpeas as they do in Apulia, where, just before serving, they often fry a little additional dried pasta at the very last minute to add another dimension of texture to the soup.

Serves 6 to 8

Vegetarian Friendly

Tips

It's worth taking the time to use dried chickpeas and soak them overnight. Canned chickpeas are often overcooked.

The rosemary is not traditional but works well with the chickpeas.

If using smaller canned plum tomatoes, add 2 to 3 more.

2 cups	dried chickpeas, soaked over-night in cold water to cover	500 mL
1	bay leaf	1
3 cups	vegetable stock or chicken stock	750 mL
¼ cup	olive oil	60 mL
1	onion, chopped	1
3	cloves garlic, finely chopped	3
1	whole branch rosemary	1
3	large ripe plum tomatoes, peeled, seeded and chopped	3
	Salt and freshly ground black pepper to taste	
8 oz	pappardelle (or tagliatelle or fettuccine)	250 g
½ cup	chopped flat-leaf parsley	125 mL

1. In a large saucepan, combine drained chickpeas and bay leaf. Add cold water to cover by 2 inches (5 cm); bring to a boil. Reduce heat to simmer and cook for 1 hour or until chickpeas are tender. Drain, reserving cooking liquid. Wipe saucepan clean and return cooking liquid to saucepan. Add stock; bring to a boil and reduce heat to low.

2. In another large saucepan, heat olive oil over medium heat. Add onion, garlic and rosemary; cook for 5 minutes or until vegetables are softened. Stir in tomatoes; cook 5 minutes longer. Stir in stock mixture and chickpeas. Season to taste with salt and pepper. Bring to a boil; stir in pasta, reduce heat to simmer and cook, stirring occasionally, for 10 minutes or until pasta is tender. Remove rosemary. Serve sprinkled with parsley.

Quick Chickpea and Pasta Soup

Soup's on! Your fridge may be bare, but chances are you'll have the basic ingredients in your pantry to make this sustaining main-course soup for a quick-fix dinner.

Serves 4

Vegetarian Friendly

Tip

Other types of canned beans or lentils can be used instead of chickpeas.

1 tbsp	olive oil	15 mL
1	medium onion, chopped	1
2	cloves garlic, finely chopped	2
½ tsp	dried basil or Italian herbs	2 mL
2 tbsp	tomato paste	30 mL
5 cups	chicken stock or vegetable stock (approximate)	1.25 L
¾ cup	small pasta shapes such as shells	175 mL
1	can (19 oz/540 mL) chickpeas, rinsed and drained	1
	Salt and pepper	
	Grated Parmesan cheese	

1. In a large saucepan, heat oil over medium heat. Add onion, garlic and basil; cook, stirring, for 2 minutes or until softened. Add tomato paste; cook, stirring, for 30 seconds.

2. Add stock; bring to a boil. Stir in pasta and chickpeas; cook, partially covered and stirring occasionally, for 8 to 10 minutes or until pasta is just tender. Season with salt and pepper to taste. Ladle soup into bowls and serve sprinkled with Parmesan cheese.

Variation

Chickpea, Pasta and Spinach Soup: Increase stock to 6 cups (1.5 L). Stir in 4 cups (1 L) shredded fresh spinach or Swiss chard along with chickpeas and pasta.

Chickpea Soup with Chorizo and Garlic

We love the spicy sausage and the tender, meaty beans in this soup. Best of all, it comes together fast enough for Tuesday night dinner before the soccer game.

Serves 6

Tip

For a thicker soup, mash some of the beans in the pot with a potato masher.

¼ cup	olive oil	60 mL
1	onion, chopped	1
1	carrot, chopped	1
1	stalk celery, chopped	1
1	zucchini, chopped	1
1 lb	fresh chorizo sausage (bulk or with casings removed)	500 g
3 tbsp	finely chopped garlic	45 mL
1 tsp	dried thyme	5 mL
6 cups	chicken or vegetable stock	1.5 L
2 tbsp	tomato paste	30 mL
1 tsp	paprika	5 mL
2	cans (each 14 to 19 oz/398 to 540 mL) chickpeas, drained and rinsed	2
½ tsp	salt	2 mL
¼ tsp	freshly ground black pepper	1 mL
2 tbsp	minced fresh flat-leaf (Italian) parsley	30 mL

1. In a large pot, heat oil over medium heat. Add onion, carrot, celery and zucchini; sauté until softened, about 6 minutes. Add chorizo, garlic and thyme; sauté, breaking chorizo up with the back of a wooden spoon, until no longer pink, about 5 minutes.

2. Add stock, tomato paste and paprika; bring to a simmer. Add chickpeas and simmer until heated through, about 10 minutes. Season with salt and pepper.

3. Ladle into heated bowls and garnish with parsley.

Variation

If you prefer smoked chorizo sausage instead of fresh, cut it into 1-inch (2.5 cm) pieces, or crumble, and reduce the sautéing time to 2 minutes.

Harira

This traditional Moroccan soup, often made with lamb, is usually served during Ramadan at the end of a day of fasting. This vegetarian version is finished with a dollop of harissa, a spicy North African sauce, which adds flavor and punch. Served with whole-grain bread, harira makes a great light meal. A salad of shredded carrots topped with a sprinkling of currants adds color to the meal and complements the Middle Eastern flavors.

Serves 6

Vegan Friendly

Tip

If you prefer, you can use 1 cup (250 mL) dried chickpeas, soaked, cooked and drained (see pages 6 to 10), instead of the canned chickpeas.

Make Ahead

Complete Step 1. Cover and refrigerate for up to 2 days. When you're ready to cook, continue with the recipe.

• **Large (minimum 5-quart) slow cooker**

1 tbsp	olive oil	15 mL
4	stalks celery, diced	4
2	onions, coarsely chopped	2
2	cloves garlic, minced	2
1 tbsp	ground turmeric	15 mL
1 tbsp	grated lemon zest	15 mL
1/2 tsp	cracked black peppercorns	2 mL
1	can (28 oz/796 mL) diced tomatoes, with juice	1
4 cups	vegetable or chicken stock	1 L
1 cup	dried red lentils, rinsed	250 mL
1	can (14 to 19 oz/398 to 540 mL) chickpeas, drained and rinsed (see Tip, left)	1
1/2 cup	finely chopped fresh parsley	125 mL
	Harissa	

1. In a skillet, heat oil over medium heat for 30 seconds. Add celery and onions; cook, stirring, until celery is softened, about 5 minutes. Add garlic, turmeric, lemon zest and peppercorns; cook, stirring, for 1 minute. Add tomatoes with juice and bring to a boil. Transfer to slow cooker stoneware.

2. Stir in stock, lentils and chickpeas. Cover and cook on Low for 6 to 8 hours or on High for 3 to 4 hours, until mixture is hot and bubbly and lentils are tender. Stir in parsley.

3. Ladle into bowls and pass the harissa at the table.

Hearty Potato and Leek Soup

Tomato is an unusual ingredient in potato and leek soup but in the fall when tomatoes are abundant, they add a cheery note to this winter favorite. Omit them in the winter when fresh ripe organic tomatoes are not available.

Serves 6 to 8

Vegan Friendly

Tip

You can use 2 cups (500 mL) cooked chickpeas, drained and rinsed, instead of canned.

2 tbsp	olive oil	30 mL
3	onions, chopped	3
2	leeks, white and green parts, sliced	2
3	cloves garlic, finely chopped	3
2	tomatoes, seeded and chopped, optional	2
4 cups	vegetable stock or water (approx.)	1 L
4 to 5	potatoes, cut into 1-inch (2.5 cm) cubes (about 4 cups/1 L)	4 to 5
1 tsp	crushed dried rosemary	5 mL
	Sea salt and freshly ground pepper	
1	can (14 to 19 oz/398 to 540 mL) chickpeas with liquid, optional (see Tip, left)	1
2 cups	fresh spinach, optional	500 mL

1. In a large saucepan, heat oil over medium heat. Add onions and cook, stirring occasionally, for 3 minutes or until slightly soft. Stir in leeks and cook, stirring occasionally, for 6 minutes or until soft. Add garlic and cook, stirring occasionally, for 3 minutes. Add tomatoes, if using.

2. Add vegetable stock, potatoes and rosemary. Stir and bring to a boil over medium-high heat. Cover, reduce heat to low and cook for 20 minutes or until potatoes are tender when pierced with the tip of a knife.

3. Using a ladle, transfer 3 cups (750 mL) of the soup mixture to a blender. Blend until mixture is smooth. Return to saucepan and season to taste with salt and pepper. Stir in chickpeas with liquid and spinach, if using. Cook over low heat for about 2 minutes, until chickpeas are heated and spinach is wilted. Add more vegetable stock or water if a thinner soup is desired.

Coconut Curried Chickpea Soup

Fragrant and hearty, this vegetarian soup is sure to satisfy. Coconut milk adds flavor and richness, while the curry powder gives it a unique complexity found only in Indian-inspired dishes. If you like it hot, add a pinch or two of cayenne pepper.

Serves 6

Vegan Friendly

Tip

To toast coconut, add it to a dry skillet and cook over medium heat, stirring constantly, until golden brown. Transfer to a heatproof plate to cool.

2 tbsp	olive oil	30 mL
1	onion, finely chopped	1
2	cloves garlic, minced	2
1 tbsp	curry powder	15 mL
1 lb	small red-skinned potatoes, cut into $\frac{1}{2}$-inch (1 cm) dice	500 g
4 cups	vegetable stock	1 L
1 cup	unsweetened coconut milk	250 mL
$\frac{1}{2}$ tsp	salt	2 mL
2	cans (each 14 to 19 oz/398 to 540 mL) chickpeas, drained and rinsed	2
1	zucchini, cut into $\frac{1}{2}$-inch (1 cm) dice	1
1 tbsp	packed light brown sugar	15 mL
1 tbsp	freshly squeezed lime juice	15 mL
2 cups	packed baby spinach (about 3 oz/90 g)	500 mL
	Salt and freshly ground black pepper	
	Toasted sweetened shredded coconut (see Tip, left)	

1. In a large pot, heat oil over medium heat. Add onion and sauté until softened, about 6 minutes. Add garlic and sauté for 1 minute. Add curry powder and sauté for 10 seconds. Add potatoes and stir to coat.

2. Add stock and coconut milk; cook for 10 minutes. Add chickpeas and zucchini; cook for 10 minutes, or until potatoes and zucchini are tender. Stir in brown sugar and lime juice. Add spinach and stir until wilted. Season with salt and pepper to taste.

3. Ladle into heated bowls and garnish with coconut.

Zuppa di lenticchie

Lentil Soup with Rice

If you can find them, use the small brown Italian lentils from Umbria or the dark green Puy lentils —
they don't break up during cooking, and they will nicely absorb any aromatics cooked with them,
yet retain their attractive shape. Health food markets are good sources for a wide range of quality
pulses, including organic varieties.

Serves 6

1 tbsp	butter	15 mL
1 tbsp	olive oil	15 mL
2	cloves garlic, finely chopped	2
1	small onion, finely chopped	1
1	stalk celery, finely chopped	1
1	small carrot, finely chopped	1
4 oz	pancetta, finely chopped	125 g
2 tbsp	finely chopped fresh marjoram	30 mL
1½ cups	lentils, rinsed and drained	375 mL
1½ cups	canned plum tomatoes with juices, finely chopped	375 mL
6 cups	beef stock	1.5 L
½ cup	short-grained Italian Arborio rice	125 mL
	Salt and freshly ground black pepper to taste	
½ cup	grated Parmigiano-Reggiano	125 mL
2 tbsp	chopped celery leaves	30 mL

1. In a saucepan with a lid, melt butter with olive oil over medium heat. Add garlic, onion, celery, carrot, pancetta and marjoram; sauté for 5 minutes or until vegetables have softened.

2. Stir in lentils and tomatoes; cook for 3 minutes. Add beef stock and bring to a boil. Reduce heat to low and cook, covered, for 30 minutes or until lentils are almost tender.

3. Stir in rice, replace cover and simmer, stirring occasionally, for another 20 minutes or until rice and lentils are tender. Season to taste with salt and pepper.

4. Serve sprinkled with Parmigiano-Reggiano and celery leaves.

Curried Squash and Red Lentil Soup with Coconut

Delicious, slightly exotic and hearty enough to anchor a soup-and-salad dinner, this soup has everything going for it. This timing ensures that the red lentils dissolve into the broth, creating creaminess, but if you prefer your lentils to be firmer, reduce the cooking time to about 6 hours on Low.

Serves 6 to 8

Vegan Friendly

Tips

For best results, toast and grind cumin and coriander seeds yourself. *To toast cumin and coriander seeds:* Place in a dry skillet over medium heat, and cook, stirring, until fragrant, about 3 minutes. Immediately transfer to a spice grinder or mortar and grind finely.

If you prefer, use frozen diced squash when making this soup because it is so convenient.

If you don't have fresh chile peppers, stir in your favorite hot pepper sauce, to taste, just before serving.

Make Ahead

Complete Step 1. Cover and refrigerate for up to 2 days. When you're ready to cook, complete the recipe.

- **Medium to large (4 to 5 quart) slow cooker**

1 tbsp	olive or coconut oil	15 mL
2	onions, finely chopped	2
4	cloves garlic, minced	4
2 tsp	minced gingerroot	10 mL
1 tbsp	ground cumin (see Tips, left)	15 mL
2 tsp	ground coriander	10 mL
1 tsp	salt	5 mL
1 tsp	cracked black peppercorns	5 mL
1 cup	red lentils, rinsed	250 mL
1	can (28 oz/796 mL) diced tomatoes with juice	1
4 cups	vegetable broth	1 L
2 cups	diced winter squash, such as butternut (see Tips, left)	500 mL
2 tsp	curry powder, dissolved in 2 tbsp (30 mL) freshly squeezed lemon juice	10 mL
1	can (14 oz/400 mL) coconut milk, divided	1
1	long red chile pepper or 2 Thai chile peppers, seeded and minced (see Tips, left)	1
	Thin lemon slices, optional	
	Finely chopped cilantro, optional	

1. In a skillet, heat oil over medium heat. Add onions and cook, stirring, until softened, about 3 minutes. Add garlic, ginger, cumin, coriander, salt and peppercorns and cook, stirring, for 1 minute. Add lentils and toss to coat. Stir in tomatoes with juice. Transfer to slow cooker stoneware.

2. Add broth and squash. Cover and cook on Low for 8 hours or on High for 4 hours, until lentils are tender.

3. In a small bowl, combine curry powder solution and about ¼ cup (60 mL) of the coconut milk. Stir until curry powder dissolves. Add to soup. Add remaining coconut milk and chile pepper and stir well. Cover and cook on High for 15 minutes, until heated through. When ready to serve, ladle into bowls and top with lemon slices and cilantro, if using.

Savory Red Lentil Soup

Lentils were once considered "poor man's food" but that poor person could have done worse. This prehistoric legume is extremely high in protein and is also rich in minerals. Red lentils are often used in Indian dal, croquettes and curries. Here they make a hearty soup delicious. Organically grown lentils, and many other organic legumes, are widely available.

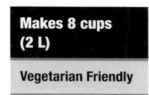

Makes 8 cups (2 L)

Vegetarian Friendly

¼ cup	olive oil	60 mL
1	large onion, chopped	1
1	large carrot, sliced	1
2	cloves garlic, chopped	2
1 tsp	dried thyme	5 mL
1 tbsp	dried marjoram	15 mL
¼ tsp	curry powder, optional	1 mL
5 cups	vegetable stock	1.25 L
1½ cups	red lentils	375 mL
¼ cup	chopped parsley	60 mL
3	medium tomatoes, chopped	3
	Salt and pepper to taste	
¼ cup	red wine	60 mL
1 cup	grated sharp Cheddar cheese (optional)	250 mL

1. In a large heavy-bottomed pot with a lid, heat oil over medium heat. Add onion, carrot, garlic, thyme, marjoram and, if using, curry; sauté for 6 minutes or until onion is transparent.

2. Add vegetable stock, red lentils, parsley and tomatoes. Season to taste with salt and pepper. Cover and simmer for 1 hour. (Add more stock, if necessary, to achieve desired consistency.)

3. Add red wine just before serving. Garnish with grated sharp Cheddar cheese, if desired.

Green Lentil Soup

Small green lentils, also known as Puy lentils, are common in France and are now easy to get everywhere else. They are slightly smaller and more delicate than the typical brown lentil, and are a nice change of pace, but brown lentils will work well in this soup too.

Serves 6 to 8

Tip

San Marzano tomatoes, imported from Italy, are thought by many to be the best canned tomatoes in the world. They hail from a small town of the same name near Naples, whose volcanic soil is thought to filter impurities from the water and render tomatoes with a thick flesh, fewer seeds and a stronger taste. Look for the words "San Marzano" on the label to be sure you're getting the best.

4	slices bacon, chopped	4
4	cloves garlic, minced	4
2	stalks celery, chopped	2
1	onion, chopped	1
1	carrot, chopped	1
2	small bay leaves	2
1 tsp	dried thyme	5 mL
2¼ cups	dried green lentils, rinsed	550 mL
10 cups	chicken stock (approx.)	2.5 L
1	can (14 oz/398 mL) diced tomatoes, with juice	1
	Salt and freshly ground black pepper	

1. In a large pot, sauté bacon over medium heat until browned and crispy, about 5 minutes. Remove with a slotted spoon to a plate lined with paper towels. Set aside.

2. Add garlic, celery, onion, carrot, bay leaves and thyme to the pot; sauté until vegetables are softened, about 6 minutes. Add lentils, stock and tomatoes with juice; bring to a boil. Reduce heat and simmer until lentils are tender, about 45 minutes. Thin with a little more stock, if necessary, and simmer for 5 minutes, or until hot. Discard bay leaves. Season with salt and pepper to taste.

3. Ladle into heated bowls and garnish with reserved bacon.

Roasted Garlic and Lentil Soup

Use fresh tomatoes in season and substitute 1 cup (250 mL) of crushed canned tomatoes in winter. Best if served immediately. When stored, even in the refrigerator, this soup thickens, absorbing the liquid.

Serves 6

Vegan Friendly

Tips

Designer rice (mahogany, black, red; short- and long-grain varieties) is becoming very popular and widely available. Look for red rice in gourmet food or natural food stores.

You can use 2 cups (500 mL) cooked lentils plus ½ cup (125 mL) vegetable stock, instead of canned.

- **Preheat oven to 375°F (190°C)**
- **10-inch (25 cm) pie plate or baking dish**

10	small (2 inch/5 cm diameter) tomatoes	10
12	cloves garlic	12
4 tbsp	olive oil, divided	60 mL
1 tbsp	chopped fresh rosemary	15 mL
1 cup	chopped onion	250 mL
1 tsp	ground cumin	5 mL
½ tsp	crushed fennel seeds	2 mL
½ tsp	sea salt	2 mL
Pinch	ground ginger	Pinch
Pinch	ground nutmeg	Pinch
1 cup	red or brown rice (see Tips, left)	250 mL
3 cups	vegetable stock or water, divided (approx.)	750 mL
1	can (19 oz/540 mL) lentils with liquid (see Tips, left)	1

1. In pie plate, combine tomatoes and garlic and toss with 2 tbsp (30 mL) of the oil and rosemary. Bake in preheated oven for 40 minutes or until garlic is soft. Let cool.

2. Meanwhile, in a large saucepan, heat remaining oil over medium heat. Add onion and cook, stirring occasionally, for 6 to 8 minutes or until soft. Add cumin, fennel, salt, ginger, nutmeg and rice. Cook, stirring constantly, for 1 minute. Add 2 cups (500 mL) of the vegetable stock. Increase heat to high and bring to a boil. Cover, reduce heat to low and simmer for 40 minutes or until rice is tender.

3. When tomatoes and garlic are cool enough to handle, transfer to a blender and add remaining vegetable stock. Blend until smooth. Add tomato purée and lentils with liquid to rice in saucepan. Bring to a simmer and cook for 1 to 2 minutes or until heated through. Add more vegetable stock or water if a thinner soup is desired.

Moroccan Spiced Lentil Soup

Most Mediterranean countries have their own version of this satisfying soup — a wonderful concoction of legumes, herbs and spices. Here's how it's made in North Africa. Serve with focaccia or pita bread and follow it with a lighter main course.

Serves 6

Make Ahead

Soup can be refrigerated, covered, for up to 3 days. Reheat over medium heat until piping hot, adding a little extra stock if soup has become too thick.

1 tbsp	olive oil	15 mL
2	onions, chopped	2
1	clove garlic, minced	1
1 tsp	ground ginger	5 mL
1 tsp	paprika	5 mL
1 tsp	turmeric	5 mL
¼ tsp	cayenne pepper	1 mL
1 cup	red lentils, rinsed and drained	250 mL
4 cups	beef or chicken stock	1 L
1	can (28 oz/796 mL) diced tomatoes	1
1	can (19 oz/540 mL) chickpeas, rinsed and drained	1
⅓ cup	chopped fresh cilantro	75 mL
¼ tsp	salt	1 mL
¼ tsp	black pepper	1 mL

1. In a large saucepan or Dutch oven, heat oil over medium-high heat. Add onions and garlic; cook, stirring, for 3 to 5 minutes or until onions are soft but not brown. Add ginger, paprika, turmeric and cayenne; cook, stirring, for about 1 minute. Add lentils; stir to coat with onion-and-spice mixture.

2. Add stock and tomatoes. Bring to a boil over high heat, stirring occasionally. Reduce heat to medium-low; simmer, covered, for 30 to 40 minutes or until lentils are very soft and have started to break up.

3. Stir in chickpeas, cilantro, salt and pepper; simmer, uncovered, for 10 minutes to allow flavors to blend. If desired, season to taste with additional salt and pepper. Ladle into warm soup bowls. Serve at once.

Salads and Dressings

Tuscan White Bean and Tomato Salad . . . 74

White Bean Salad with Lemon-Dill
   Vinaigrette 75

Bean Salad with Mustard-Dill
   Dressing. 76

Greek Bean and Tomato Salad 77

Grilled Corn and Lima Bean Salad. 78

Corn and Three-Bean Salad 79

Tex-Mex Rotini Salad 80

Italian Bean Pasta Salad. 81

Potluck Bean and Pasta Salad 82

Black Bean and Rice Salad. 83

Black Bean and Bulgur Salad with
   Orange and Pepperoni 84

Chickpea and Roasted Pepper Salad. . . . 84

Tortilla Bean Salad with
   Creamy Salsa Dressing. 85

Black-Eyed Pea Salad with
   Tomato and Feta 86

Southwestern Bean and Barley Salad
   with Roasted Peppers 87

Roasted Vegetable Salad 88

Cajun Blackened Potato and
   Mung Bean Salad 89

Grilled Mediterranean Vegetable
   and Lentil Salad 90

Cajun Potato and Red Lentil Salad 91

Lentil Salad with Feta Cheese. 92

Lentil Salad with Dried Cranberries
   and Pistachios 93

Marinated Lentil Salad 94

Tabbouleh with Lentils 95

Dressings, etc.

Sesame Tofu Vinaigrette. 95

Dijon Vinaigrette. 96

Asian Tofu Dressing 96

Red Wine Vinaigrette 97

Tofu Mayonnaise 97

Cajun Black Spice 98

Yogurt Cheese. 98

Tuscan White Bean and Tomato Salad

A simple, excellent salad that is very quick to prepare when using good-quality canned white beans. We like to add variety and texture by making this salad with different varieties of dried beans or fava beans cooked in the kitchen.

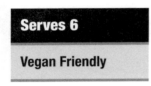

Serves 6

Vegan Friendly

Tip

For speed and convenience, replace dried beans with 1 can (14 to 19 oz/398 to 540 mL) white beans, rinsed and drained.

1 cup	dried white navy beans (see Tip, left)	250 mL
	Kosher or sea salt	
¼ cup	olive oil	60 mL
2 tsp	finely chopped garlic	10 mL
	Freshly ground black pepper	
2 cups	diced seeded ripe tomatoes	500 mL
¼	red onion, diced	¼
1 tbsp	coarsely chopped oregano	15 mL
2 tbsp	balsamic vinegar	30 mL

1. Place beans in a bowl and add water to cover. Set aside to soak overnight in the refrigerator. Drain beans.

2. In a saucepan over medium heat, add beans and cover with cold water, about 4 cups (1 L). Bring to a boil and cook until soft, 40 to 45 minutes. Remove from heat. Add a pinch of salt and let stand for 5 minutes. Drain and set aside.

3. In a large skillet, heat oil over medium-low heat. Add garlic and sauté until soft and just beginning to caramelize, 1 to 2 minutes. Add beans and toss to combine with garlic-infused oil. Season lightly with salt and pepper. Let cool.

4. In a large bowl, combine cooled beans, tomatoes, red onion, oregano and vinegar. Toss to combine well. Season with black pepper to taste.

White Bean Salad with Lemon-Dill Vinaigrette

Bean salads can be so disappointing. But this one is fresh-tasting and holds up well for several hours without refrigeration — perfect for a buffet table.

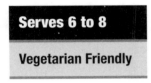

Serves 6 to 8

Vegetarian Friendly

Tip

Dill is one of the few fresh herbs that freeze well. Simply place in a plastic bag and freeze for up to 6 months. To use, just break off what you need from the frozen bunch. For best results, add to cooked dishes rather than salads.

Make Ahead

The bean salad can be refrigerated for up to 8 hours. Let stand at room temperature for 30 minutes before serving.

2	cans (each 19 oz/540 mL) white kidney beans, drained and rinsed	2
2	small tomatoes, chopped	2
1/2 cup	finely chopped red onion	125 mL
1/4 cup	chopped fresh dill, divided	60 mL
1/4 cup	olive oil	60 mL
2 tbsp	fresh lemon juice	30 mL
1 tbsp	liquid honey	15 mL
1/4 tsp	salt	1 mL
1/4 tsp	black pepper	1 mL

1. In a large serving bowl, combine beans, tomatoes, onion and 3 tbsp (45 mL) dill.
2. In a small bowl, whisk together olive oil, lemon juice, honey, salt and pepper. Add to beans; toss well. If desired, season to taste with additional salt and pepper. Serve garnished with remaining dill.

Bean Salad with Mustard-Dill Dressing

Bean salad is another staple we've grown up with over the years. Originally this salad used canned string beans, but fresh beans give it a new lease on taste, as does the addition of fiber-packed chickpeas.

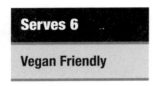

Serves 6

Vegan Friendly

Tip

Instead of chickpeas, you can try canned mixed beans. This includes a combination of chickpeas, red and white kidney beans and black-eyed peas. It's available in supermarkets.

1 lb	green beans	500 g
1	can (19 oz/540 mL) chickpeas, rinsed and drained	1
1/3 cup	chopped red onions	75 mL
2 tbsp	finely chopped fresh dill	30 mL
2 tbsp	olive oil	30 mL
2 tbsp	red wine vinegar	30 mL
1 tbsp	Dijon mustard	15 mL
1 tbsp	granulated sugar	15 mL
1/4 tsp	salt	1 mL
1/4 tsp	pepper	1 mL

1. Trim ends of beans; cut into 1-inch (2.5 cm) lengths. In a large pot of boiling salted water, cook beans for 3 to 5 minutes (count from time water returns to a boil) or until tender-crisp. Drain; rinse under cold water to chill. Drain well.

2. In a serving bowl, combine green beans, chickpeas, onions and dill.

3. In a small bowl, whisk together oil, vinegar, mustard, sugar, salt and pepper until smooth. Pour over beans and toss well. Refrigerate until serving time.

Variation

French Salad Dressing: In a bowl, stir together 2 tbsp (30 mL) red wine vinegar and 1 1/2 tsp (7 mL) Dijon mustard. Add 1/3 cup (75 mL) olive oil (or use part vegetable oil), 1 minced clove garlic and 1 tsp (5 mL) dried fine herbs. Season with a pinch of granulated sugar, salt and pepper to taste. Store in covered jar in the refrigerator. Makes 1/2 cup (125 mL).

Greek Bean and Tomato Salad

Vine-ripened tomatoes, arguably the greatest gastronomic pleasure of summer, add the necessary sweetness to this substantial salad. It makes a wonderful lunch or starting course for a dinner, as well as a very useful addition to buffets since it lives nicely for a couple of hours after it's assembled. Feel free to use up to twice as much olive oil as called for in the recipe — that is, if calories aren't a problem — and you'll have a richer taste sensation.

Serves 4 to 6

2 cups	cooked white kidney beans or 1 can (19 oz/540 mL), rinsed and drained	500 mL
2	ripe medium tomatoes, cut into $\frac{1}{2}$-inch (1 cm) wedges	2
$\frac{1}{2}$ cup	thinly sliced red onions	125 mL
4	black olives, pitted and halved	4
	Few sprigs fresh parsley, chopped	
2 tbsp	red wine vinegar	30 mL
2 tbsp	extra virgin olive oil	30 mL
$\frac{1}{2}$ tsp	salt	2 mL
$\frac{1}{4}$ tsp	freshly ground black pepper	1 mL
4 oz	feta cheese in big crumbles	125 g
1 tsp	olive oil	5 mL
$\frac{1}{2}$	red bell pepper, cut into thin strips	$\frac{1}{2}$

1. Put beans into a bowl. Add tomatoes, red onions, olives and parsley. Do not toss.

2. In a small bowl, whisk together vinegar, 2 tbsp (30 mL) olive oil, salt and pepper until slightly emulsified. Sprinkle on beans; toss and fold until well mixed, but without mashing beans. Transfer the salad to a serving bowl. Distribute the feta crumbles decoratively on top.

3. In a small frying pan, heat 1 tsp (5 mL) oil over high heat; cook red pepper, turning often, for 3 to 4 minutes or until charred slightly and wilting. Decorate salad with the red peppers. Serve immediately, or cover and keep unrefrigerated for up to 2 hours.

Grilled Corn and Lima Bean Salad

Of the hundreds of salads we have created over the years, this has proven to be a runaway bestseller! We thought of keeping the recipe a secret, but it's too good not to share. It's a colorful, refreshing salad and makes a satisfying lunch all by itself.

Serves 4 to 6

Vegetarian Friendly

Tip

Slicing kernels from a cob of corn: Make a slice across the bottom of the corncob so that it stands upright on a large cutting board. Hold the blade of a sharp knife against the cob at the top and slice downwards, firmly following the shape of the cob and releasing the kernels as you go.

• **Preheated barbecue or indoor grill**

2	ears corn, husk and silk removed	2
3 tbsp	olive oil, divided	45 mL
	Kosher or sea salt	
2 cups	frozen lima beans	500 mL
1 cup	halved cherry tomatoes	250 mL
1	shallot, diced	1
¼ cup	kalamata olives, pitted and roughly chopped	60 mL
2 tbsp	apple cider vinegar	30 mL
	Freshly ground black pepper	
1 cup	baby arugula	250 mL
½ cup	crumbled feta cheese	125 mL

1. Brush corn lightly with 1 tbsp (15 mL) of the oil and sprinkle with salt. Place on a lightly oiled grill over medium-high heat and grill until lightly charred on all sides. Let cool and slice kernels from the cob (see Tip, left). Transfer to a large bowl and set aside.

2. In a saucepan of boiling lightly salted water, blanch lima beans until tender, 3 to 5 minutes. Drain and let cool. Add to corn with tomatoes, shallot and olives.

3. In a small bowl, whisk vinegar with remaining oil and season with salt and pepper to taste.

4. Pour dressing over vegetables and mix together well. Taste and adjust seasoning. Gently fold in arugula and feta.

Corn and Three-Bean Salad

Tip

Use any combination of cooked beans.

For a sweeter salad, try balsamic vinegar.

Make Ahead

Prepare salad and dressing separately up to a day ahead. Pour dressing over top just before serving.

8 oz	pasta wheels or small shell pasta	250 g
1 cup	canned black beans or chickpeas, drained and rinsed	250 mL
¾ cup	canned red kidney beans, drained and rinsed	175 mL
¾ cup	canned white kidney beans, drained and rinsed	175 mL
¾ cup	canned corn niblets, drained and rinsed	175 mL
1¼ cups	diced red bell peppers	300 mL
¾ cup	diced carrots	175 mL
½ cup	diced red onions	125 mL

Dressing

¼ cup	lemon juice	60 mL
3 tbsp	vegetable oil	45 mL
3 tbsp	red wine or cider vinegar	45 mL
2 tsp	crushed garlic	10 mL
½ cup	chopped cilantro or parsley	125 mL

1. Cook pasta in boiling water according to package instructions or until firm to the bite. Rinse with cold water. Drain and place in a serving bowl.

2. Add black beans, red kidney beans, white kidney beans, corn niblets, red peppers, carrots and onions.

3. *Make the dressing:* In a small bowl, combine lemon juice, oil, wine, garlic and cilantro. Pour over dressing and toss.

Tex-Mex Rotini Salad

Tortilla chips are a great snack food — but only if they're baked! The traditional deep-fried variety is much higher in fat and calories.

Tip

For a great snack, melt some light Cheddar cheese over tortilla chips. Kids love them!

8 oz	rotini	250 g
1½ cups	diced ripe plum tomatoes	375 mL
1 cup	canned red kidney beans, drained and rinsed	250 mL
1 cup	canned corn kernels, drained and rinsed	250 mL
½ cup	chopped fresh cilantro	125 mL
½ cup	chopped green onions	125 mL

Dressing

⅓ cup	barbecue sauce	75 mL
2½ tbsp	cider vinegar	37 mL
2 tsp	molasses	10 mL
1 tsp	minced jalapeño pepper (optional)	5 mL
1 oz	baked tortilla chips (about 12)	30 g

1. In a large pot of boiling water, cook rotini for 8 to 10 minutes or until tender but firm; drain. Rinse under cold running water; drain. In a serving bowl combine pasta, tomatoes, kidney beans, corn, cilantro and green onions.

2. In a bowl combine barbecue sauce, cider vinegar, molasses and jalapeño pepper, if using; whisk well. Pour dressing over salad; toss to coat well. Garnish with crumbled tortilla chips. Serve.

Italian Bean Pasta Salad

Serves 6 to 8 as an appetizer

Vegetarian Friendly

Tip

Use any combination of cooked beans. Try black beans or lima beans.

Make Ahead

Prepare salad and dressing early in the day. Toss up to 2 hours ahead.

12 oz	medium shell pasta	375 g
2½ cups	chopped tomatoes	625 mL
¾ cup	diced green bell peppers	175 mL
¾ cup	diced red onions	175 mL
⅔ cup	canned red kidney beans, drained	150 mL
⅔ cup	canned white kidney beans, drained	150 mL
⅔ cup	canned chickpeas, drained	150 mL
3 oz	feta cheese, crumbled	90 g

Dressing

¼ cup	lemon juice	60 mL
3 tbsp	olive oil	45 mL
1 tbsp	red wine vinegar	15 mL
2 tsp	crushed garlic	10 mL
2½ tsp	dried basil	12 mL
1½ tsp	dried oregano	7 mL

1. Cook pasta in boiling water according to package instructions or until firm to the bite. Rinse with cold water. Drain and place in a serving bowl. Add tomatoes, green peppers, onions, red kidney beans, white kidney beans, chickpeas and feta cheese.

2. *Make the dressing:* In a small bowl, whisk together lemon juice, oil, vinegar, garlic, basil and oregano. Pour over pasta and toss.

Potluck Bean and Pasta Salad

Bean salads and macaroni salads are standard fare at Western hoedowns and prairie picnics. Here's a recipe that combines the best of both with a few new twists, a favorite for summer barbecues and potluck dinners.

Serves 8

Tip

For convenience, use 1 can (14 oz/398 mL) kidney beans and 1 can (14 oz/398 mL) chickpeas, rinsed and drained.

Dressing

2 tbsp	red wine vinegar	30 mL
1 tbsp	fresh lemon juice	15 mL
1 tbsp	Dijon mustard	15 mL
2 tsp	Worcestershire sauce	10 mL
1 tsp	granulated sugar	5 mL
1/2 tsp	salt	2 mL
1/4 tsp	freshly ground black pepper	1 mL
2	cloves garlic	2
1/2 cup	extra virgin olive oil	125 mL
2 tbsp	minced fresh parsley	30 mL
1 tbsp	basil pesto or minced fresh basil	15 mL
3 cups	short pasta (small shells, rotini or radiatore)	750 mL
1 1/2 cups	cooked kidney beans	375 mL
1 1/2 cups	cooked chickpeas	375 mL
1 cup	diced yellow peppers	250 mL
1/2 cup	sliced black olives	125 mL
3	large plum tomatoes, seeded and chopped	3
1/2	red onion, diced	1/2
	Salt and pepper to taste	

1. *Make the dressing:* In a small glass measuring cup, whisk together vinegar, lemon juice, mustard, Worcestershire sauce, sugar, salt and pepper; set aside. In a food processor, chop garlic. Add vinegar mixture and process until well mixed. With machine running, slowly pour olive oil, parsley and pesto through feed tube. Set aside.

2. In a large pot of boiling, salted water, cook pasta for 8 to 10 minutes or until al dente; drain. Rinse under cold running water; drain again, shaking well to remove any excess water.

3. In a large bowl, toss together pasta, kidney beans, chickpeas and dressing. Add yellow peppers, olives, chopped tomatoes and red onion. Chill well. Season to taste with salt and pepper.

Black Bean and Rice Salad

This colorful salad makes a great summer meal or portable potluck offering. It's also very Western, with Tex-Mex overtones and earthy black beans.

Serves 8

1 cup	dried black beans, soaked overnight in water to cover	250 mL
1	onion, halved	1
2	cloves garlic, chopped	2
1	small carrot	1
1	sprig fresh parsley	1
1 cup	white rice	250 mL
1 tbsp	canola oil	15 mL
1 tsp	turmeric	5 mL
½ tsp	ground cumin	2 mL
½ tsp	salt	2 mL

Dressing

3 tbsp	olive oil	45 mL
3 tbsp	fresh lime juice	45 mL
½ tsp	ground cumin	2 mL
2	tomatoes, seeded and diced	2
1	small red onion, diced	1
1	red bell pepper, diced	1
1	jalapeño pepper, seeded and minced	1
¼ cup	chopped cilantro	60 mL
	Cayenne pepper to taste	

1. In a saucepan combine drained beans with 8 cups (2 L) cold water, onion, garlic, carrot and parsley; bring to a boil. Reduce heat and simmer for 1½ hours or until tender. Drain and cool. Discard onion, carrot and parsley.

2. Meanwhile, in a small saucepan combine 1¾ cups (425 mL) cold water, rice, oil, turmeric, cumin and salt; bring to a boil. Reduce heat to low and simmer, covered, for 30 minutes. Fluff rice and cool to room temperature.

3. *Make the dressing:* In a small bowl, whisk together olive oil, lime juice and cumin. Set aside.

4. In a large bowl, toss cooled beans and rice with tomatoes, red onion, red pepper, jalapeño, cilantro and dressing. Season to taste with cayenne pepper and, if desired, additional salt. Chill.

Black Bean and Bulgur Salad with Orange and Pepperoni

1 cup	bulgur	250 mL
1¼ cups	hot water	300 mL
	Finely grated zest and juice of 1 large orange	
⅓ cup	vegetable oil	75 mL
¼ cup	cider vinegar	60 mL
	Salt and freshly ground black pepper	
2 cups	canned black beans, drained and rinsed	500 mL
½	onion, finely chopped	½
1	small chile pepper, minced	1
1	cucumber, peeled, seeded and diced	1
4 oz	pepperoni, finely diced	125 g

1. Soak bulgur in water until tender, about 15 minutes; drain. Whisk together orange zest, orange juice, oil, vinegar and salt and pepper, to taste. Add bulgur, beans, onion, chile pepper, cucumber and pepperoni; toss to coat. Cover and refrigerate for several hours to mingle flavors.

Chickpea and Roasted Pepper Salad

This salad is quick and easy to prepare, tastes good and travels well. It's a perfect stand-by for summer picnics.

Tip

We periodically taste test various brands of canned goods and are always amazed at the differences in taste and texture. In this case we find a quality brand of organic legumes is superior.

1	roasted red bell pepper, diced	1
1	carrot, grated	1
2	cans (each 14 to 19 oz/398 to 540 mL) chickpeas, rinsed and drained	2
½ cup	Red Wine Vinaigrette (page 97)	125 mL
2 tbsp	chopped flat-leaf parsley	30 mL
2 tsp	chopped oregano	10 mL
	Salt and freshly ground black pepper	

1. In a large bowl, combine roasted pepper, carrot and chickpeas.
2. Add vinaigrette, parsley and oregano and toss to combine. Season with salt and pepper to taste.

Tortilla Bean Salad with Creamy Salsa Dressing

Tips

Southwestern all the way, this salad is low in fat — thanks to the light dressing.

Use a mild or hot salsa, whichever you prefer.

Vary beans and vegetables to your taste.

To prevent salad from wilting, do not pour dressing over until ready to serve.

Make Ahead

Prepare salad and dressing early in the day. Toss just before serving.

Salad

3 cups	romaine lettuce, washed, dried and torn into pieces	750 mL
1 cup	canned chickpeas, drained and rinsed	250 mL
1 cup	canned red kidney beans, drained and rinsed	250 mL
1 cup	shredded carrots	250 mL
1 cup	chopped red bell peppers	250 mL
¾ cup	chopped red onions	175 mL
⅓ cup	chopped fresh cilantro	75 mL

Dressing

3 tbsp	salsa	45 mL
3 tbsp	light sour cream	45 mL
2 tbsp	light mayonnaise	30 mL
1 tsp	minced garlic	5 mL
¾ to 1 tsp	chili powder	3 to 5 mL
1 oz	tortilla chips, crushed (about 12)	30 g

1. In a large bowl, combine lettuce, chickpeas, kidney beans, carrots, red peppers, red onions and cilantro.

2. *Make the dressing:* In a small bowl, whisk together salsa, sour cream, mayonnaise, garlic and chili powder.

3. Just before serving, pour dressing over salad. Toss to coat. Sprinkle with tortilla chips. Serve immediately.

Black-Eyed Pea Salad with Tomato and Feta

Double up the ingredients in this colorful salad and take along to a summer potluck. If the salad has to travel, combine black-eyed peas, onion and olives with the dressing and pack tomato, herbs and feta in small containers to add before serving.

Serves 4 to 6

Vegetarian Friendly

Tip

For speed and convenience, replace dried beans with 1 can (14 to 19 oz/398 to 540 mL) black-eyed peas, rinsed and drained.

1 cup	dried black-eyed peas (see Tip, left)	250 mL
	Kosher or sea salt	
1	large ripe tomato, seeded and diced	1
1/2	red onion, chopped	1/2
1/4 cup	kalamata olives, pitted and halved	60 mL
1/4 cup	Red Wine Vinaigrette (page 97)	60 mL
2 tbsp	coarsely chopped flat-leaf parsley	30 mL
1 tbsp	finely chopped oregano	15 mL
1/2 cup	crumbled feta cheese	125 mL
	Freshly ground black pepper	

1. Place black-eyed peas in a bowl and add water to cover. Set aside to soak overnight in the refrigerator. Drain peas.

2. In a saucepan over medium heat, place black-eyed peas and cover with cold water, about 4 cups (1 L). Bring to a boil and cook until soft, 35 to 45 minutes. Remove from heat. Add a pinch of salt and let stand for 5 minutes. Drain. Transfer to a large bowl. Let cool.

3. Add tomato, red onion and olives. Add vinaigrette, parsley and oregano and toss to mix well. Season with salt to taste. Garnish with feta and a few grindings of black pepper.

Southwestern Bean and Barley Salad with Roasted Peppers

Ingredients traditionally associated with the American Southwest, such as beans, corn and peppers, combine with hearty barley to produce this deliciously robust salad. Packed with nutrients, it is particularly high in dietary fiber. It makes a great addition to a buffet or potluck dinner. Keep leftovers in the fridge for a nutritious lunch or after-school snacks.

Makes 8 side servings

Vegan Friendly

Tips

For this quantity of beans, soak and cook 1 cup (250 mL) dried beans (pages 6 to 10) or use 1 can (14 to 19 oz/398 to 540 mL) red kidney beans, drained and rinsed.

Poblano peppers are a mild chile pepper. If you are a heat seeker, you might want to add an extra one, or even a minced seeded jalapeño pepper for some real punch. The suggested quantity produces a mild result, which most people will enjoy. If you're heat averse, use bell peppers instead.

1 cup	whole (hulled) barley	250 mL

Dressing

3 tbsp	red wine vinegar	45 mL
1/2 tsp	salt	2 mL
	Freshly ground black pepper	
1/2	clove garlic, finely grated or put through a press	1/2
1/2 cup	extra virgin olive oil	125 mL
2 cups	cooked red kidney beans (see Tips, left)	500 mL
2 cups	cooked corn kernels	500 mL
2	roasted poblano or roasted red bell peppers, peeled, seeded and diced (see Tips, left)	2
2	whole sun-dried tomatoes, packed in olive oil, finely chopped	2
1	small red onion, diced	1
1/4 cup	finely chopped parsley	60 mL

1. In a heavy saucepan, bring 2 1/2 cups (625 mL) water or stock to a rapid boil. Add barley and return to a rapid boil. Reduce heat to low. Cover and place a heat diffuser under the pot, if necessary. Cook until barley is tender, about 1 hour. Allow to cool.

2. *Dressing:* In a small bowl, combine vinegar, salt and pepper to taste, stirring until salt dissolves. Stir in garlic. Gradually whisk in olive oil. Set aside.

3. In a serving bowl, combine barley, kidney beans, corn, roasted peppers, sun-dried tomatoes and onion. Add dressing and toss well. Garnish with parsley. Chill until ready to serve.

Variations

Substitute an equal quantity of cooked wheat, spelt or Kamut berries or farro for the barley.

Roasted Vegetable Salad

In summer the grill is easy and fast for grilling vegetables. Use an oiled basket or skewer the veggies whole to grill, then cut into serving-size bites. When combined with balsamic vinegar, the plums morph into a tart-sweet self-basting dressing.

Tip

You can use 2 cups (500 mL) cooked chickpeas, drained and rinsed, instead of canned.

- **Preheat oven to 375°F (190°C)**
- **Rimmed baking sheet, lightly oiled**

2	black plums, cut into eighths	2
1	red bell pepper, cut into eighths	1
1	carrot, cut in half lengthwise and then crosswise into eighths	1
1	onion, cut into eighths	1
2	cauliflower florets, thinly sliced	2
	Sea salt and freshly ground pepper	
4 tbsp	olive oil, divided	60 mL
2 cups	packed seasonal greens	500 mL
2 tbsp	balsamic vinegar	30 mL
1	can (14 to 19 oz/398 to 540 mL) chickpeas, drained and rinsed (see Tip, left)	1

1. On prepared baking sheet, combine plums, red pepper, carrot, onion and cauliflower. Season to taste with salt and pepper. Toss with 2 tbsp (30 mL) of the oil and arrange in a single layer. Bake in preheated oven for 30 to 40 minutes or until tender when pierced with the tip of a knife.

2. In a salad bowl, toss greens with roasted vegetables and pan juices. Add remaining oil, vinegar and chickpeas. Taste and add more salt and pepper, if required.

Cajun Blackened Potato and Mung Bean Salad

Indian food stores often have many different varieties of lentils and beans. Mung beans, also known as moong beans, are delicate and small — perfect for this unusual potato salad.

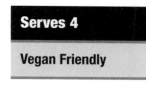

Serves 4

Vegan Friendly

Tip

If using store-bought Cajun spice, start with 1 1/2 tsp (7 mL) because it may be stronger than the homemade version. Taste and add more as required.

1/2 cup	yellow mung beans, rinsed	125 mL
1 1/2 cups	water	375 mL
6	medium potatoes, scrubbed	6
3 tbsp	olive oil	45 mL
1 tbsp	freshly squeezed lemon juice	15 mL
1 to 2 tbsp	Cajun Black Spice (page 98) or store-bought (see Tip, left)	15 to 30 mL
1 tsp	salt	5 mL
1 cup	fresh or frozen corn kernels, cooked	250 mL

1. In a saucepan, combine beans and water. Bring to a boil over medium-high heat. Reduce heat and simmer gently for 20 minutes or until tender. Drain and rinse in a colander. Let cool slightly.

2. Meanwhile, in a saucepan, cover potatoes with water. Bring to a boil over high heat. Cover, reduce heat and simmer for about 20 minutes or until tender. Drain and rinse with cold water. Let cool and slip off skins.

3. In a large bowl, whisk together olive oil, lemon juice, 1 tbsp (15 mL) of the Cajun spice and salt. Slice potatoes directly into the oil mixture. Stir in beans and corn. Taste and add more Cajun seasoning or salt, if required.

Variation

Substitute any lentil for the mung beans or use 1 cup (250 mL) cooked fava beans or flageolets in place of the beans and add in Step 3.

Grilled Mediterranean Vegetable and Lentil Salad

Using the grill keeps the kitchen cool in the summertime, but the vegetables may be roasted in the oven (see Tip, below).

Serves 4 to 6

Vegan Friendly

Tip

To roast vegetables in the oven, place on a lightly oiled rimmed baking sheet and roast in a 400°F (200°C) oven for 30 minutes or until soft.

- **Preheat barbecue grill to High**
- **2 grilling baskets, lightly oiled**

1	red bell pepper, cut in half	1
2	small zucchini	2
2 tbsp	olive oil, divided	30 mL
1	eggplant, cut into ½-inch (1 cm) rounds	1

Dressing

¼ cup	olive oil	60 mL
1 tbsp	freshly squeezed lemon juice	15 mL
1 tbsp	balsamic vinegar	15 mL
1 tbsp	tamari or soy sauce	15 mL
1	clove garlic, minced	1
1 tbsp	chopped fresh oregano	15 mL
1 tbsp	chopped fresh mint or tarragon	15 mL

Salad

½	red onion, thinly sliced	½
½	cucumber, diced	½
1 cup	cooked lentils or black-eyed peas, drained and rinsed	250 mL
	Sea salt and freshly ground pepper	

1. Arrange red pepper halves and zucchini in a prepared grilling basket. Brush with 1 tbsp (15 mL) of the oil and grill for 8 to 10 minutes or until tender when pierced with the tip of a knife. Arrange eggplant in remaining basket and brush with remaining oil. Grill for 3 to 4 minutes or until tender. Let vegetables cool enough to handle. Peel and slice red pepper and cut zucchini and eggplant into chunks.

2. *Dressing:* Meanwhile, in a large bowl, whisk together oil, lemon juice, vinegar, tamari, garlic, oregano and mint.

3. *Assemble Salad:* Add red onion, cucumber and lentils to dressing. Add grilled vegetables and stir to combine well. Taste and season with salt and pepper, if required.

Cajun Potato and Red Lentil Salad

Tips

Double the amounts for a summer picnic or barbecue.

If not accustomed to cayenne pepper, start with $\frac{1}{4}$ tsp (1 mL) and gradually add more to taste.

Large sprouts such as broccoli or sunflower work well in this recipe, but you can use any type available.

$\frac{1}{2}$ cup	red lentils, rinsed	125 mL
$1\frac{1}{2}$ cups	water	375 mL
4	large potatoes, scrubbed and halved	4
$\frac{1}{3}$ cup	flaxseed oil	75 mL
3 tbsp	raspberry vinegar	45 mL
2 tbsp	sesame seeds	30 mL
2 tbsp	poppy seeds	30 mL
2 tbsp	flax seeds	30 mL
$\frac{1}{3}$ cup	plain yogurt	75 mL
1 tsp	cayenne powder	5 mL
	Salt and black pepper	
$\frac{1}{4}$ cup	chopped scapes (see Variations, below)	60 mL
3	hard-boiled eggs, cut into wedges	3
$\frac{1}{4}$ cup	large sprouts (see Tips, left)	60 mL

1. In a saucepan combine lentils with water. Bring to a boil; reduce heat and simmer gently for 20 minutes or until lentils are tender. Allow to cool in a colander.

2. Meanwhile, in a medium saucepan, cover potatoes with cold water. Bring to a boil, reduce heat and simmer for 20 to 25 minutes or until just tender. Drain and rinse with cold water. When cool enough to handle, cut into 1-inch (2.5 cm) pieces.

3. In a small bowl, whisk together oil, raspberry vinegar, sesame seeds, poppy seeds, flax seeds, yogurt and cayenne. Season to taste with salt and pepper.

4. In a large salad bowl, combine cooled lentils, potatoes and scapes. Gently stir in dressing. Garnish with egg wedges and sprouts.

Variations

Substitute green onions for the scapes; sour cream for the yogurt; and/or more or less cayenne pepper, to taste.

Lentil Salad with Feta Cheese

There are countless versions of this healthful salad served along the Mediterranean from North Africa and Spain all the way to Turkey and beyond. Not only is it delicious and good for you, but the flavors are bright with lemon and mint, while the tomatoes and feta cheese add color and punch.

Serves 6

Vegetarian Friendly

Hands-on time:
20 minutes

Start to finish:
30 minutes

Tip

Use a combination of green French Puy lentils, orange or red Indian lentils and the easy-to-find brown lentils. The colors are very pretty.

Make Ahead

The salad can be made up to 1 day ahead, covered and refrigerated. Add feta cheese just before serving.

1 cup	lentils, washed and picked over	250 mL
1 tsp	salt, divided	5 mL
1	shallot, minced	1
1	clove garlic, minced	1
¼ cup	white wine vinegar	60 mL
1 tsp	liquid honey	5 mL
¼ tsp	freshly ground black pepper	1 mL
⅓ cup	extra virgin olive oil	75 mL
2 cups	grape tomatoes, halved	500 mL
¼ cup	chopped fresh mint	60 mL
2 tsp	freshly squeezed lemon juice, optional	10 mL
½ cup	crumbled feta cheese	125 mL

1. In a medium saucepan over medium heat, cover lentils and ¼ tsp (1 mL) of the salt with water by 2 inches (5 cm) and bring to a boil. Reduce heat to low, cover and simmer lentils for 15 minutes or until tender. Drain and set aside.

2. In a large bowl, combine shallot, garlic, vinegar, honey, ¼ tsp (1 mL) salt and pepper. Let stand for a few minutes for flavors to blend. Whisk in olive oil. Taste and adjust flavor with more salt or pepper, if necessary.

3. Add warm lentils and remaining ½ tsp (2 mL) salt to bowl with dressing and toss to mix. Add tomatoes and mint. Taste and add lemon, if desired. Refrigerate if not eating right away. Bring to room temperature before serving and top with feta cheese.

Lentils

Lentils come in quite a few shapes and sizes. There are the usual brown lentils at most grocery stores, the green lentils from France (*lentils du Puy*), lentils from India (dal) and the black beluga lentils at specialty markets. Like a mother with many children, we love them all equally, but sometimes prefer one type over another depending on the occasion. They all cook in basically the same way, so use whichever lentil strikes your fancy.

Lentil Salad with Dried Cranberries and Pistachios

You will be surprised at how the addition of cranberries, celery, carrot and pistachios adds sweetness and crunch to this salad. The colors in this mélange remind us of bright and breezy Lilly Pulitzer dresses from the '60s. The flavors, however, are very today.

Serves 6

Hands-on time:
30 minutes

Start to finish:
30 minutes

Tip

It is easier than ever to find shelled pistachios. You should look for unsalted natural (green) pistachios. If you can't find them, slivered almonds will work in a pinch.

Make Ahead

The salad can be made up to 1 day ahead, covered and refrigerated. Stir in pistachios and sprinkle with feta just before serving.

½ cup	dried cranberries	125 mL
1	recipe Lentil Salad with Feta Cheese (page 92)	1
½ cup	finely diced carrot	125 mL
½ cup	finely diced celery	125 mL
½ cup	pistachios	125 mL
	Zest of 1 lemon	
1 tbsp	freshly squeezed lemon juice	15 mL
1	8-oz (250 g) empty can with both ends removed, optional	1

1. In a bowl, soak dried cranberries in hot water for 10 minutes. Drain.

2. Make Lentil Salad with Feta Cheese recipe, adding cranberries, carrot, celery, pistachios, lemon zest and lemon juice in Step 3.

3. For a more structured look on your plate, place an empty 8-oz (250 g) can with both ends removed on the plate. Spoon salad into can and compress lightly with back of a fork. Lift can directly up and it will leave a lovely disk of molded salad on the plate. Garnish with feta.

Variations

Substitute raisins or dried cherries for the cranberries.

Marinated Lentil Salad

Serves 4

¼ cup	extra-virgin olive oil, divided	60 mL
1	large onion, chopped	1
2	bay leaves	2
1	clove garlic, minced	1
8 cups	water	2 L
3 cups	dried brown lentils	750 mL
¼ tsp	hot pepper flakes	1 mL
	Salt	
3 tbsp	freshly squeezed lemon juice	45 mL
½ cup	Dijon Vinaigrette (page 96)	125 mL
¼ cup	chopped fresh Italian (flat-leaf) parsley	60 mL
	Freshly ground black pepper to taste	
12	oil-cured black olives, pitted	12
1	large tomato, cut into wedges	1

1. In a large skillet, heat half the oil over medium heat. Sauté onion until tender. Add bay leaves, garlic, water, lentils, hot pepper flakes and salt, to taste; simmer until lentils are tender, about 1 hour. Drain.

2. Stir in lemon juice and the remaining oil; let cool. Toss with vinaigrette, parsley, pepper and additional salt. Discard bay leaves. Cover and refrigerate for about 1 hour, until chilled. Serve garnished with olives and tomato wedges. Store in an airtight container in the refrigerator for up to 4 days.

Tabbouleh with Lentils

1 cup	dried brown lentils	250 mL
5 cups	water, divided	1.25 mL
¾ cup	medium-grain bulgur, rinsed thoroughly	175 mL
½ tsp	salt	2 mL
Pinch	ground allspice	Pinch
3	green onions, finely chopped	3
2	cloves garlic, minced	2
1	cucumber, peeled, seeded and diced	1
1 cup	diced seeded tomato	250 mL
¼ cup	chopped fresh mint	60 mL
¼ cup	chopped fresh Italian (flat-leaf) parsley	60 mL
¼ cup	freshly squeezed lemon juice	60 mL
¼ cup	olive oil	60 mL
	Lettuce leaves	
	Lemon wedges	

1. Boil lentils in 4 cups (1 L) of the water for 40 minutes; drain.

2. Combine bulgur and lentils in a large bowl. Bring the remaining water, salt and allspice to a boil; add to bulgur mixture and let stand until water is absorbed. Toss with green onions, garlic, cucumber, tomato, mint, parsley, lemon juice and olive oil. Serve on lettuce leaves, garnished with lemon wedges.

Sesame Tofu Vinaigrette

Serve this vinaigrette with poached vegetable salads, Chinese cabbage coleslaw or fish and seafood salads.

1	small clove garlic	1
6 tbsp	canola oil	90 mL
¼ cup	cubed silken tofu	60 mL
3 tbsp	rice vinegar	45 mL
2 tbsp	dark sesame oil	30 mL
1 tsp	soy sauce	5 mL
¼ cup	toasted sesame seeds	60 mL

1. In a blender or food processor, purée garlic, canola oil, tofu, vinegar, sesame oil and soy sauce, thinning with a few drops of water, if necessary. Stir in sesame seeds.

Dijon Vinaigrette

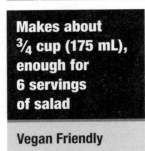

**Makes about
¾ cup (175 mL),
enough for
6 servings
of salad**

Vegan Friendly

1	clove garlic, minced	1
3 tbsp	red wine vinegar	45 mL
2 tbsp	Dijon mustard	30 mL
⅓ cup	canola oil	75 mL
⅓ cup	extra-virgin olive oil	75 mL
	Salt and freshly ground black pepper	

1. Combine garlic, vinegar and mustard. Whisk in canola oil and olive oil in a slow, steady stream. Season with salt and pepper, to taste.

Variation

Tarragon Mustard Vinaigrette: Follow recipe for Dijon Vinaigrette, but add 2 tsp (10 mL) dried tarragon or 2 tbsp (30 mL) chopped fresh tarragon.

Asian Tofu Dressing

**Makes about
¾ cup (175 mL)**

Vegan Friendly

½	clove garlic	½
4 oz	silken tofu, drained	125 g
2 tbsp	rice wine vinegar	30 mL
1 tsp	soy sauce	5 mL
	Salt and freshly ground white pepper to taste	
¼ cup	canola oil	60 mL
3 tbsp	dark sesame oil	45 mL

1. In a food processor, purée garlic, tofu, vinegar, soy sauce, salt and pepper. With the motor running, through the feed tube, add canola oil and sesame oil in a slow, steady stream and process until incorporated.

Variation

Tofu Tuna Sandwich Spread: Prepare Asian Tofu Dressing. Toss with 2 cans (each 6 oz/170 g) water-packed tuna, drained and crumbled, 1 carrot, shredded, and 1 stalk celery, diced. Serves 4.

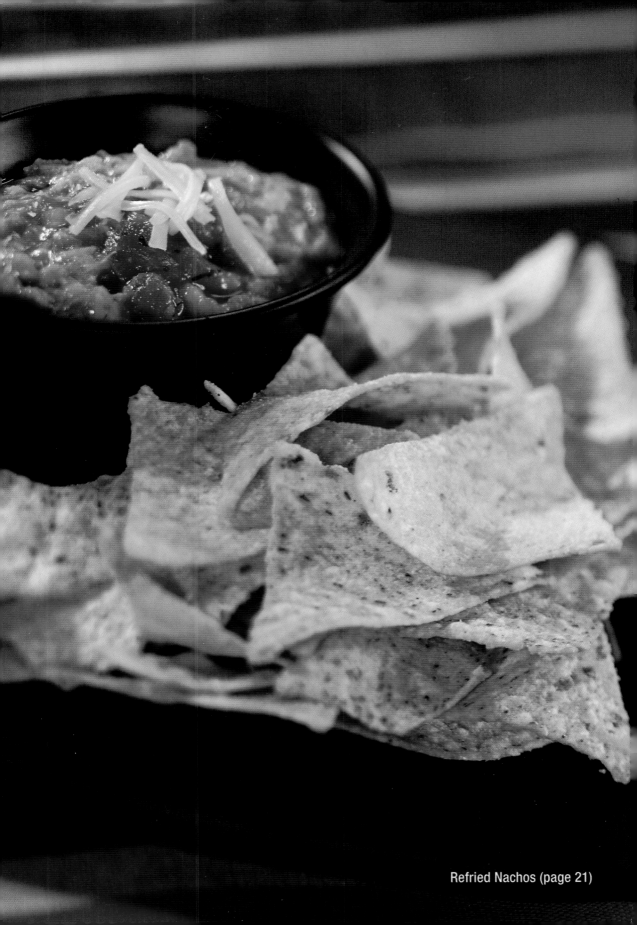

Refried Nachos (page 21)

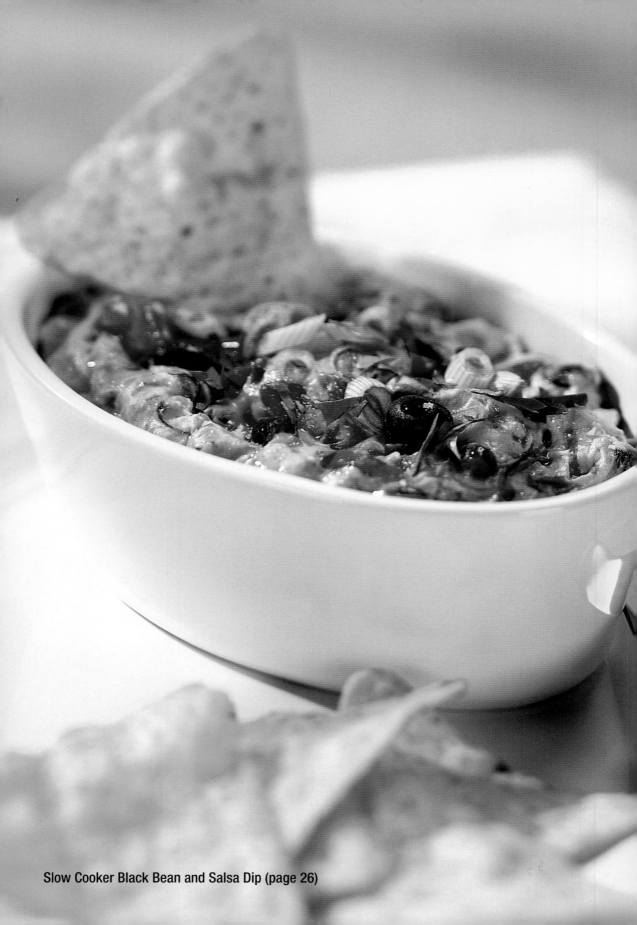

Slow Cooker Black Bean and Salsa Dip (page 26)

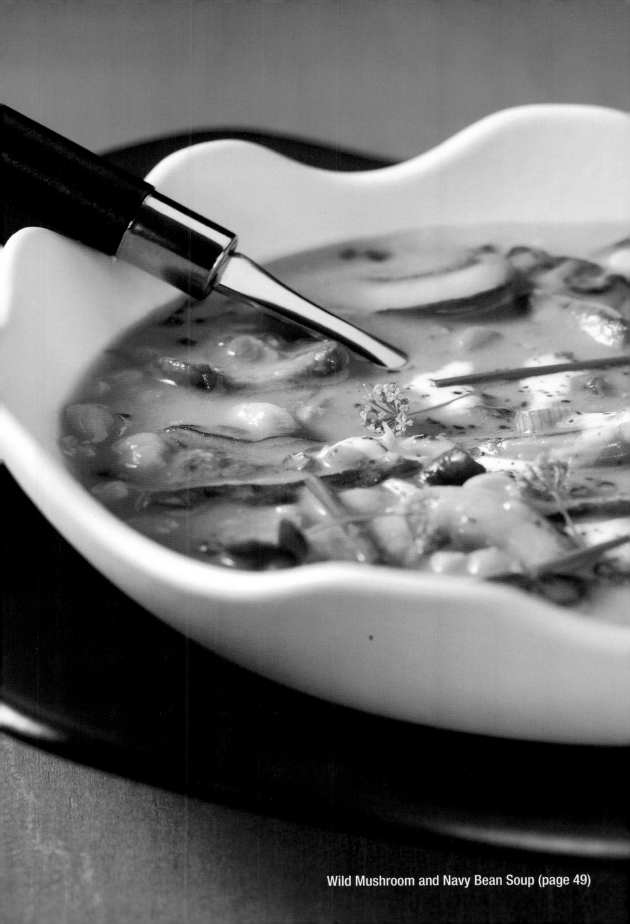

Wild Mushroom and Navy Bean Soup (page 49)

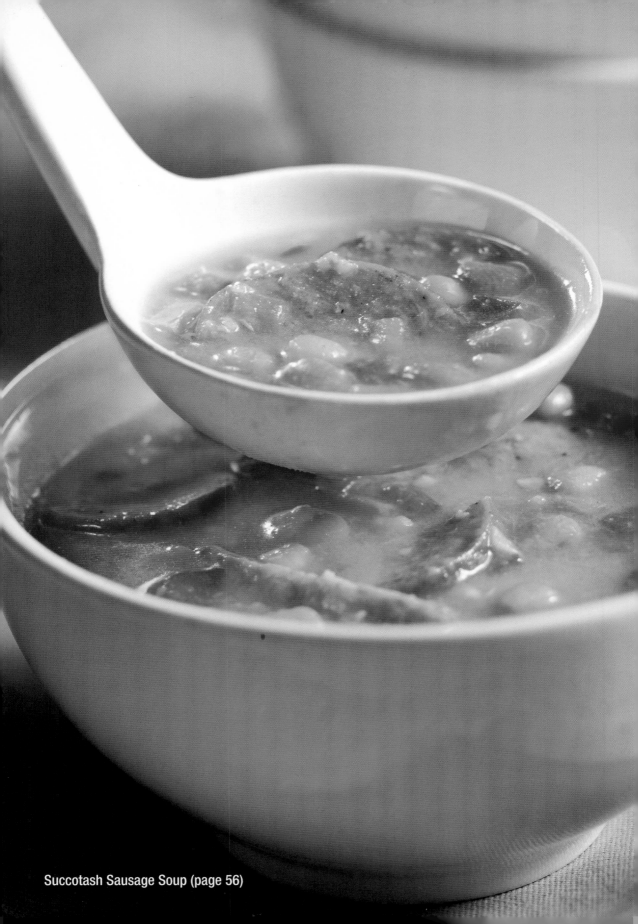

Succotash Sausage Soup (page 56)

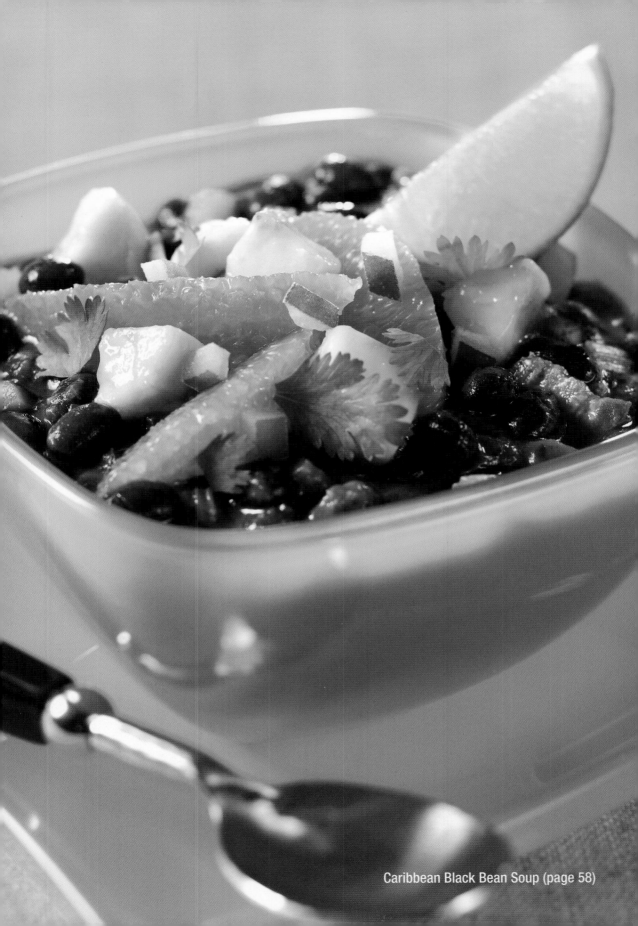

Caribbean Black Bean Soup (page 58)

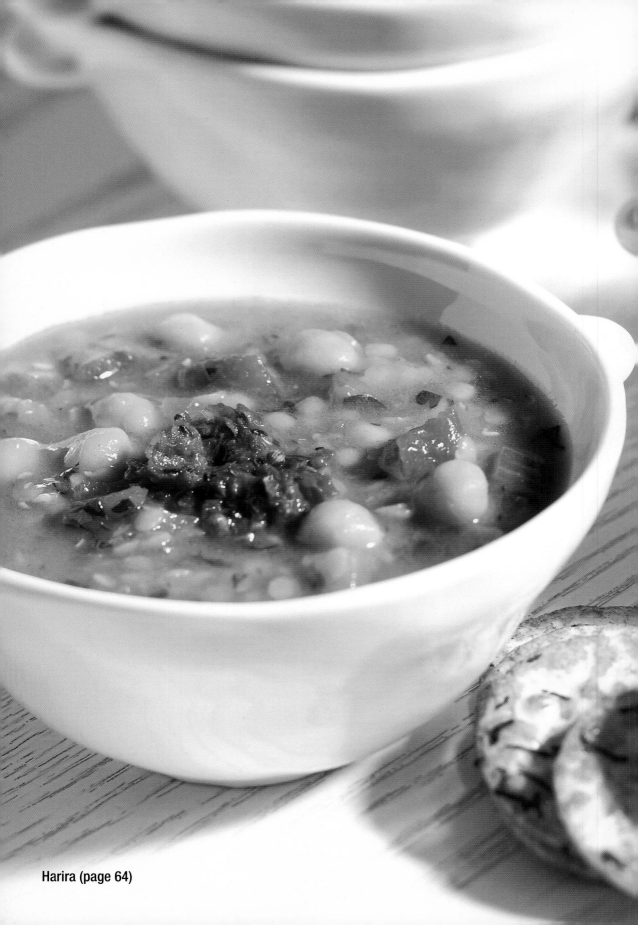
Harira (page 64)

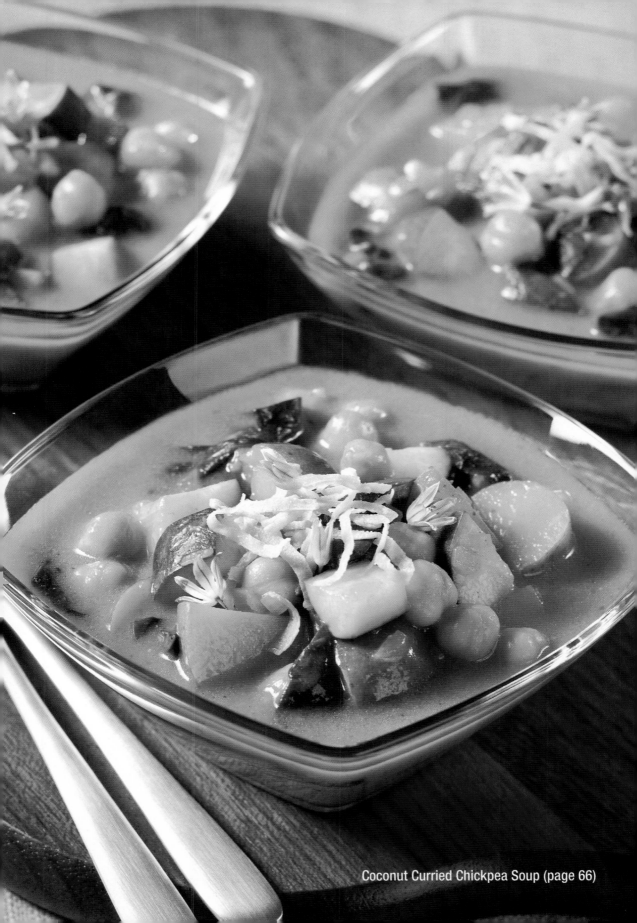

Coconut Curried Chickpea Soup (page 66)

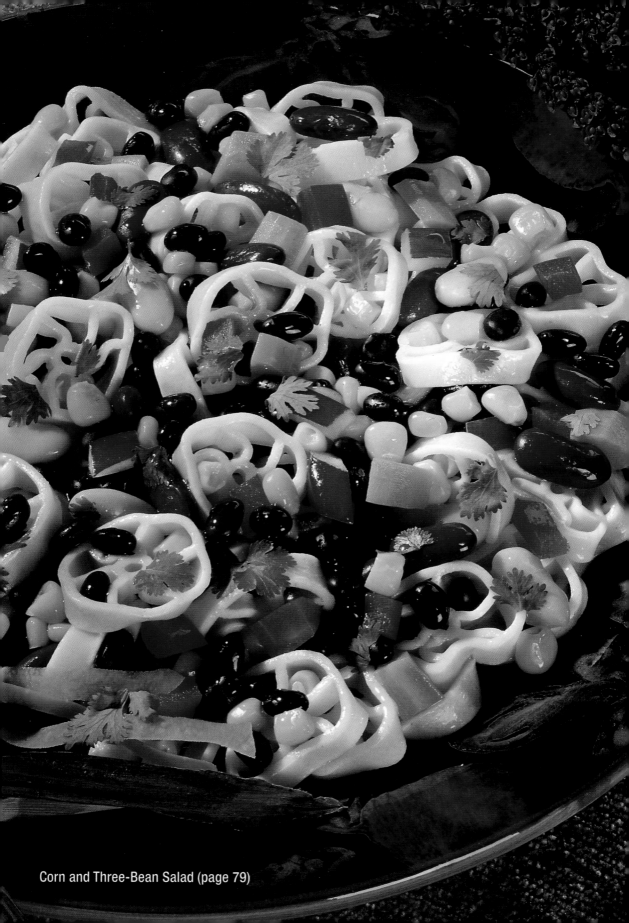

Corn and Three-Bean Salad (page 79)

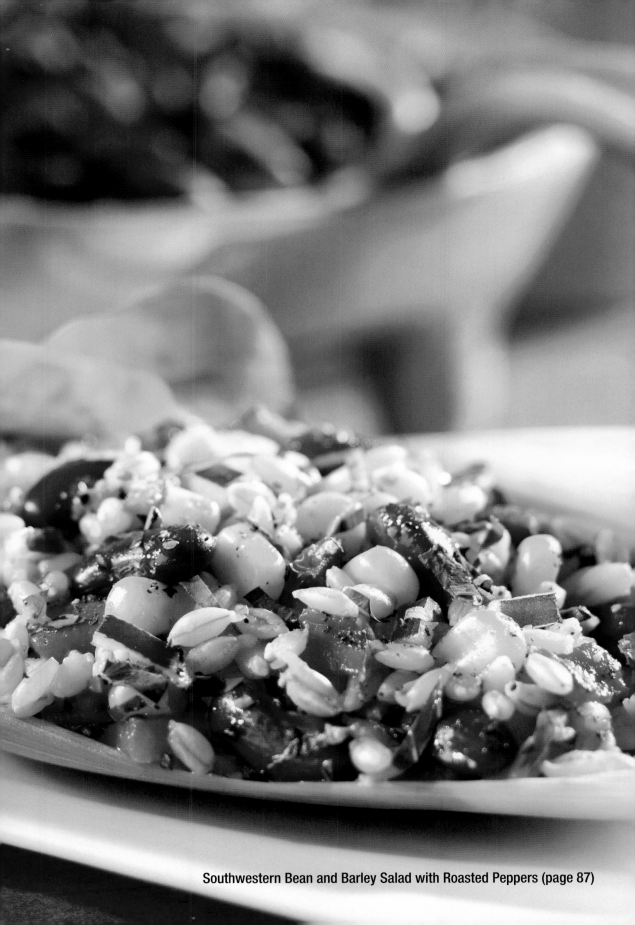

Southwestern Bean and Barley Salad with Roasted Peppers (page 87)

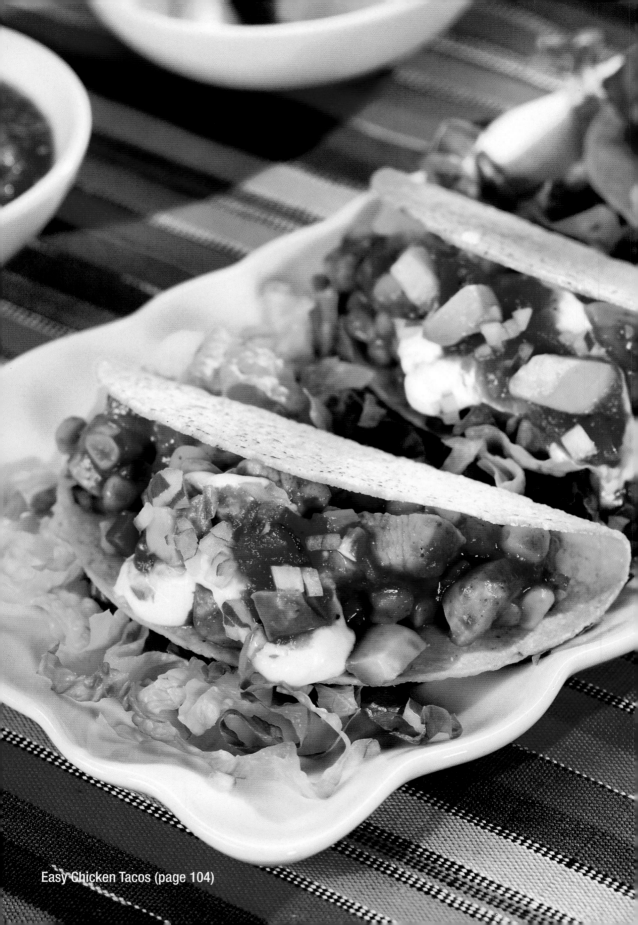

Easy Chicken Tacos (page 104)

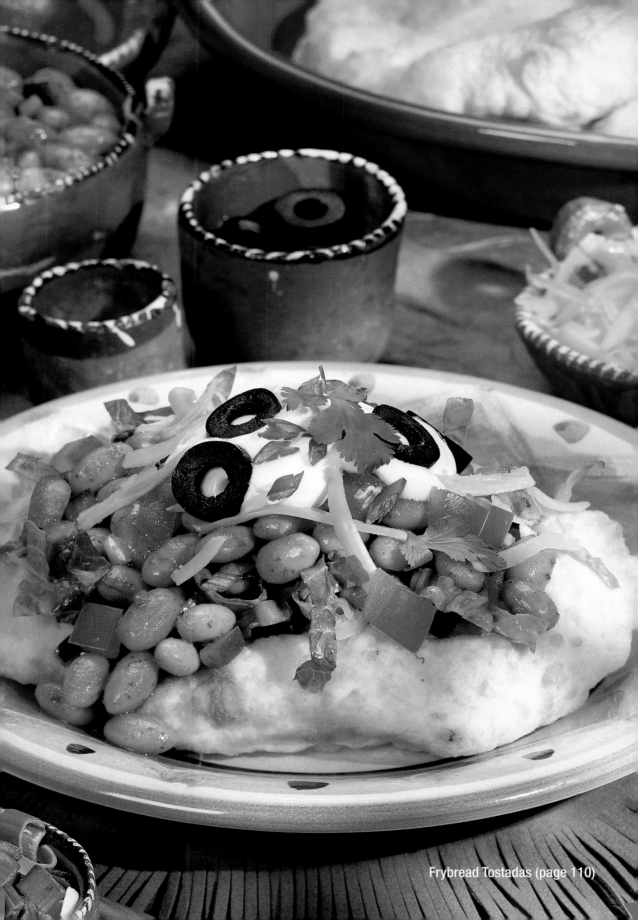

Frybread Tostadas (page 110)

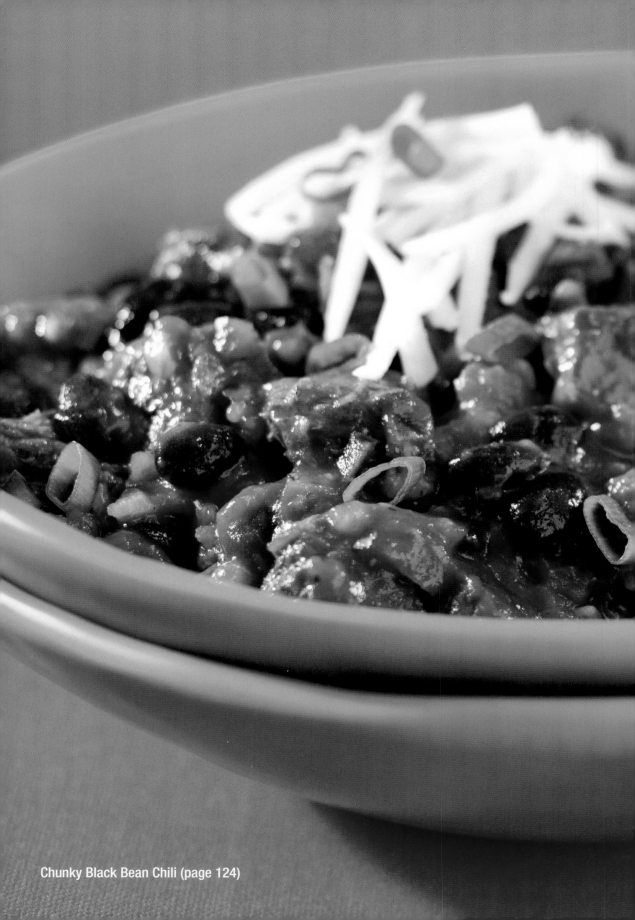

Chunky Black Bean Chili (page 124)

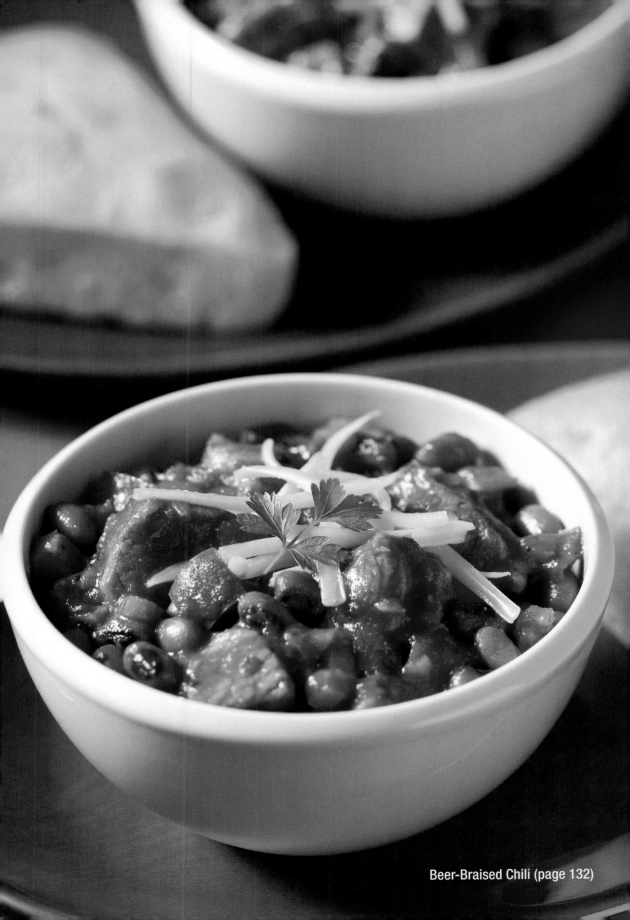

Beer-Braised Chili (page 132)

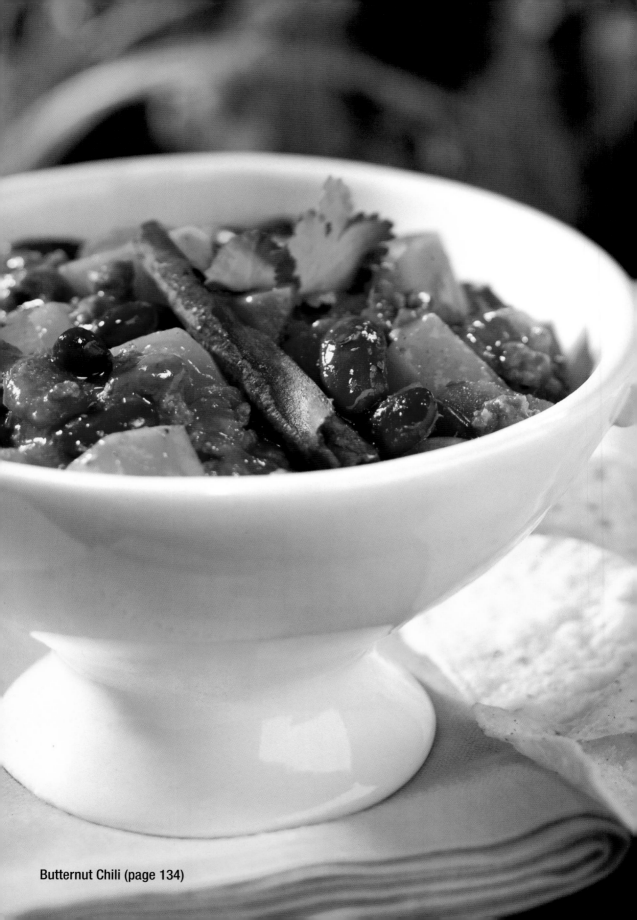

Butternut Chili (page 134)

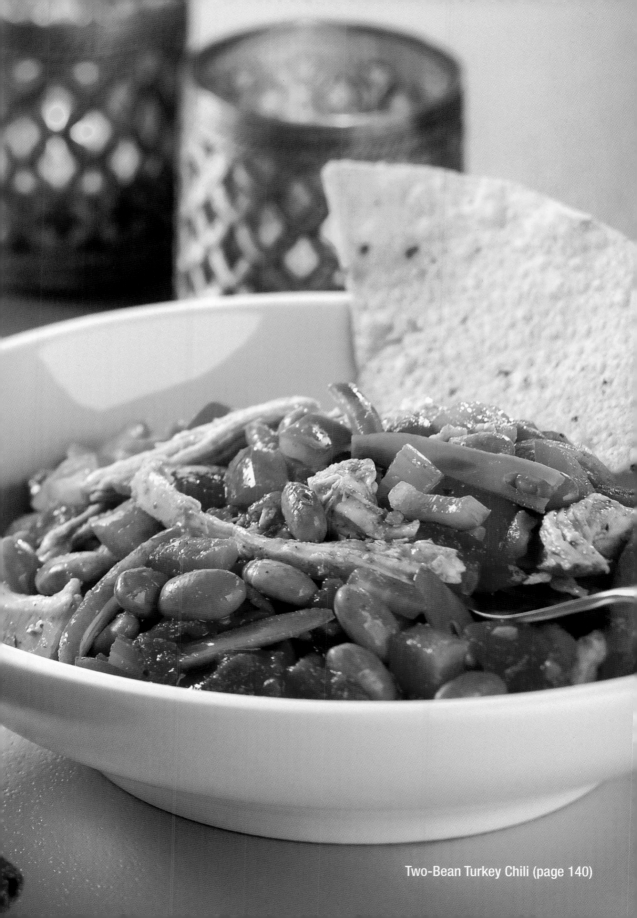

Two-Bean Turkey Chili (page 140)

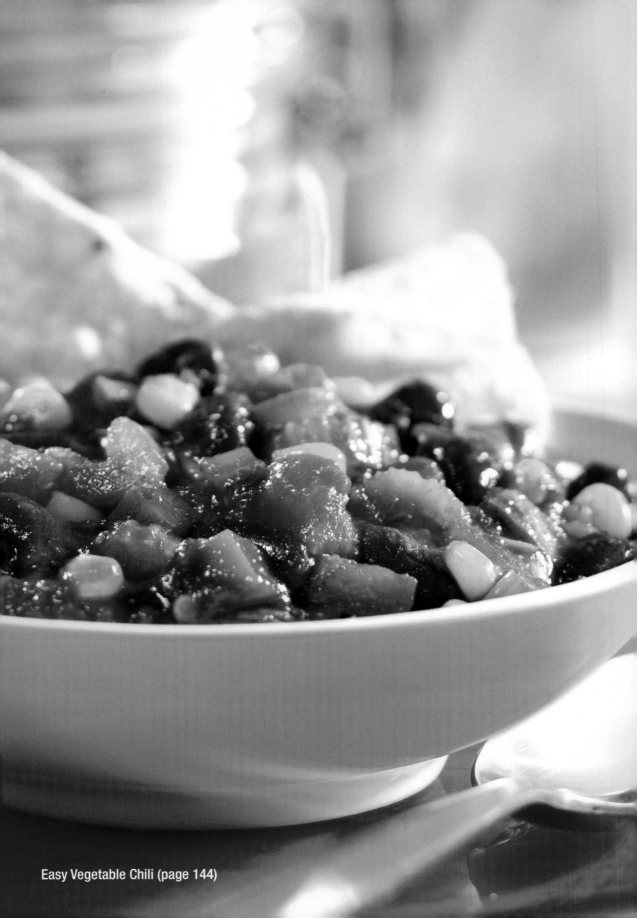

Easy Vegetable Chili (page 144)

Red Wine Vinaigrette

We most frequently use the proportion of three parts oil to one part acidic ingredient (vinegar or citrus juice or a combination) in our salad dressings. However, the proportion may be adjusted to taste and will vary according to the individual characteristics of the oil and vinegar being used and the salad ingredients (e.g., bean salads benefit from a splash more acidity).

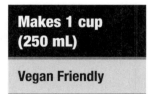

**Makes about
½ cup (125 mL)**

Vegan Friendly

Tips

Read the ingredient label on most commercial salad dressings and you will see sugar fairly high on the list.

Our collective taste buds obviously favor sweetness. If you find your homemade dressing too acidic to your taste, add a pinch of sugar or drizzle of honey.

1 tsp	finely chopped garlic, optional	5 mL
1 tsp	Dijon mustard	5 mL
¼ tsp	kosher or sea salt	1 mL
2 tbsp	red wine vinegar	30 mL
6 tbsp	extra virgin olive oil	90 mL
Pinch	freshly ground black pepper	Pinch
1 tbsp	freshly squeezed lemon juice, optional	15 mL

1. In a small bowl, mash together garlic, if using, mustard and salt. Add vinegar. Slowly whisk in oil. Season with pepper to taste. Add lemon juice for a little fruity acidity, if needed.

Variation

White Wine Vinaigrette: Substitute white wine vinegar for the red wine vinegar and proceed as above.

Tofu Mayonnaise

Even though it's not a true mayonnaise, this dressing is a delicious lower-fat alternative.

**Makes 1 cup
(250 mL)**

Vegan Friendly

Tip

Store, tightly covered, in the refrigerator for up to 3 days.

1	clove garlic	1
8 oz	soft tofu, drained	250 g
2 tbsp	freshly squeezed lemon juice	30 mL
1 tsp	Dijon mustard	5 mL
	Salt and freshly ground pepper	

1. In a blender or food processor, chop garlic. Add tofu, lemon juice and mustard and process for 20 seconds or until smooth. Add salt and pepper, to taste. Process for 5 seconds to blend.

Cajun Black Spice

Makes ⅓ cup (75 mL)

Vegan Friendly

2	dried cayenne peppers	2
1 tbsp	whole brown mustard seeds	15 mL
1 tbsp	whole black peppercorns	15 mL
1 tbsp	whole allspice berries	15 mL
1 tbsp	whole fennel seeds	15 mL
1 tsp	whole cloves	5 mL

1. Using scissors, cut cayenne pepper pods into small pieces. In a small spice wok or dry cast-iron skillet, combine pepper pieces and their seeds with mustard, peppercorns, allspice, fennel and cloves. Toast over medium-high heat for 2 to 3 minutes or until the seeds begin to pop and their fragrance is released. Let cool.

2. In a mortar (using pestle) or small electric grinder, pound or grind toasted spices until coarsely or finely ground.

Yogurt Cheese

The longer the yogurt drains, the thicker the resulting "cheese" will be. This is a healthy, low-fat alternative for the mayonnaise and cream cheese in dips and spreads.

Makes 1⅓ cups (325 mL)

Vegetarian Friendly

Tip

Store cheese, tightly covered, in the refrigerator for up to 2 days.

2 cups	natural yogurt	500 mL

1. Spoon yogurt into a sieve lined with cheesecloth; cover with plastic wrap. Set over a bowl to drain. Refrigerate for 2 to 3 hours or until yogurt is thick and reduced to about 1⅓ cups (325 mL).

Wraps, Rolls, Sandwiches and Burgers

Cuban-Style Tofu Sandwich 100

Black Bean Quesadillas 101

Sirloin and Chorizo Frijole Tacos 102

Oven-Fried Beef and Bean
    Chimichangas. 103

Easy Chicken Tacos 104

Oaxaca Chicken Tacos 105

Three-Bean Tacos 106

Red Chili con Carne Soft Tacos 107

Red Beans and Rice Soft Tacos
    with Cajun Sauce 108

Cajun Sauce 108

Chicken Tortillas. 109

Frybread Tostadas 110

Easy Tostadas 111

Chicken Enchilada Casserole
    with Teriyaki Sauce 112

Hummus and Sautéed Vegetable
    Wraps 113

Cracked Wheat and Lima Bean
    Wrap 114

Falafel in Pita. 115

Chickpea-Herb Burgers 116

Falafel Burgers with Creamy
    Sesame Sauce 117

Chickpea Tofu Burgers with
    Cilantro Mayonnaise 118

Taco Burgers 119

Bean Burgers with Dill Sauce 120

Black Bean Burgers 121

Lentil Burgers with Yogurt Sauce. 122

Cuban-Style Tofu Sandwich

Tofu is a wonderful protein source that is high in vitamins and minerals and low in calories and saturated fat. Grilling brings out its great flavor.

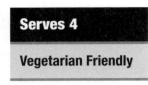

Serves 4

Vegetarian Friendly

Tip

Feel free to freeze firm or extra-firm tofu. To use, just thaw and squeeze dry.

- **Preheat lightly greased barbecue grill to medium-high**

⅓ cup	freshly squeezed orange juice	75 mL
2 tbsp	freshly squeezed lime juice	30 mL
2	cloves garlic, minced	2
2 tbsp	chopped fresh cilantro	30 mL
1 tsp	ground cumin	5 mL
¼ tsp	salt	1 mL
¼ tsp	freshly ground black pepper	1 mL
1 lb	extra-firm tofu, drained (see Tip, left)	500 g
8	slices Italian bread	8
1 tbsp	butter	15 mL
4	lettuce leaves	4
4	tomato slices	4
	Low-fat mayonnaise, optional	

1. In a small bowl, combine orange juice, lime juice, garlic, cilantro, cumin, salt and pepper. Cut tofu horizontally into four ½-inch (1 cm) thick slices. Pour orange juice mixture over tofu and refrigerate for 30 minutes.

2. Place tofu on grill for 5 minutes per side or until thoroughly heated.

3. Place bread slices on a work surface. Brush one side of each bread slice with butter. Place bread on grill, buttered side down, for 1 to 2 minutes or until toasted. Serve tofu on bread with lettuce, tomato and mayonnaise, if using. Serve immediately.

Black Bean Quesadillas

This is the perfect hearty vegetarian appetizer, filled with black beans, bell peppers and spices.

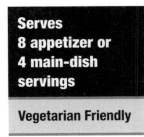

**Serves
8 appetizer or
4 main-dish
servings**

Vegetarian Friendly

Tip

To make ahead,
chop bell peppers,
red onions and
mushrooms and
refrigerate in a tightly
sealed container for
up to 8 hours.

1 tbsp	olive oil	15 mL
1 cup	sliced mushrooms	250 mL
1 cup	chopped red onion (about 1 medium)	250 mL
1/2 cup	diced red bell pepper	125 mL
1/2 cup	diced yellow bell pepper	125 mL
1	can (14 to 19 oz/398 to 540 mL) black beans, rinsed and drained	1
1/2 cup	chopped tomatoes	125 mL
1/4 cup	salsa	60 mL
2 tbsp	sliced black olives	30 mL
1/4 tsp	ground cumin	1 mL
4	8-inch (20 cm) flour tortillas	4
1 cup	shredded pepper Jack or Monterey Jack cheese	250 mL

Toppings, optional

Sour cream
Salsa or pico de gallo
Chopped green onions

1. In a large skillet, heat oil over medium heat. Sauté mushrooms, red onion and red and yellow bell peppers for 5 minutes or until tender. Add beans, tomatoes, salsa, olives and cumin. Sauté for 2 minutes or until heated through. Remove from pan.

2. In same skillet, heat tortillas over medium heat. Spread bean mixture equally over center of each tortilla. Top each with 1/4 cup (60 mL) of the cheese. Fold tortilla over and cook for 2 minutes or until lightly browned and cheese is melted. Repeat with remaining quesadillas. Cut each quesadilla into 6 wedges and garnish with desired toppings.

Variation

Chicken and Black Bean Quesadillas: Add 1 1/2 cups (375 mL) cooked chicken for a heartier appetizer or main-dish quesadilla.

Sirloin and Chorizo Frijole Tacos

Chorizo, a spicy Mexican sausage, blends well with frijoles (refried beans) and sirloin.

Makes 8 tacos

Tips

To warm corn tortillas in a skillet, place a dry nonstick or cast-iron skillet over medium heat. Place tortilla in a skillet and heat each side by turning once until warm and pliable, about 1 minute per side. Place in a tortilla warmer or wrap in foil to keep warm until ready to use.

To warm flour tortillas in a skillet follow the same instructions but place in a griddle or skillet over medium-high heat.

1 tbsp	olive oil	15 mL
1 lb	boneless beef sirloin steak, cut into bite-size pieces	500 g
4 oz	fresh chorizo sausage, removed from casings	125 g
1 cup	refried beans (page 276), warmed	250 mL
8	6- to 8-inch (15 to 20 cm) corn or flour tortillas, skillet-warmed (see Tips, left)	8
1 cup	shredded Monterey Jack cheese	250 mL
1 cup	shredded lettuce	250 mL

1. In a large skillet, heat oil over medium-high heat. Sauté steak until well browned and all juices have evaporated, 6 to 8 minutes. Add chorizo and sauté until sirloin is slightly charred and chorizo is slightly browned. Drain excess grease.

2. To build taco, spread refried beans equally on one side of each tortilla. Top with meat mixture, cheese and lettuce. Fold tortillas in half.

Oven-Fried Beef and Bean Chimichangas

These oven-fried chimichangas are just as tasty as the full-fat version. They are simple to prepare, and kids love them.

Tip

To warm tortillas, place on a plate, layered with paper towels, alternating paper towels and tortillas and covering top layer with a towel. Microwave on High for 10 to 20 seconds or until warm.

- **Preheat oven to 350°F (180°C)**
- **Baking sheet, coated with cooking spray**

1 lb	lean ground beef	500 g
1	can (16 oz/500 g) fat-free refried beans	1
1 cup	shredded reduced-fat sharp (aged) Cheddar cheese	250 mL
1	can (4 1/2 oz/127 mL) chopped green chiles, drained	1
1/4 cup	mild salsa	60 mL
8	9-inch (23 cm) reduced-fat flour tortillas, warmed (see Tip, left)	8

Toppings, optional

Shredded lettuce
Nonfat sour cream or Greek yogurt
Pico de gallo

1. In a large skillet, brown beef for 4 minutes or until meat is no longer pink inside.
2. In a large bowl, combine beef, refried beans, cheese, green chiles and salsa.
3. Place warmed tortillas on a work surface. Place 1/3 cup (75 mL) of the bean mixture just below center of each tortilla. Fold opposite sides of tortillas over filling, forming rectangles. Secure with wooden toothpicks. Place on prepared baking sheet.
4. Bake in preheated oven for 8 minutes. Turn and bake for 5 minutes more or until lightly browned. Remove toothpicks, and serve with desired toppings.

Variation

Chicken Chimichangas: Omit beef, add 1 1/2 cups (375 mL) chopped cooked chicken with the beans in Step 2 and proceed as directed.

Easy Chicken Tacos

Kids love this tactile dish, and adults enjoy its Tex-Mex flavors and ease of preparation. The spicing is mild to appeal to young palates, but the heat is easily bumped up with the addition of a jalapeño or chipotle pepper (see Variations, below) or spicy salsa as a garnish.

Serves 4

Tips

If desired, use 8 oz (250 g) precooked sliced chicken breast in this recipe. Chop and add to the pan along with the beans.

The consistency of refried beans varies among brands. If yours are almost solid when removed from the can, you may need to add as much as 1/4 cup (60 mL) water along with the beans to facilitate integration of the ingredients. Or, you can make your own (see page 276).

1 tbsp	vegetable oil	15 mL
8 oz	skinless boneless chicken breasts, cut into 1/2-inch (1 cm) cubes (see Tips, left)	250 g
1/2 tsp	chili powder	2 mL
	Freshly ground black pepper	
1 cup	drained canned corn kernels or thawed corn kernels	250 mL
1	roasted red pepper, finely chopped	1
1	can (14 oz/398 mL) refried beans (see Tips, left)	1
1 cup	shredded Tex-Mex cheese mix or Monterey Jack cheese	250 mL
12	taco shells	12
	Salsa	
	Shredded lettuce	
	Chopped tomato	
	Finely chopped red or green onion	
	Cubed avocado	
	Sour cream	

1. In a skillet, heat oil over medium heat. Add chicken and cook, stirring, until lightly browned and no longer pink inside, about 5 minutes. Sprinkle with chili powder, and black pepper to taste. Cook, stirring, for 1 minute. Add corn, red pepper and beans and bring to a boil.

2. Reduce heat to low and simmer for 2 to 3 minutes. Add cheese and stir until melted.

3. Warm taco shells according to package directions. Fill with bean mixture and garnish with any combination of salsa, lettuce, tomato, onion, avocado and/or sour cream.

Variations

For a spicier result, add 1 finely chopped jalapeño pepper or chipotle pepper in adobo sauce along with the chili powder.

Oaxaca Chicken Tacos

This is a quick version of a classic that you will find in Mexican kitchens. Refried beans teamed with roasted chicken are among the simple flavors of Mexico.

Makes 8 tacos

Tips

Lard adds an authentic flavor to taco fillings. It actually has less cholesterol and saturated fat than butter. But you can substitute 1 tbsp (15 mL) vegetable oil or olive oil for the lard.

Cotija is a crumbly, sharp Mexican cheese. You could substitute freshly grated Parmesan or a milder feta or goat cheese.

Serve with Pico de Gallo (page 29).

1 tbsp	lard (see Tips, left)	15 mL
3 cups	diced roasted chicken	750 mL
4	green onions, trimmed and finely chopped	4
3	jalapeños, seeded and minced	3
1 ½ cups	refried beans, warmed (page 276)	375 mL
8	6-inch (15 cm) corn tortillas, skillet-warmed (see Tips, page 102)	8
1 cup	crumbled Cotija cheese (see Tip, left)	250 mL

1. In a large skillet, heat lard over medium heat. Sauté chicken, green onions and jalapeños until vegetables are tender-crisp, 4 to 6 minutes.

2. To build tacos, spread beans equally on one side of each tortilla. Divide chicken mixture equally among tortillas. Top with cheese. Fold tortillas in half.

Variation

Substitute feta cheese for the Cotija cheese.

Three-Bean Tacos

Fresh garden herbs add superb flavor to this bean taco. Enjoy a healthy taco filled with veggies full of fiber.

Tips

If you are pressed for time, use canned pinto beans, rinsed and drained.

Panela is a fresh Mexican cheese that tastes like a combination of Monterey Jack and mozzarella cheese. Its main characteristic is that it does not melt but will get soft when warmed.

1 tbsp	olive oil	15 mL
¾ cup	cooked pinto beans (see Tips, left)	175 mL
½ cup	canned red beans, drained and rinsed	125 mL
½ cup	canned black beans, drained and rinsed	125 mL
¼ cup	diced seeded tomato	60 mL
⅓ cup	minced seeded jalapeño	75 mL
¼ cup	chopped fresh cilantro	60 mL
2 tbsp	chopped fresh basil	30 mL
	Salt and freshly ground black pepper	
8	6-inch (15 cm) corn tortillas, skillet-warmed (see Tips, page 102)	8
2 cups	chopped salad mix	500 mL
1 cup	crumbled panela or shredded Monterey Jack cheese (see Tips, left)	250 mL

1. In a large skillet, heat oil over medium-high heat. Sauté pinto, red and black beans, tomato, jalapeño, cilantro and basil until beans are heated through, 8 to 10 minutes. Season with salt and pepper to taste. Drain off excess liquid.

2. To build tacos, divide bean mixture equally among tortillas. Top with salad mix and cheese. Fold tortillas in half.

Red Chili con Carne Soft Tacos

Fun Tex-Mex tacos get everyone's attention. Good old-fashioned chili and beans layered with flavor is a crowd pleaser.

Tips

There are a variety of beans on the market. Beans in chili sauce or red beans are the best selection.

Serve chili con carne family style, in a large bowl, with warmed flour tortillas. Offer bowls of lettuce, cheese, onions and tomatoes.

1 lb	lean ground beef	500 g
1 tsp	garlic powder	5 mL
1 tsp	ground cumin	5 mL
3 tbsp	chili powder	45 mL
1	can (15 oz/425 mL) chili beans (see Tips, left)	1
12	6- to 8-inch (15 to 20 cm) flour tortillas, skillet-warmed (see Tips, page 102)	12
2 to 3 cups	shredded lettuce	500 to 750 mL
1½ cups	shredded Cheddar cheese	375 mL
1 to 2	onions, minced	1 to 2
1 to 2	tomatoes, chopped	1 to 2

1. In a large skillet over medium heat, sauté beef, garlic powder and cumin, breaking up meat with a spoon, until meat is browned and no longer pink, 10 to 12 minutes. Drain off excess fat. Reduce heat to medium-low. Add chili powder, $\frac{1}{2}$ cup (125 mL) water and beans and boil gently, stirring often, until well blended and heated through.

2. To build taco, place 2 heaping tbsp (30 mL) of chile mixture in a tortilla. Top with lettuce, cheese, onion and tomato.

Red Beans and Rice Soft Tacos with Cajun Sauce

Cajun cooking is so popular and this regional favorite makes the best tacos. Enjoy tasty beans and tender rice loaded in fresh tortillas.

Makes 8 tacos

Vegetarian Friendly

1 tbsp	olive oil	15 mL
1	clove garlic, minced	1
1½ cups	canned or cooked red beans, rinsed and drained	375 mL
1 cup	cooked white rice	250 mL
¼ cup	minced green bell pepper	60 mL
Pinch	cayenne pepper	Pinch
	Salt and freshly ground black pepper	
8	6- to 8-inch (15 to 20 cm) flour tortillas, skillet-warmed (see Tips, page 102)	8
2 cups	chopped romaine lettuce	500 mL
1	onion, chopped	1
	Cajun Sauce (see below)	

1. In a large skillet, heat oil over medium-high heat. Sauté garlic, beans, rice, bell pepper and cayenne pepper until vegetables are tender and beans are heated through, 10 to 12 minutes. Season with salt and pepper to taste.
2. To build tacos, divide bean mixture equally among tortillas. Top with lettuce, onion and Cajun Sauce. Fold tortillas in half.

Cajun Sauce

Cajun seasoning is made up of three different chile flavors, adding a savory, spicy taste to this creamy sauce.

Makes 1 cup (250 mL)

- **Blender or food processor**

½ cup	plain yogurt	125 mL
½ cup	mayonnaise	125 mL
1 tsp	Cajun or Creole seasoning	5 mL

1. In a blender, pulse yogurt, mayonnaise and seasoning until smooth and well blended. Serve immediately or transfer to an airtight container or squeeze bottle and refrigerate, stirring occasionally, for up to 4 days.

Chicken Tortillas

Serves 4

Tips

Boneless turkey breast, pork or veal scallopini can replace the chicken.

The cheese adds a creamy texture to the tortillas. Mozzarella can also be used.

Make Ahead

Prepare filling early in the day and gently reheat before stuffing tortillas. Add extra stock if sauce is too thick.

- **Preheat oven to 375°F (190°C)**
- **Baking sheet sprayed with vegetable spray**

6 oz	skinless boneless chicken breast, diced	175 g
1 tsp	vegetable oil	5 mL
1 tsp	crushed garlic	5 mL
1 cup	chopped onions	250 mL
½ cup	finely chopped carrots	125 mL
1 cup	tomato pasta sauce	250 mL
1 cup	canned red kidney beans, drained	250 mL
½ cup	chicken stock	125 mL
1 tsp	chili powder	5 mL
8	small 6-inch (15 cm) flour tortillas	8
½ cup	shredded Cheddar cheese (optional)	125 mL

1. In a nonstick skillet sprayed with vegetable spray, cook chicken over high heat for 2 minutes or until done in the center. Remove from skillet and set aside.

2. Reduce heat to medium and add oil to pan. Respray with vegetable spray and cook garlic, onions and carrots for 10 minutes or until browned and softened, stirring often. Add some water if vegetables start to burn. Add tomato sauce, beans, stock and chili powder and cook for 10 to 12 minutes or until carrots are tender, mixture has thickened and most of the liquid is absorbed. Stir in chicken and remove from heat.

3. Put ⅓ cup (75 mL) mixture on each tortilla; sprinkle with cheese (if using) and roll up. Put on prepared baking sheet and bake in preheated oven for 10 minutes or until heated through.

Frybread Tostadas

Frybread or bannock is always found at Native powwows and at rodeos like the Calgary Stampede, where you can have it hot and sprinkled with sugar. Natives throughout the West, from prairie Blackfoot tribes to the Navajo in Arizona, rely on frybread as a daily staple. This dish is a kind of tostada, with beans (or you can use ground beef), lettuce, tomatoes, cheese and guacamole piled high on a piece of warm frybread.

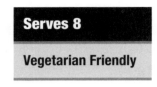

Serves 8

Vegetarian Friendly

Frybread

3 cups	all-purpose flour (or half white and half whole wheat)	750 mL
1 tsp	baking powder	5 mL
1 tsp	salt	5 mL
Pinch	granulated sugar (optional)	Pinch
1 cup	warm milk	250 mL
1 tsp	canola oil	5 mL
	Canola oil for frying	

Toppings

1 tbsp	canola oil	15 mL
2	cloves garlic, minced	2
1	onion, chopped	1
1	green bell pepper, chopped	1
2	cans (each 19 oz/540 mL) pinto beans, rinsed and drained	2
1/4 cup	tomato sauce or ketchup or bottled barbecue sauce	60 mL
1 tbsp	chili powder	15 mL
1 tsp	ground cumin	5 mL
1 cup	shredded lettuce	250 mL
1 cup	chopped tomato	250 mL
1 cup	shredded sharp Cheddar cheese	250 mL
1/2 cup	low-fat sour cream	125 mL
1/4 cup	sliced black olives	60 mL
1/4 cup	chopped cilantro	60 mL
1/4 cup	chopped green onions	60 mL

1. *Frybread:* In a large bowl, stir together flour, baking powder, salt and, if using, sugar. Stir in the warm milk and oil, mixing with a wooden spoon. Stir in just enough warm water to make a soft but not sticky dough, up to 1/2 cup (125 mL). Divide dough into 8 equal pieces. Shape each piece into a 6-inch (15 cm) round, stretching and flattening dough with your hands.

2. In a heavy frying pan, heat $\frac{1}{2}$ inch (1 cm) canola oil over medium-high heat. One at a time, fry dough rounds for 1 to 2 minutes per side or until golden brown. Drain on paper towels.

3. *Topping:* In a frying pan, heat oil over medium-high heat. Add garlic, onion and green pepper; cook for 5 minutes or until tender. Stir in beans, tomato sauce, chili powder and cumin; cook, stirring, for 2 minutes or until heated through.

4. Place frybreads on individual plates. Pile some shredded lettuce on each piece of frybread, then top with some warm bean mixture, chopped tomato and Cheddar cheese. Place a dollop of sour cream on top of the tostadas, and sprinkle each with some sliced black olives, cilantro and green onions.

Easy Tostadas

Tostadas *means "toasted" in Spanish. They are usually flat or bowl-shaped and filled with an array of Mexican ingredients.*

Serves 4

Vegetarian Friendly

Tip
To cut calories, decrease the amount of refried beans, use low-fat sour cream and use less cheese.

• **Preheat broiler**

4	8-inch (20 cm) corn tortillas	4
1 cup	refried beans	250 mL
1 cup	canned or cooked black beans, drained and rinsed	250 mL
1 cup	shredded Monterey Jack cheese	250 mL
1 cup	shredded iceberg lettuce	250 mL
1 cup	chopped avocado	250 mL
1 cup	chopped tomato	250 mL

Toppings, optional
Salsa

Sour cream

Chopped jalapeños

1. Place tortillas on a baking sheet. Spread $\frac{1}{4}$ cup (60 mL) each refried beans, black beans and cheese over each tortilla. Broil for 2 minutes or until cheese is melted and edges are browned. Top equally with lettuce, avocado, tomato and desired toppings. Cut each tortilla into 4 wedges and serve immediately.

Variations
Feel free to add chopped cooked chicken, beef or shrimp to this recipe.

Chicken Enchilada Casserole with Teriyaki Sauce

East meets West in this flavorful chicken enchilada dish. The added heat is tamed by the cheese and sour cream.

Makes 6 servings

Tip

Visit www. intensityacademy.com to find Carrot Karma Hot Sauce, Chai Thai Teriyaki and more! They're absolutely fantastic in this dish.

- **Preheat oven to 350°F (180°C)**
- **13- by 9-inch (33 by 23 cm) glass baking dish, greased**

1 tbsp	olive oil	15 mL
1	onion, chopped	1
2 cups	shredded cooked chicken breasts	500 mL
¼ cup	spicy barbecue sauce, such as Carrot Karma Hot Sauce (see Tip, left)	60 mL
¾ cup	teriyaki sauce, such as Chai Thai Teriyaki (see Tip, left)	175 mL
8	6-inch (15 cm) corn tortillas	8
1	can (14 to 19 oz/398 to 540 mL) kidney beans, drained	1
2 cups	shredded Cheddar cheese	500 mL
2 cups	salsa	500 mL
½ cup	sour cream	125 mL

1. In a large skillet, heat oil over medium heat. Sauté onion for 5 to 7 minutes or until softened. Remove from heat and stir in chicken, barbecue sauce and teriyaki sauce.

2. Arrange 4 tortillas in prepared baking dish, overlapping as necessary. Top with chicken mixture, beans and half the cheese. Arrange the remaining tortillas on top. Top with salsa and the remaining cheese.

3. Bake in preheated oven for 30 to 35 minutes or until cheese is melted. Serve topped with sour cream.

Hummus and Sautéed Vegetable Wraps

Tips

Flavored tortillas — such as pesto, sun-dried tomato, herb or whole wheat — are now appearing in many supermarkets. The different colors make these wraps an attractive dish for entertaining.

Try substituting other herbs — such as cilantro, basil or parsley — for the dill.

If tahini is unavailable, use peanut butter.

Make Ahead

Prepare hummus up to 3 days in advance.

Sauté vegetables early in the day and reheat before serving.

- **Food processor**

1 cup	canned chickpeas, rinsed and drained	250 mL
1/4 cup	tahini	60 mL
1/4 cup	water	60 mL
2 tbsp	freshly squeezed lemon juice	30 mL
4 tsp	olive oil	20 mL
1 tbsp	chopped fresh parsley	15 mL
3/4 tsp	minced garlic	3 mL
2 tsp	vegetable oil	10 mL
1 cup	diced onions	250 mL
1 1/4 cups	diced red bell peppers	300 mL
1 1/4 cups	chopped snow peas	300 mL
1/4 cup	chopped fresh dill (or 2 tsp/10 mL dried)	60 mL
4	10-inch (25 cm) flour tortillas, preferably different flavors, if available	4

1. *Make the hummus:* In a food processor, combine chickpeas, tahini, water, lemon juice, oil, parsley and garlic; process until creamy and smooth. Transfer to a bowl and set aside.

2. In a large nonstick saucepan, heat oil over medium-high heat. Add onions and sauté 4 minutes or until soft and browned. Add red peppers and sauté for 4 minutes or until soft. Add snow peas and sauté for 2 minutes or until tender-crisp. Stir in dill and remove from heat.

3. Divide hummus equally among tortillas, spreading to within 1/2 inch (1 cm) of edge. Divide vegetable mixture between tortillas. Form each tortilla into a packet by folding bottom edge over filling, then sides, then top, to enclose filling completely.

Cracked Wheat and Lima Bean Wrap

Tip

This makes enough filling for 10 large wraps so if you don't have a large crowd to feed, make half the recipe or freeze leftover filling.

2 tbsp	olive oil	30 mL
1 cup	chopped onions	250 mL
2	cloves garlic, minced	2
1 cup	chopped celery	250 mL
2 tbsp	finely chopped preserved ginger	30 mL
1 tsp	ground cumin	5 mL
1 tbsp	ground turmeric	15 mL
1 cup	cracked wheat	250 mL
3 tbsp	fresh lemon juice	45 mL
1	can (28 oz/796 mL) stewed tomatoes	1
1	can (19 oz/540 mL) lima beans, drained and coarsely chopped	1
	Salt and black pepper	
2/3 cup	plain yogurt	150 mL
10	large flour tortillas	10
1 cup	sliced black olives	250 mL
2 cups	shredded lettuce	500 mL

1. In a large skillet, heat oil over medium-low heat. Cook onions and garlic for 10 minutes or until soft. Add celery; cook, stirring often, for 3 minutes. Add ginger, cumin and turmeric; cook for 2 minutes.

2. Stir in cracked wheat, lemon juice and tomatoes, breaking up tomatoes with back of a spoon. Simmer over low heat, covered, for 20 minutes or until liquid is absorbed and wheat is tender.

3. Remove from heat; stir in lima beans. Season to taste with salt and pepper. Allow to cool to room temperature or store in refrigerator for up to 3 days.

4. Spread 1 tbsp (15 mL) yogurt on each tortilla. Spoon about 1/2 cup (125 mL) filling down center of each wrap. Top with 1 rounded tbsp (20 mL) olives and 3 tbsp (45 mL) lettuce. Fold bottom up and both sides in, leaving top open. Fold in half. Serve slightly warm.

Variations

Substitute sour cream for yogurt and 1 1/2 cups (375 mL) cooked lentils or chickpeas for the lima beans.

Omit olives and lettuce, if desired.

Falafel in Pita

These tasty treats are a gift from the Middle East, where they are eaten the way hamburgers are in North America. Liberally garnished, they make a great lunch or light dinner.

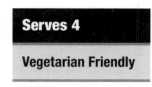

Serves 4

Vegetarian Friendly

Tip

For this quantity of chickpeas, use 1 can (14 to 19 oz/398 to 540 mL) drained and rinsed, or cook 1 cup (250 mL) dried chickpeas.

• Food processor

2 cups	drained cooked chickpeas (see Tip, left)	500 mL
1/2 cup	sliced green onions	125 mL
2 tbsp	freshly squeezed lemon juice	30 mL
1 tbsp	minced garlic	15 mL
1 to 2 tsp	curry powder	5 to 10 mL
1	egg	1
2 tbsp	oil	30 mL
1/2 cup	all-purpose flour	125 mL
4	pita breads	4
	Chopped peeled cucumber	
	Chopped tomato	
	Shredded lettuce	
	Plain yogurt or soy yogurt	

1. In a food processor fitted with metal blade, process chickpeas, green onions, lemon juice, garlic, and curry powder to taste, until blended but chickpeas retain their texture, about 30 seconds. Using your hands, shape into 4 large patties.

2. In a shallow bowl, lightly beat egg. In a skillet, heat oil over medium heat. Dip each patty into the egg, then into the flour, coating both sides well. Fry until golden and heated through, about 2 minutes per side.

3. Fill each pita bread with a falafel and garnish with cucumber, tomato, lettuce and yogurt, as desired.

Variation

Pepper-Spiked Falafel in Pita: Add 1 or 2 roasted red peppers to the chickpeas before processing.

Chickpea-Herb Burgers

Tip

Whether grilled on the barbecue or baked in the oven, these burgers are great with all the trimmings.

- **Preheat oven to 375°F (190°C) or grill to high**
- **Parchment-lined baking sheet or greased grill**
- **Food processor or blender**

1 tbsp	vegetable oil	15 mL
1	can (19 oz/540 mL) chickpeas, drained	1
1/2 cup	grated onions	125 mL
2	cloves garlic, minced	2
3 cups	shredded carrots	750 mL
1/2 cup	spelt flakes	125 mL
1/4 cup	unblanched almonds	60 mL
1/4 cup	sunflower seeds	60 mL
2 tbsp	flax seeds	30 mL
2 tbsp	chopped parsley	30 mL
2 tbsp	basil leaves	30 mL
1 tbsp	fresh thyme leaves	15 mL
1	egg	1
	Salt and black pepper	

1. In a food processor or blender, purée oil, chickpeas, onions, garlic and carrots until well combined.
2. Add spelt flakes, almonds, sunflower seeds, flax seeds, parsley, basil, thyme and egg. Process until finely chopped and holding together. Season to taste with salt and pepper if desired.
3. Form mixture into 6 patties. Arrange patties on prepared baking sheet or grill. Bake in preheated oven or grill for 3 minutes per side, being careful to turn burgers gently.

Variation

Substitute rolled oats for the spelt flakes.

Falafel Burgers with Creamy Sesame Sauce

Tips

Replace cilantro with dill or parsley.

Peanut butter can replace tahini.

Make Ahead

Prepare burgers early in the day and refrigerate until ready to cook. Prepare sauce up to a day ahead.

• **Food processor**

2 cups	drained canned chickpeas	500 mL
1/4 cup	chopped green onions	60 mL
1/4 cup	chopped cilantro	60 mL
1/4 cup	finely chopped carrots	60 mL
1/4 cup	bread crumbs	60 mL
3 tbsp	lemon juice	45 mL
3 tbsp	water	45 mL
2 tbsp	tahini (puréed sesame seeds)	30 mL
2 tsp	minced garlic	10 mL
1/4 tsp	ground black pepper	1 mL

Sauce

1/4 cup	light sour cream	60 mL
2 tbsp	tahini	30 mL
2 tbsp	chopped cilantro	30 mL
2 tbsp	water	30 mL
2 tsp	lemon juice	10 mL
1/2 tsp	minced garlic	2 mL
2 tsp	vegetable oil, divided	10 mL

1. Put chickpeas, green onions, cilantro, carrots, bread crumbs, lemon juice, water, tahini, garlic and black pepper in food processor; pulse on and off until finely chopped. With wet hands, form each 1/4 cup (60 mL) into a patty.

2. In a small bowl, whisk together sour cream, tahini, cilantro, water, lemon juice and garlic.

3. In a nonstick skillet sprayed with vegetable spray, heat 1 tsp (5 mL) of the oil over medium heat. Add 4 patties and cook for 3 1/2 minutes or until golden; turn and cook for 3 1/2 minutes longer or until golden and hot inside. Remove from pan. Heat remaining 1 tsp (5 mL) oil and cook remaining patties. Serve with sesame sauce.

Chickpea Tofu Burgers with Cilantro Mayonnaise

Tips

Serve in pita breads or on rolls, with lettuce, tomatoes and onions.

Tofu is found in the vegetable section of your grocery store. If desired, it can be replaced with 5% ricotta cheese.

Tahini is a sesame paste, usually found in the international section of your grocery store. If unavailable, try peanut butter.

The combination of chickpeas and tofu produces a rich texture in these unusual burgers.

Make Ahead

Prepare patties and sauce up to 1 day in advance. Bake just before serving.

- **Preheat oven to 425°F (220°C)**
- **Baking sheet sprayed with vegetable spray**
- **Food processor**

1 cup	canned chickpeas, rinsed and drained	250 mL
8 oz	firm tofu	250 g
1/3 cup	dry bread crumbs	75 mL
2 tbsp	tahini	30 mL
1 1/2 tbsp	freshly squeezed lemon juice	22 mL
1 tsp	minced garlic	5 mL
1	egg	1
1/4 tsp	freshly ground black pepper	1 mL
1/4 tsp	salt	1 mL
1/3 cup	chopped fresh cilantro	75 mL
1/4 cup	chopped green onions	60 mL
1/4 cup	chopped red bell peppers	60 mL

Sauce

1/4 cup	2% plain yogurt	60 mL
1/4 cup	light sour cream	60 mL
1/4 cup	chopped fresh cilantro	60 mL
1 tbsp	light mayonnaise	15 mL
1/2 tsp	minced garlic	2 mL

1. In a food processor, combine chickpeas, tofu, bread crumbs, tahini, lemon juice, garlic, egg, pepper and salt; process until smooth. Add cilantro, green onions and red peppers; pulse on and off until well-mixed. With wet hands, scoop up 1/4 cup (60 mL) of mixture and form into a patty. Put on prepared baking sheet. Repeat procedure for remaining patties. Bake in preheated oven for 20 minutes, turning burgers at halfway point.

2. *Meanwhile, make the sauce:* In a small bowl, stir together yogurt, sour cream, cilantro, mayonnaise and garlic; set aside. Serve burgers hot with sauce on the side.

Taco Burgers

This is a good twist on the usual Mexican fare, and everyone loves this combination of burgers and Mexican all in one.

Serves 4

Tip

When buying taco seasoning mix, look for the reduced-sodium version.

Make Ahead

If you want to prepare these ahead, assemble burgers, refrigerate overnight and cook the next day.

• **Instant-read thermometer**

1 lb	ground sirloin	500 g
2 tsp	taco seasoning mix (see Tip, left)	10 mL
1 cup	refried beans with chiles, divided	250 mL
¾ cup	salsa or Pico de Gallo (page 29) or store-bought, divided	175 mL
2 tbsp	chopped fresh cilantro	30 mL
4	hamburger buns, split and toasted	4
1 cup	shredded iceberg lettuce	250 mL
4	pepper Jack cheese slices	4

Toppings, optional

Avocado slices
Tomato slices
Red onion slices

1. In a large bowl, combine sirloin and seasoning mix. Shape into 4 patties, about ¾ inch (2 cm) thick. In a large nonstick skillet coated with cooking spray, fry burgers over medium heat for 4 to 5 minutes per side or until an instant-read thermometer registers 160°F (71°C).

2. In a small bowl, combine ¼ cup (60 mL) of the refried beans, salsa, and cilantro.

3. Serve patties on buns with salsa mixture, lettuce, cheese and remaining refried beans. Top with desired toppings.

Bean Burgers with Dill Sauce

Tips

Serve in a pita or tortilla with lettuce, tomatoes and onions.

Another simple topping can be made with 3 parts 2% yogurt and 1 part Dijon mustard.

Substitute black beans with another bean of your choice.

Make Ahead

Prepare mixture and sauce up to 1 day in advance. Reheat gently.

- Preheat oven to 425°F (220°C)
- Baking sheet sprayed with vegetable spray

Burgers

2 cups	canned black beans, rinsed and drained	500 mL
1/2 cup	dry seasoned bread crumbs	125 mL
1/3 cup	chopped fresh dill	75 mL
1/3 cup	chopped red onions	75 mL
1/4 cup	finely chopped carrots	60 mL
2 tbsp	cornmeal	30 mL
1	egg	1
1 1/2 tsp	minced garlic	7 mL
1/4 tsp	salt	1 mL

Sauce

3 tbsp	light sour cream	45 mL
2 tbsp	light mayonnaise	30 mL
2 tsp	freshly squeezed lemon juice	10 mL
1/4 to 1/2 tsp	minced garlic	1 to 2 mL
1 tbsp	chopped fresh dill (or 1/2 tsp/2 mL dried)	15 mL

1. In a food processor, combine black beans, bread crumbs, dill, onions, carrots, cornmeal, egg, garlic and salt. Pulse on and off until well combined. With wet hands, scoop up 1/4 cup (60 mL) of mixture and form into a patty. Put on prepared baking sheet. Repeat procedure for remaining patties. Bake in preheated oven for 15 minutes, turning at the halfway point.

2. *Meanwhile, make the sauce:* In a small bowl, stir together sour cream, mayonnaise, lemon juice, garlic and dill. Serve burgers hot with sauce on side.

Black Bean Burgers

This is a really popular recipe that is simple to prepare. Serve on a bun or in a lettuce wrap and top with your favorite toppings.

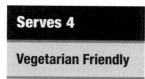

Serves 4

Vegetarian Friendly

Tip

To make these ahead of time, prep burgers and refrigerate for up to 8 hours.

- **Instant-read thermometer**

1	can (14 to 19 oz/398 to 540 mL) black beans, drained and rinsed	1
3/4 cup	panko bread crumbs	175 mL
2 tbsp	finely chopped red onion	30 mL
1/2 tsp	ground cumin	2 mL
1/2 tsp	sea salt	2 mL
1/8 tsp	hot pepper flakes	0.5 mL
1	large egg, lightly beaten	1
3 tbsp	yellow cornmeal	45 mL
3 tbsp	olive oil	45 mL
4	hamburger buns, split and toasted	4

Toppings, optional

Lettuce leaves

Salsa

Avocado

Shredded Monterey Jack cheese or slices

1. In a large bowl, mash beans with a fork. Stir in bread crumbs, red onion, cumin, salt, hot pepper flakes and egg. Shape into 4 equal patties, about 1/2 inch (1 cm) thick. Lightly coat both sides with cornmeal.

2. In a large nonstick skillet, heat olive oil over medium heat. Fry patties for 5 minutes per side or until an instant-read thermometer registers 160°F (71°C) or until hot in center and lightly browned. Place burgers on buns and serve with desired toppings.

Lentil Burgers with Yogurt Sauce

Lentils are high in fiber, protein and B vitamins and low in fat. Best of all, they taste great in this recipe.

Tips

Lentils can be found where dried beans are sold in most grocery stores.

To cook lentils, place in a small saucepan and cover with water by 1 inch (2.5 cm). Bring to a boil. Reduce heat and simmer, covered, for 15 to 20 minutes or until lentils are tender but still holding their shape. Drain well.

• **Food processor**

⅓ cup	dry bread crumbs	75 mL
2	cloves garlic, chopped	2
2 tsp	ground cumin	10 mL
½ tsp	hot pepper flakes	2 mL
¼ tsp	kosher salt	1 mL
¼ tsp	freshly ground black pepper	1 mL
¾ cup	canned or cooked lentils, rinsed, drained and cooled (see Tips, left)	175 mL
¼ cup	cooked white rice	60 mL
3 tbsp	olive oil, divided	45 mL
2	large egg whites	2
	Cilantro-Yogurt Sauce (below), optional	

1. In a food processor, pulse bread crumbs, garlic, cumin, hot pepper flakes, salt and pepper. Add lentils, rice, 1 tbsp (15 mL) of the oil and egg whites and process until coarsely chopped.

2. Divide mixture into 4 equal burgers, about ¾ inch (2 cm) thick.

3. In a large nonstick skillet, heat remaining oil over medium-low heat. Add burgers and fry for 8 to 10 minutes per side or until crisp and browned. Transfer to a paper-towel-lined plate to drain. Serve with Cilantro-Yogurt Sauce, if desired.

Cilantro-Yogurt Sauce

This cilantro sauce is wonderful on many sandwiches, especially ones with a little heat.

¾ cup	plain yogurt	175 mL
½ cup	chopped cucumber	125 mL
2 tbsp	chopped Italian flat-leaf parsley	30 mL
2 tbsp	chopped fresh cilantro	30 mL
1 tsp	freshly grated lemon zest	5 mL
¼ tsp	salt	1 mL
¼ tsp	freshly ground black pepper	1 mL

1. In a small bowl, whisk together yogurt, cucumber, parsley, cilantro, lemon zest, salt and pepper. Use immediately or cover and refrigerate for up to 2 days.

Chilies

Chunky Black Bean Chili. 124

20-Minute Chili 125

Pork and Beef Chili with Ancho Sauce . . 126

Tex-Mex Chili. 127

Red Chili with Anchos. 128

Wagon Boss Chili. 129

Easy Chili con Carne 130

Sausage and Black Bean Chili. 131

Beer-Braised Chili 132

Chili con Carne Pronto 133

Butternut Chili 134

Greek Chili with Black Olives
    and Feta Cheese. 135

Not-Too-Corny Turkey Chili
    with Sausage 136

Lime-Spiked Turkey Chili
    with Pinto Beans. 138

Chicken and Black Bean Chili 139

Two-Bean Turkey Chili 140

Vegetarian Chili 141

Hominy and Red Bean Chili. 142

Very Veggie Chili 143

Easy Vegetable Chili. 144

Black Bean Chili with Hominy
    and Sweet Corn 145

Amaranth Chili. 146

Black Bean Chili. 147

Bean and Sweet Potato Chili
    on Garlic Polenta 148

Chunky Black Bean Chili

Here's a great-tasting, stick-to-your-ribs chili that is perfect for a family dinner or a casual evening with friends. Serve this with crusty bread, a green salad and robust red wine or cold beer.

Serves 8

Tips

If you prefer, you can use 2 cups (500 mL) dried black beans, soaked, cooked and drained (see pages 6 to 10 or Basic Beans in the Slow Cooker, page 277), instead of the canned beans.

Garnish this chili with any combination of sour cream, finely chopped red or green onion, shredded Monterey Jack cheese and/or salsa.

Make Ahead

Complete Step 2, heating 1 tbsp (15 mL) oil in pan before softening the onions. Cover and refrigerate for up to 2 days. When you're ready to cook, brown the beef, or if you're pressed for time, omit this step. Continue with the recipe.

- **Large (minimum 4 quart) slow cooker**

1 tbsp	vegetable oil (approx.)	15 mL
2 lbs	stewing beef, trimmed, cut into 1-inch (2.5 cm) cubes and patted dry	1 kg
2	onions, finely chopped	2
4	cloves garlic, minced	4
1 tbsp	cumin seeds, toasted and ground (see Tip, page 130)	15 mL
1 tbsp	dried oregano, crumbled	15 mL
1 tsp	cracked black peppercorns	5 mL
1 tsp	salt	5 mL
1	can (28 oz/796 mL) diced tomatoes, with juice	1
1½ cups	flat beer or beef stock, divided	375 mL
4 cups	cooked black beans, drained and rinsed	1 L
2	dried ancho chiles	2
2	dried New Mexico chiles	2
4 cups	boiling water	1 L
1 cup	coarsely chopped fresh cilantro	250 mL
1 to 2	jalapeño peppers, chopped (optional)	1 to 2

1. In a skillet, heat oil over medium-high heat for 30 seconds. Add beef, in batches, and cook, stirring, until lightly browned, about 4 minutes per batch, adding a bit more oil between batches if necessary. Transfer to slow cooker stoneware as completed.

2. Reduce heat to medium. Add onions and cook, stirring, until softened, about 3 minutes. Add garlic, cumin, oregano, peppercorns and salt; cook, stirring, for 1 minute. Add tomatoes with juice and cook, breaking up with the back of a spoon. Add 1 cup (250 mL) of the beer and bring to a boil. Transfer to stoneware and stir well.

3. Stir in beans. Cover and cook on Low for 8 to 10 hours or on High for 4 to 5 hours, until beef is tender.

4. About an hour before recipe has finished cooking, combine ancho chiles, New Mexico chiles and boiling water in a heatproof bowl. Set aside for 30 minutes, weighing down chiles with a cup to ensure they remain submerged. Drain, discarding soaking liquid and stems, and coarsely chop chiles. Transfer to a blender and add cilantro, jalapeños (if using) and the remaining beer; purée.

5. Add chile mixture to stoneware and stir well. Cover and cook on High for 30 minutes, until mixture is hot and bubbly and flavors meld.

6. Ladle into bowls and garnish as desired (see Tips, page 124).

20-Minute Chili

Here's a streamlined version of chili that's a snap. Make a double batch and have containers stashed away in the freezer for quick microwave meals. Just ladle into bowls and, if desired, top with shredded Monterey Jack cheese. Set out a basket of crusty bread — supper is that easy.

Serves 4 to 6

Tip

Add just a pinch of red pepper flakes for a mild chili, but if you want to turn up the heat, use amount specified in the recipe.

1 lb	lean ground beef or turkey	500 g
1	large onion, chopped	1
2	large cloves garlic, finely chopped	2
1	large green bell pepper, chopped	1
4 tsp	chili powder	20 mL
1 tbsp	all-purpose flour	15 mL
1 tsp	dried basil	5 mL
1 tsp	dried oregano	5 mL
$\frac{1}{4}$ to $\frac{1}{2}$ tsp	red pepper flakes	1 to 2 mL
2 cups	tomato pasta sauce	500 mL
1$\frac{1}{3}$ cups	beef stock	325 mL
1	can (19 oz/540 mL) kidney beans or pinto beans, rinsed and drained	1
	Salt and pepper	

1. In a Dutch oven or large saucepan over medium-high heat, cook beef, breaking up with a wooden spoon, for 5 minutes or until no longer pink.

2. Reduce heat to medium. Add onion, garlic, green pepper, chili powder, flour, basil, oregano and red pepper flakes; cook, stirring, for 4 minutes or until vegetables are softened. Stir in tomato sauce and stock. Bring to a boil; cook, stirring, until thickened. Add beans; season with salt and pepper to taste. Reduce heat and simmer, covered, for 10 minutes.

Pork and Beef Chili with Ancho Sauce

Dutch ovens are cast-iron pots that can be suspended above the fire or set right down into the fire on their stubby legs and surrounded by coals. More coals are piled on the lids and the ovens left to "bake" their contents, whether they be biscuits, roasts or loaves of bread.

Cooking over a campfire in a Dutch oven is not easy. Many cowboy cooks report campfire cooking disasters, from charred biscuit and scorched stews to petrified eggs, coming from these big cast-iron pots. The best advice, says one cook, is to use good hardwood to build your fire. Oak, hickory, maple or mesquite will all provide good heat-holding coals for hours of cooking, while soft woods like cedar, aspen or poplar make for poor, inconsistent heat and bitter smoke.

Serves 8

2	dried ancho chiles	2
¼ cup	olive oil	60 mL
1 lb	pork shoulder stew meat, cut into ½-inch (1 cm) cubes	500 g
1 lb	beef chuck steak, cut into ¼- to ½-inch (5 mm to 1 cm) cubes	500 g
1	large onion, chopped	1
5	cloves garlic, minced	5
4 oz	spicy Italian sausage, casings removed	125 g
1 tbsp	ground cumin	15 mL
1 tbsp	crushed hot chiles	15 mL
2	cans (each 19 oz/540 mL) tomatoes, chopped	2
¼ cup	rye whisky	60 mL
1 tbsp	dried oregano	15 mL
1½ cups	cooked black beans	375 mL
¼ cup	tomato paste	60 mL
	Salt and pepper to taste	

1. Soak ancho chiles in hot water 20 minutes or until softened; drain. Chop, discarding stems and seeds; set aside.

2. In a large Dutch oven, heat oil over medium-high heat. In several batches, cook diced pork and beef, turning often, for 4 minutes or until well-browned. With a slotted spoon, transfer to a bowl, leaving behind as much oil as possible; set aside. Reduce heat to medium-low. Add onion, garlic and sausage; cook, stirring to break up meat, for 4 minutes or until onion is softened and meat is no longer pink. Stir in ancho chiles, cumin and crushed chiles; cook for 5 minutes or until onion is tender.

3. Stir in browned pork and beef, tomatoes, whisky and oregano. Bring to a boil. Reduce heat to low and simmer, covered, for 1½ hours.

4. Stir in beans and tomato paste. Simmer 15 minutes longer to heat through. Season to taste with salt and pepper.

Tex-Mex Chili

We use good-quality finely chopped beef instead of ground beef in our basic chili and include a mixture of chiles (jalapeños and chipotles) to boost the flavor. Begin with the smaller amount of heat and adjust to suit your taste. We prefer the texture of dried beans cooked from scratch but canned beans are just fine. Serve with hot cornbread and accompany with your favorite condiments, sour cream and shredded Cheddar cheese. A chili is great party fare, especially for a horde of ravenous teenagers.

Serves 6

Tip

For convenience, replace cooked beans with 1 can (14 to 19 oz/398 to 540 mL) red kidney or black beans, rinsed and drained.

2 tbsp	vegetable oil	30 mL
2 lbs	boneless chuck beef, finely chopped	1 kg
	Salt and freshly ground black pepper	
2	onions, chopped	2
2	cloves garlic, finely chopped	2
1	jalapeño pepper, seeded and chopped	1
1 to 2 tbsp	chili powder	15 to 30 mL
1 tsp	ground cumin	5 mL
1 tsp	paprika	5 mL
1 tsp	dried oregano	5 mL
1	chipotle pepper in adobo sauce, chopped	1
1 cup	chopped fresh or canned tomatoes	250 mL
1 cup	beer	250 mL
2 cups	beef stock (approx.)	500 mL
1½ cups	cooked red kidney or black beans (see Tip, left)	375 mL

1. In a large heavy pot, heat oil over medium-high heat. Add beef and brown well on all sides. You may need to do this in batches, adding more oil if needed. Do not crowd pan. Remove from pot. Season lightly with salt and pepper and set aside.

2. Reduce heat to medium. Add onions and sauté until soft and lightly browned, 5 to 6 minutes. Add garlic, jalapeño, chili powder to taste, cumin, paprika and oregano and cook, stirring, 1 to 2 minutes.

3. Return beef to the pot with any collected juices. Stir in chipotle, tomatoes, beer and stock to cover. Bring to a simmer. Reduce heat and simmer, partially covered, stirring occasionally, until beef is tender, 1½ to 2 hours. Add beans and heat through. Taste and adjust seasoning.

Red Chili with Anchos

This robust chili is a meal in itself. Serve it with warm whole-grain rolls and an abundance of garnishes to lighten it up.

Tip

To rehydrate ancho chiles for this recipe, about 1 hour before recipe has finished cooking, in a heatproof bowl, soak dried ancho peppers in boiling water for 30 minutes, weighing down with a cup to ensure they are submerged. Drain, reserving $\frac{1}{2}$ cup (125 mL) of the soaking liquid. Discard stems and chop chiles coarsely.

Make Ahead

Complete Steps 2 and 4. Cover and refrigerate vegetable and chile mixtures separately for up to 2 days. (The chile mixture will lose some of its vibrancy if held this long. For best results, complete Step 4 while the chili is cooking.) When you're ready to cook, brown the pork and continue with the recipe. Or, if you prefer, add the unbrowned pork to the stoneware along with the vegetable

• **Large (minimum 5 quart) slow cooker**

2 tbsp	olive oil, divided	30 mL
2 lbs	trimmed pork shoulder or blade (butt), cut into 1-inch (2.5 cm) cubes, and patted dry	1 kg
2	onions, finely chopped	2
4	stalks celery, diced	4
4	cloves garlic, minced	4
1 tbsp	dried oregano leaves	15 mL
1 tbsp	ground cumin (see Tips, page 130)	15 mL
1 tsp	salt	5 mL
1 tsp	cracked black peppercorns	5 mL
1	piece (2 inches/5 cm) cinnamon stick	1
1 tbsp	cider vinegar	15 mL
1	can (28 oz/796 mL) crushed tomatoes	1
3 cups	cooked pinto beans	750 mL
2	dried ancho chiles, rehydrated (see Tip, left)	2
2	jalapeño peppers, seeded and chopped	2
$\frac{1}{2}$ cup	celery leaves or parsley	125 mL
	Sour cream or shredded Cheddar or Jack cheese	
	Shredded lettuce	
	Finely chopped red or green onion	

1. In a skillet, heat 1 tbsp (15 mL) of the oil over medium-high heat. Add pork, in batches, and cook, stirring, until browned, about 4 minutes per batch. Transfer to stoneware as completed.

2. Reduce heat to medium. Add remaining 1 tbsp (15 mL) of oil to the pan. Add onions and celery and cook, stirring, until softened, about 5 minutes. Add garlic, oregano, cumin, salt, peppercorns and cinnamon stick and cook, stirring, for 1 minute. Add vinegar and boil until evaporated, about 10 seconds. Add tomatoes and bring to a boil, scraping up brown bits from bottom of pan.

3. Transfer to stoneware. Add beans and stir well. Cover and cook on Low for 8 hours or on High for 4 hours, until meat is tender.

mixture, being aware that the result will not be as flavorful as that produced using browned meat.

4. In a blender, combine rehydrated chiles, jalapeños, celery leaves and reserved soaking liquid (see Tip, page 128). Purée.

5. Add chile mixture to stoneware and stir well. Cover and cook on High for 30 minutes, until hot and bubbly and flavors meld. Pass sour cream, shredded lettuce and chopped onion at the table and let people help themselves.

Wagon Boss Chili

This chili is served at an Alberta guest ranch where you can recall the days of the big cattle drives, complete with thousands of head of cattle and mounted cowboys, led by the wagon boss. When cowboy cooks first put meat and peppers together, the seeds of modern-day chili were sown and the West became the official domain of chili, hot sauces, searing salsas and chiliheads.

Serves 6

Tip

Substitute Romano beans or red kidney beans if you can't find pinto beans.

2 tbsp	canola oil	30 mL
2 lbs	lean round steak, cut into ½-inch (1 cm) cubes	1 kg
3	cloves garlic, minced	3
2 cups	chopped onions	500 mL
2 cups	beef broth	500 mL
2 cups	canned tomatoes with juices, chopped	500 mL
2 tbsp	chili powder	30 mL
1 tsp	dried oregano	5 mL
1 tsp	ground cumin	5 mL
½ tsp	cayenne pepper	2 mL
½ tsp	salt	2 mL
¼ tsp	freshly ground black pepper	1 mL
1	can (19 oz/540 mL) pinto beans, rinsed and drained	1
3 tbsp	cornmeal	45 mL

1. In a Dutch oven, heat oil over medium-high heat. In several batches, cook beef, turning occasionally, for 5 minutes or until well-browned. Return all beef to saucepan, along with garlic and onions; cook for 5 minutes or until onions are tender.

2. Stir in 1 cup (250 mL) water, beef broth, tomatoes, chili powder, oregano, cumin, cayenne pepper, salt and pepper. Bring to a boil, reduce heat to low and simmer, covered, for 2 hours or until meat is very tender.

3. Stir in beans and cornmeal; simmer for another 20 minutes or until mixture is heated through and thickened.

Easy Chili con Carne

Simple and classic. Chili made with ground beef is among the easiest to prepare and has a delicious homestyle flavor. Make extra because you'll enjoy the leftovers. To highlight the retro vibe, serve in Fiestaware bowls, accompanied with buttered whole-grain toast.

Serves 6 to 8

Tips

To maximize flavor, instead of using ground cumin, toast and grind whole cumin seeds yourself. Place seeds in a dry skillet over medium heat, stirring until fragrant, about 3 minutes. Using a mortar and pestle or a spice grinder, pound or grind as finely as you can.

For this quantity, use canned beans and rinse them well, or soak and cook 1 1/2 cups (375 mL) dried beans.

Make Ahead

Complete Step 1. Cover mixture, ensuring it cools promptly, and refrigerate for up to 2 days. When you're ready to cook, complete the recipe.

• **Medium to large (3 1/2 to 5 quart) slow cooker**

2 tbsp	olive oil	30 mL
1 1/2 lbs	lean ground beef	750 g
2	onions, finely chopped	2
4	stalks celery, diced	4
4	cloves garlic, minced	4
2 tbsp	ground cumin (see Tips, left)	30 mL
1 tbsp	dried oregano leaves	15 mL
1 tsp	salt	5 mL
1 tsp	cracked black peppercorns	5 mL
1 tsp	caraway seeds	5 mL
1 tbsp	packed brown sugar	15 mL
1	can (28 oz/796 mL) crushed tomatoes	1
3 cups	cooked red kidney beans, drained (see Tips, left)	750 mL
2 tbsp	Mexican chili powder	30 mL
1 tbsp	apple cider vinegar	15 mL
1 tbsp	water	15 mL
1	green bell pepper, seeded and diced	1

1. In a large skillet, heat oil over medium-high heat. Add beef, onions and celery and cook, stirring, until beef is no longer pink, about 7 minutes. Add garlic, cumin, oregano, salt, peppercorns and caraway seeds and cook, stirring, for 1 minute. Add brown sugar and tomatoes and bring to a boil.

2. Transfer to slow cooker stoneware. Add kidney beans and stir well. Cover and cook on Low for 6 to 8 hours or on High for 3 to 4 hours, until hot and bubbly.

3. In a small bowl, combine chili powder, vinegar and water. Mix until blended. Add to stoneware and stir well. Add bell pepper and stir well. Cover and cook on High about 20 minutes, until pepper is tender.

Sausage and Black Bean Chili

This nutritious family dinner is packed with flavor and ready in no time. It's delicious over hot white rice or with crusty rolls, accompanied by a crisp green salad.

Serves 4

Tips

If you prefer a less spicy version of this dish, substitute 1 green bell pepper, thinly sliced, or 1 cup (250 mL) frozen mixed bell pepper strips for the jalapeño.

Use hot or sweet Italian sausage, depending upon your preference.

1 lb	Italian sausage, removed from casings	500 g
1 cup	diced onion	250 mL
1 to 2	jalapeño peppers, finely chopped (see Tips, left)	1 to 2
1/2 tsp	salt	2 mL
	Freshly ground black pepper	
3/4 cup	tomato-based chili sauce	175 mL
2 tbsp	Dijon mustard	30 mL
1 tbsp	Worcestershire sauce	15 mL
1	can (19 oz/540 mL) black beans, drained and rinsed	1

1. In a skillet over medium heat, cook sausage, breaking up with a spoon, until lightly browned and no longer pink inside, about 5 minutes. Drain off all but 1 tbsp (15 mL) fat.

2. Add onion to pan and cook, stirring, until softened, about 3 minutes. Add jalapeño pepper, salt, and black pepper to taste. Cook, stirring, for 1 minute. Add chili sauce, Dijon mustard and Worcestershire sauce. Bring to a boil. Stir in beans.

3. Reduce heat to low and simmer until mixture is bubbling and flavors are combined, about 10 minutes. Taste and adjust seasoning.

Variations

Add 1 green bell pepper, thinly sliced, or 1 cup (250 mL) frozen mixed bell pepper strips along with the jalapeño.

Sausages: Sausages are a quick way of adding flavor to many dishes. They can speed up food preparation because the chopping, seasoning and sometimes even cooking have already been completed. Uncooked or cured, they are widely available in many different forms. Uncooked sausage cooks quickly and blends well with a wide variety of foods. Fresh uncooked sausage will keep for 3 days in the refrigerator and can be frozen for as long as 2 months.

Beer-Braised Chili

If you're tired of beef-based chilies with red beans, try this equally delicious but lighter version. It makes a great potluck dish or the centerpiece for a casual evening with friends. For a special occasion, serve with hot cornbread.

Tips

For this quantity of beans, use 2 cans (14 to 19 oz/398 to 540 mL) drained and rinsed black-eyed peas, or soak and cook 2 cups (500 mL) dried beans yourself (see pages 6 to 10 or Basic Beans in the Slow Cooker, page 277).

Many butchers sell cut-up pork stewing meat, which is fine to use in this recipe.

For best results, toast and grind the cumin and coriander seeds yourself. Place seeds in a dry skillet over medium heat, stirring until fragrant, about 3 minutes. Using a mortar and pestle or a spice grinder, pound or grind as finely as you can.

Make Ahead

Complete Step 2. Cover and refrigerate mixture for up to 2 days. When you're ready to cook, complete the recipe.

• **Large (minimum 5 quart) slow cooker**

4 cups	cooked black-eyed peas (see Tips, left)	1 L
2 tbsp	olive oil, divided	30 mL
4 oz	chunk bacon, diced	125 g
2 lbs	trimmed pork shoulder or blade (butt), cut into 1-inch (2.5 cm) cubes, and patted dry (see Tips, left)	1 kg
2	onions, finely chopped	2
4	stalks celery, diced	4
4	cloves garlic, minced	4
2 tsp	ground cumin (see Tips, left)	10 mL
2 tsp	ground coriander	10 mL
2 tsp	dried oregano leaves, crumbled	10 mL
1 tsp	salt	5 mL
1 tsp	cracked black peppercorns	5 mL
1	piece (2 inches/5 cm) cinnamon stick	1
1 cup	flat beer	250 mL
1	can (14 oz/398 mL) crushed tomatoes	1
1	each red and green bell peppers, seeded and diced	1
1 to 2	chipotle peppers in adobo sauce, minced	1 to 2
	Sour cream	
	Finely chopped red onion	
	Shredded Monterey Jack cheese	

1. In a skillet, heat 1 tbsp (15 mL) of the oil over medium-high heat. Add bacon and cook, stirring, until browned and crisp, about 4 minutes. Using a slotted spoon, transfer to slow cooker stoneware. Add pork, in batches, and cook, stirring, until browned, about 4 minutes per batch. Transfer to stoneware as completed.

2. Reduce heat to medium. Add remaining 1 tbsp (15 mL) of oil to pan. Add onions and celery and cook, stirring, until softened, about 5 minutes. Add garlic, cumin, coriander, oregano, salt, peppercorns and cinnamon and cook, stirring, for 1 minute. Add beer, bring to a boil and boil for 1 minute, scraping up brown bits. Stir in tomatoes.

3. Transfer to stoneware. Stir in peas. Cover and cook on Low for 6 hours or on High for 3 hours. Stir in bell peppers and chipotles. Cover and cook on High for about 20 minutes, until peppers are tender. Garnish with any combination of sour cream, onion and/or cheese.

Chili con Carne Pronto

Here's a tasty old-fashioned chili that is quick and easy to make. Serve with hot buttered toast. If you prefer a spicier version, add a jalapeño or chipotle pepper (see Variations, below).

Serves 4

Tip

If you have celery in your crisper, substitute 2 stalks, peeled and diced, for the celery seed. Cook with the onion and beef, until the celery is softened, about 6 minutes.

1 tbsp	vegetable oil	15 mL
1 lb	lean ground beef, thawed if frozen	500 g
1 cup	diced onion	250 mL
1 tbsp	minced garlic	15 mL
1 tbsp	chili powder	15 mL
½ tsp	celery seed (see Tip, left)	2 mL
2 cups	spicy tomato sauce, such as arrabbiata	500 mL
1	can (19 oz/540 mL) kidney beans, drained and rinsed	1

1. In a skillet, heat oil over medium-high heat. Add beef and onion and cook, breaking up meat with a spoon, until beef is no longer pink inside, about 5 minutes. Add garlic, chili powder and celery seed and cook, stirring, for 1 minute. Add tomato sauce and beans. Bring to a boil.

2. Reduce heat to low and simmer until beans are heated through and flavors are combined, about 10 minutes.

Variations

Add ½ cup (125 mL) diced bell pepper along with the garlic.

For a spicier version, add 1 finely chopped jalapeño pepper or, if you prefer a bit of smoke, 1 finely chopped chipotle pepper in adobo sauce, along with the garlic.

Celery Seed: Keep celery seed in your pantry: it is an easy way to impart a celery flavor to soups and stews. Because it has a very strong taste that some people don't like, use it cautiously, as it can easily overpower a dish, leaving an unpleasant bitterness. It is not to be confused with celery salt, which is usually a blend of ground celery seed, salt and other herbs.

Butternut Chili

This combination of beef, butternut squash, ancho chiles and cilantro is a real winner. Don't be afraid to make extra — it's great reheated.

Tips

Use 1 cup (250 mL) dried kidney beans, soaked, cooked and drained (see pages 6 to 10), or 1 can (14 to 19 oz/398 to 540 mL) canned kidney beans, drained and rinsed.

If you prefer, you can soak and purée the chiles while preparing the chili and refrigerate until you're ready to add them to the recipe.

Make Ahead

Complete Steps 1 and 3. Cover and refrigerate tomato and chile mixtures separately overnight. The next morning, continue with the recipe.

- **Large (minimum 4 quart) slow cooker**

1 tbsp	vegetable oil	15 mL
1 lb	lean ground beef	500 g
2	onions, finely chopped	2
4	cloves garlic, minced	4
1	stick cinnamon, about 2 inches (5 cm) long	1
1 tbsp	cumin seeds, toasted and ground (see Tips, page 136)	15 mL
2 tsp	dried oregano	10 mL
1 tsp	salt	5 mL
1/2 tsp	cracked black peppercorns	2 mL
1	can (28 oz/796 mL) diced tomatoes, with juice	1
3 cups	cubed butternut squash (1-inch/2.5 cm cubes)	750 mL
2 cups	cooked kidney beans (see Tips, left)	500 mL
2	dried New Mexico, ancho or guajillo chiles	2
2 cups	boiling water	500 mL
1/2 cup	coarsely chopped fresh cilantro	125 mL

1. In a skillet, heat oil over medium-high heat for 30 seconds. Add beef and onions; cook, stirring and breaking meat up with a spoon, until beef is no longer pink, about 10 minutes. Add garlic, cinnamon stick, cumin, oregano, salt and peppercorns; cook, stirring, for 1 minute. Add tomatoes with juice and bring to a boil.

2. Place squash and beans in slow cooker stoneware and cover with beef mixture. Cover and cook on Low for 6 to 8 hours or on High for 3 to 4 hours, until squash is tender.

3. About an hour before recipe has finished cooking, combine dried chiles and boiling water in a heatproof bowl. Set aside for 30 minutes, weighing down chiles with a cup to ensure they remain submerged. Drain, reserving 1/2 cup (125 mL) of the soaking liquid. Discard stems and coarsely chop chiles. Transfer to a blender and add cilantro and reserved soaking liquid; purée.

4. Add chile mixture to stoneware and stir well. Cover and cook on High for 30 minutes, until mixture is hot and bubbly and flavors meld. Discard cinnamon stick.

Greek Chili with Black Olives and Feta Cheese

Tips

Leave the skin on zucchini and eggplant for extra fiber.

Other canned beans can be used, such as chickpeas, white navy beans or black beans.

Another cheese can replace the feta, such as goat, Cheddar or mozzarella.

Great as leftovers.

Make Ahead

Prepare up to a day ahead and gently reheat, adding more stock if too thick.

1 tsp	vegetable oil	5 mL
2 tsp	minced garlic	10 mL
1 cup	chopped onions	250 mL
1 cup	chopped zucchini	250 mL
1 cup	sliced mushrooms	250 mL
1 cup	chopped green bell peppers	250 mL
1½ cups	chopped eggplant	375 mL
8 oz	lean ground beef or lamb	250 g
1 cup	canned red kidney beans, drained	250 mL
1 cup	canned white kidney beans, drained	250 mL
1	can (19 oz/540 mL) tomatoes, puréed	1
1½ cups	beef or chicken stock	375 mL
⅓ cup	sliced black olives	75 mL
1 tbsp	chili powder	15 mL
1½ tsp	dried basil	7 mL
1½ tsp	dried oregano	7 mL
2 oz	feta cheese, crumbled	60 g

1. In a large nonstick saucepan sprayed with vegetable spray, heat oil over medium heat. Add garlic, onions, zucchini, mushrooms, green peppers and eggplant; cook for 8 minutes or until softened. Add beef and cook, stirring to break up, for 2 minutes or until no longer pink. Drain any excess fat.

2. Mash ½ cup (125 mL) of the red kidney beans and ½ cup (125 mL) of the white kidney beans. Add tomatoes, stock, mashed and whole beans, olives, chili powder, basil and oregano to saucepan; bring to a boil. Reduce heat to low and simmer, covered, for 30 minutes. Sprinkle with cheese before serving.

Not-Too-Corny Turkey Chili with Sausage

Loaded with vegetables and the complex flavors of a variety of hot peppers, this yummy chili is mild enough to be enjoyed by all family members, even with the addition of a chipotle pepper in adobo sauce.

Serves 6 to 8

Tips

Use 1 cup (250 mL) dried pinto beans, soaked, cooked and drained (see pages 6 to 10 or Basic Beans in the Slow Cooker, page 277) or 1 can (14 to 19 oz/ 398 to 540 mL) pinto beans, drained and rinsed.

Toasting the cumin seeds intensifies their flavor. Stir the seeds in a dry skillet over medium heat until fragrant, about 3 minutes. Transfer to a mortar or spice grinder and grind.

Make Ahead

Complete Steps 1 and 3. Cover and refrigerate tomato and chile mixtures (see Tips, page 144) separately for up to 2 days. When you're ready to cook, continue with the recipe.

- **Large (minimum 4 quart) slow cooker**

1 tbsp	oil	15 mL
1 lb	mild Italian sausage, removed from casings	500 g
4	stalks celery, diced	4
2	onions, finely chopped	2
6	cloves garlic, minced	6
1 tbsp	cumin seeds, toasted and ground (see Tips, left)	15 mL
1 tbsp	dried oregano	15 mL
1 tsp	salt	5 mL
1	can (28 oz/796 mL) diced tomatoes, with juice	1
1 lb	boneless skinless turkey, cut into ½-inch (1 cm) cubes	500 g
2 cups	cooked pinto beans (see Tips, left)	500 mL
2	dried ancho, guajillo or New Mexico chiles	2
2 cups	boiling water	500 mL
1 cup	coarsely chopped fresh cilantro	250 mL
½ cup	chicken broth	125 mL
2 tsp	chili powder	10 mL
1	chipotle chile in adobo sauce (optional)	1
1	red bell pepper, diced	1
2 cups	corn kernels, thawed if frozen	500 mL

1. In a skillet, heat oil over medium heat for 30 seconds. Add sausage, celery and onions; cook, stirring and breaking meat up with a spoon, until sausage is no longer pink, about 10 minutes. Add garlic, cumin, oregano and salt; cook, stirring, for 1 minute. Add tomatoes with juice and bring to a boil. Transfer to slow cooker stoneware.

2. Stir in turkey and beans. Cover and cook on Low for 6 hours or on High for 3 hours, until turkey is no longer pink inside.

3. About an hour before recipe has finished cooking, combine dried chiles and boiling water in a heatproof bowl. Set aside for 30 minutes, weighing chiles down with a cup to ensure they remain submerged. Drain, discarding soaking liquid and stems, and coarsely chop chiles. Transfer to a blender and add cilantro, broth, chili powder and chipotle pepper (if using); purée.

4. Add chile mixture to stoneware, along with red pepper and corn, and stir well. Cover and cook on High for 30 minutes, until pepper is tender and flavors meld.

Lime-Spiked Turkey Chili with Pinto Beans

Surprisingly light, with a mild hit of hot pepper, this chili is a universal favorite. Serve it with buttered whole wheat toast.

Tips

If you are halving this recipe, be sure to use a small (2 to 3 quart) slow cooker.

For best results, toast and grind the cumin yourself. Place seeds in a dry skillet over medium heat and cook, stirring, until fragrant, about 3 minutes. Using a mortar and pestle or a spice grinder, pound or grind as finely as you can.

Make Ahead

Complete Step 1. Cover and refrigerate mixture for up to 2 days. When you're ready to cook, complete the recipe.

- **Medium to large (3½ to 5 quart) slow cooker**

2 tbsp	olive oil	30 mL
1 lb	ground turkey	500 g
2	onions, finely chopped	2
4	stalks celery, diced	4
4	cloves garlic, minced	4
1 tbsp	ground cumin (see Tips, left)	15 mL
1 tbsp	dried oregano leaves	15 mL
2 tsp	grated lime zest	10 mL
1 tsp	dried thyme leaves	5 mL
1 tsp	ground allspice	5 mL
1 tsp	salt	5 mL
1 tsp	cracked black peppercorns	5 mL
1	piece (2 inches/5 cm) cinnamon stick	1
1	can (5½ oz/156 mL) tomato paste	
2 tsp	brown sugar	10 mL
2 cups	chicken or turkey stock	500 mL
3 cups	cooked pinto beans	750 mL
½ tsp	cayenne pepper, dissolved in 2 tbsp (30 mL) freshly squeezed lime juice	2 mL
1	can (4½ oz/127 mL) minced mild green chiles	1
	Finely chopped cilantro, optional	
	Shredded lettuce, optional	
	Finely chopped red or green onion, optional	
	Shredded Cheddar or Jack cheese, optional	
	Sour cream, optional	

1. In a skillet, heat oil over medium heat. Add turkey, onions and celery and cook until turkey is no longer pink and vegetables are soft, about 7 minutes. Add garlic, cumin, oregano, lime zest, thyme, allspice, salt, peppercorns and cinnamon stick and cook, stirring, for 1 minute. Stir in tomato paste and brown sugar. Add stock and bring to a boil.

2. Transfer to stoneware. Stir in beans. Cover and cook on Low for 6 hours or on High for 3 hours. Stir in cayenne solution and chiles. Cover and cook on High for 10 minutes. Serve garnished with any one or a combination of cilantro, lettuce, onion, cheese or sour cream.

Variation

Lime-Spiked Chicken Chili with Pinto Beans: Substitute an equal quantity of ground chicken for the turkey.

Chicken and Black Bean Chili

Serve this tasty chili, which is lighter than one made with beef, with hot crusty bread and a steamed green vegetable.

Serves 4

1 tbsp	vegetable oil	15 mL
1 lb	skinless boneless chicken breasts, cut into $1/2$-inch (1 cm) cubes	500 g
1 tbsp	minced garlic	15 mL
1 tbsp	chili powder	15 mL
1 tsp	cumin seeds, crushed	5 mL
$1^1/_2$ cups	spicy tomato sauce, such as arrabbiata	375 mL
1	can (19 oz/540 mL) black beans, drained and rinsed	1
1 tbsp	lemon or lime juice	15 mL

1. In a skillet, heat oil over medium heat. Add chicken and cook, stirring, until it begins to brown and is no longer pink inside, about 3 minutes. Add garlic, chili powder and cumin seeds and cook, stirring, for 1 minute.

2. Add tomato sauce, beans and lemon juice. Stir to combine. Reduce heat to low and simmer for 10 minutes to allow flavors to combine.

Variation

Chicken, Sausage and Black Bean Chili: Stir in 4 oz (125 g) kielbasa, cut into $1/2$-inch (1 cm) slices and quartered, along with the tomato sauce.

Two-Bean Turkey Chili

This tasty chili, which has just a hint of heat, is perfect for family get-togethers. Add a tossed green salad, sprinkled with shredded carrots, and whole-grain rolls.

Tips

You'll need about 3 cups (750 mL) cubed turkey breast to make this chili.

You can also use leftover turkey. Use 3 cups (750 mL) shredded cooked turkey and add along with the bell peppers.

Add the jalapeño pepper if you're a heat seeker; add the chipotle in adobo sauce if you like a hint of smoke as well.

Toasting the cumin seeds intensifies their flavor. Stir the seeds in a dry skillet over medium heat until fragrant, about 3 minutes. Transfer to a mortar or spice grinder and grind.

Make Ahead

Complete Step 1. Cover and refrigerate for up to 2 days. When you're ready to cook, continue with the recipe.

• **Large (minimum 4 quart) slow cooker**

1 tbsp	olive oil	15 mL
4	stalks celery, diced	4
2	onions, finely chopped	2
6	cloves garlic, minced	6
1 tbsp	cumin seeds, toasted and ground (see Tips)	15 mL
2 tsp	dried oregano	10 mL
1/2 tsp	cracked black pepper	2 mL
	Zest of 1 lime	
2 tbsp	fine cornmeal	30 mL
1 cup	chicken or turkey stock	250 mL
1	can (28 oz/796 mL) tomatoes, with juice, coarsely chopped	1
2 lbs	skinless boneless turkey breast, cut into 1/2-inch (1 cm) cubes	1 kg
2	cans (each 14 to 19 oz/398 to 540 mL) pinto beans, drained and rinsed	2
2 cups	frozen sliced green beans	500 mL
1 tbsp	New Mexico or ancho chili powder, dissolved in 2 tbsp (30 mL) lime juice	15 mL
1	green bell pepper, diced	1
1	red bell pepper, diced	1
1	can (4 1/2 oz/127 mL) diced mild green chiles	1
1	jalapeño pepper or chipotle pepper in adobo sauce, diced (optional)	1

1. In a skillet, heat oil over medium heat for 30 seconds. Add celery and onions; cook, stirring, until celery is softened, about 5 minutes. Add garlic and cook, stirring, for 1 minute. Add cumin, oregano, pepper and lime zest; cook, stirring, for 1 minute. Add cornmeal and toss to coat. Add stock and cook, stirring, until mixture boils, about 1 minute. Add tomatoes with juice and return to a boil. Transfer to slow cooker stoneware.

2. Stir in turkey, pinto beans and green beans. Cover and cook on Low for 8 hours or on High for 4 hours, until turkey is tender and mixture is bubbly. Add chili powder solution, green and red peppers, mild green chiles and jalapeño (if using). Cover and cook on High for 30 minutes, until bell peppers are tender.

Vegetarian Chili

This recipe comes from a café in Calgary called The Breadline. It's easy to make and chock full of healthy vegetables. Although you probably won't find many vegetarian cowboys, this is a very tasty chili, very low in fat, and excellent as a meatless dinner or side dish.

Serves 6 to 8

Vegan Friendly

1/3 cup	olive oil	75 mL
1 lb	zucchini, cut into 1/2-inch (1 cm) dice	500 g
1 lb	onions, cut into 1/2-inch (1 cm) dice	500 g
4	cloves garlic, minced	4
1	large red bell pepper, chopped	1
2	cans (each 28 oz/796 mL) tomatoes, crushed	2
1 1/2 lbs	cubed ripe tomatoes (about 4 cups/ 1 L, chopped)	750 g
4 tsp	chili powder	20 mL
1 tbsp	ground cumin	15 mL
1 tbsp	dried basil	15 mL
1 tbsp	dried oregano	15 mL
1 1/2 tsp	freshly ground pepper	7 mL
1 tsp	salt	5 mL
1 tsp	fennel seed	5 mL
2 tbsp	chopped fresh parsley	30 mL
1	can (19 oz/540 mL) red kidney beans, rinsed and drained	1
1	can (14 oz/398 mL) chickpeas, rinsed and drained	1
1 tbsp	chopped fresh dill	15 mL
1 tbsp	lemon juice	15 mL
3/4 tsp	granulated sugar	3 mL

1. In a large saucepan, heat olive oil over medium-high heat. Add zucchini, onions, garlic and bell pepper; cook, stirring often, for 8 minutes or until starting to soften. Stir in canned and fresh tomatoes, chili powder, cumin, basil, oregano, pepper, salt, fennel seed and parsley; bring to a boil. Reduce heat to medium and simmer, uncovered and stirring often, for 30 minutes.

2. Stir in kidney beans, chickpeas, dill, lemon juice and sugar; cook for 15 minutes.

Hominy and Red Bean Chili

This tasty chili is brimming with flavorful vegetables. For a change, try finishing with Avocado Topping (see Tips, below) instead of the usual fixings.

Serves 6 to 8

Vegan Friendly

Tips

Use any red bean such as small red Mexican beans, kidney beans or even pink pinto beans in this recipe.

You can also use 1 cup (250 mL) dried red beans, soaked, cooked and drained (see pages 6 to 10 or Basic Beans in the Slow Cooker, page 277), instead of the canned beans.

To make Avocado Topping: In a bowl, combine 2 tbsp (30 mL) each finely chopped green onion and cilantro. Add 1 tbsp (15 mL) lime juice and 1 avocado, chopped into ½-inch (1 cm) cubes. Toss to combine. This topping makes a nice finish for many chilies.

For convenience, use frozen diced squash in this recipe.

• **Large (approx. 5 quart) slow cooker**

2 tsp	cumin seeds	10 mL
4	whole allspice	4
1 tbsp	vegetable oil	15 mL
2	onions, finely chopped	2
2	carrots, peeled and chopped	2
4	cloves garlic, minced	4
1 tsp	chili powder	5 mL
1 tsp	dried oregano leaves	5 mL
1	can (28 oz/796 mL) tomatoes, including juice, coarsely chopped	1
1 cup	vegetable stock	250 mL
1	can (14 to 19 oz/398 to 540 mL) red kidney beans, drained and rinsed (see Tips, left)	1
1	can (15 oz/475 mL) hominy, drained and rinsed	1
2 cups	cubed (½ inch/1 cm) peeled celery root	500 mL
2 cups	diced yellow squash (see Tips, left)	500 mL
1 to 2	chipotle chiles in adobo sauce, finely chopped	1 to 2
	Shredded lettuce (optional)	
	Finely chopped green onion (optional)	
	Finely chopped cilantro	
	Sour cream (optional)	

1. In a large dry skillet, toast cumin seeds and allspice, stirring, until they release their aroma. Transfer to a spice grinder or mortar, or use the bottom of a measuring cup or wine bottle, to coarsely grind. Set aside.

2. In same skillet, heat oil over medium heat. Add onions and carrots and cook, stirring, until carrots are softened, about 7 minutes. Add garlic, chili powder, oregano and reserved cumin and allspice and cook, stirring, for 1 minute. Add tomatoes with juice and vegetable stock and bring to a boil. Transfer to slow cooker stoneware. Add beans, hominy, celery root and squash and stir to combine.

Make Ahead

This dish can be assembled before it is cooked, without adding the chipotle chiles. Complete Steps 1 and 2. Cover and refrigerate. When you are ready to cook, continue with Step 3.

3. Cover and cook on Low for 8 hours or on High for 4 hours, until vegetables are tender. Stir in chipotle chiles. Cover and cook on High for 15 minutes, to blend flavors. Ladle into bowls and garnish with shredded lettuce and green onion, if using, and cilantro. Top each serving with a dollop of sour cream, if using.

Variation

Hominy and Chickpea Chili: Substitute an equal quantity of chickpeas for the beans.

Very Veggie Chili

Here's a tasty vegetarian chili that uses chili powder and tomato sauce spiked with hot peppers to quickly achieve an authentic chili flavor. If made with frozen diced butternut squash (see Variation below), the zucchini chopping is eliminated and the result is even speedier. Serve this the old-fashioned way — with toast — and top with a dollop of sour cream, if desired.

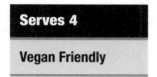

Serves 4

Vegan Friendly

1 tbsp	vegetable oil	15 mL
1 cup	diced onion	250 mL
2	medium zucchini, cut into $\frac{1}{2}$-inch (1 cm) cubes (about 1 lb/500 g)	2
1 tbsp	minced garlic	15 mL
1 tbsp	chili powder	15 mL
1	can (12 oz/341 mL) corn kernels, drained, or $1\frac{1}{2}$ cups (375 mL) frozen corn kernels, thawed	1
1	can (19 oz/540 mL) red kidney beans, drained and rinsed	1
2 cups	spicy tomato sauce, such as arrabbiata	500 mL
	Sour cream (optional)	

1. In a skillet, heat oil over medium heat. Add onion and zucchini and cook, stirring occasionally, until zucchini is tender, about 8 minutes. Add garlic and chili powder and cook, stirring, for 1 minute.

2. Add corn, kidney beans and tomato sauce. Bring to a boil. Reduce heat to low and simmer for 10 minutes to combine flavors. Ladle into bowls and top with sour cream, if desired.

Variation

Squash and Black Bean Chili: Substitute 3 cups (750 mL) diced butternut squash for the zucchini and 1 can (19 oz/540 mL) black beans for the kidney beans.

Easy Vegetable Chili

Not only is this chili easy to make, it is also delicious. The mild dried chiles add interesting flavor, along with a nice bit of heat. Add the jalapeño only if you're a heat seeker.

Serves 4 to 6

Vegan Friendly

Tips

Use 1 cup (250 mL) dried red kidney beans, soaked, cooked and drained (see pages 6 to 10 or Basic Beans in the Slow Cooker, page 277) or 1 can (14 to 19 oz/ 398 to 540 mL) red kidney beans, drained and rinsed.

Be aware that if you make the chili mixture (Step 3) ahead of time it will lose some of its vibrancy. For best results, complete Step 3 while the chili is cooking or no sooner than the night before you plan to cook.

Make Ahead

Complete Steps 1 and 3. Cover and refrigerate tomato and chile mixtures separately for up to 2 days. When you're ready to cook, continue with the recipe.

• **Large (minimum 4 quart) slow cooker**

1 tbsp	oil	15 mL
4	stalks celery, diced	4
2	onions, chopped	2
4	cloves garlic, minced	4
2 tsp	cumin seeds, toasted and ground (see Tips, page 145)	10 mL
2 tsp	dried oregano	10 mL
1 tsp	salt	5 mL
1	can (14 oz/398 mL) diced tomatoes, with juice	1
2 cups	cooked red kidney beans (see Tips, left)	500 mL
2	dried New Mexico, ancho or guajillo chiles	2
2 cups	boiling water	500 mL
1 cup	coarsely chopped fresh cilantro	250 mL
1 cup	vegetable broth, tomato juice or water	250 mL
1	jalapeño pepper, coarsely chopped (optional)	1
1	green bell pepper, chopped	1
2 cups	corn kernels, thawed if frozen	500 mL

1. In a skillet, heat oil over medium heat for 30 seconds. Add celery and onions; cook, stirring, until celery is softened, about 5 minutes. Add garlic, cumin, oregano and salt; cook, stirring, for 1 minute. Add tomatoes with juice and bring to a boil. Transfer to slow cooker stoneware.

2. Stir in beans. Cover and cook on Low for 6 to 8 hours or on High for 3 to 4 hours, until hot and bubbly.

3. About an hour before recipe has finished cooking, combine dried chiles and boiling water in a heatproof bowl. Set aside for 30 minutes, weighing chiles down with a cup to ensure they remain submerged. Drain, discarding soaking liquid and stems, and coarsely chop chiles. Transfer to a blender and add cilantro, broth and jalapeño (if using); purée.

4. Add chile mixture to stoneware, along with green pepper and corn, and stir well. Cover and cook on High for 20 minutes, until pepper is tender and mixture is hot and bubbly.

Black Bean Chili with Hominy and Sweet Corn

This is a particularly thick and luscious chili, rich with the goodness of corn. It doesn't need much more than a simple green salad and perhaps some whole-grain bread to complete the meal.

Tips

For best results, toast and grind the cumin yourself. Place seeds in a dry skillet over medium heat and cook, stirring, until fragrant, about 3 minutes. Using a mortar and pestle or a clean spice grinder, pound or grind as finely as you can.

For this quantity of black beans, use 2 cans (14 to 19 oz/ 398 to 540 mL), drained and rinsed, and set excess aside for another use, or soak and cook 1½ cups (375 mL) dried black beans (see pages 6 to 10 or Basic Beans in the Slow Cooker, page 277).

Make Ahead

Complete Step 1. Cover and refrigerate mixture for up to 2 days. When you're ready to cook, complete the recipe.

• **Large (approx. 5 quart) slow cooker**

1 tbsp	olive oil	15 mL
2	onions, finely chopped	2
4	stalks celery, diced	4
2	carrots, peeled and diced	2
4	cloves garlic, minced	4
1 tbsp	ground cumin (see Tips, left)	15 mL
2 tsp	dried oregano leaves	10 mL
1 tsp	salt	5 mL
1 tsp	cracked black peppercorns	5 mL
1	can (28 oz/796 mL) crushed tomatoes	1
3 cups	cooked black beans (see Tips, left)	750 mL
1	can (14 oz/398 mL) hominy, drained	1
1 to 2 tbsp	ancho or New Mexico chili powder	15 to 30 mL
1 cup	corn kernels	250 mL
1 to 2	jalapeño peppers, seeded and diced	1 to 2

1. In a skillet, heat oil over medium heat. Add onions, celery and carrots and cook, stirring, until softened, about 7 minutes. Add garlic, cumin, oregano, salt and peppercorns and cook, stirring, for 1 minute. Stir in tomatoes and bring to a boil.

2. Transfer to slow cooker stoneware. Add beans and hominy and stir well. Cover and cook on Low for 6 hours or on High for 3 hours, until hot and bubbly. Add ancho chili powder and stir well. Stir in corn and jalapeño to taste. Cover and cook on High for 20 minutes, until corn is tender.

Amaranth Chili

Amaranth is the only grain known to provide the human system with the most effective balance of protein; it is matched only by milk.

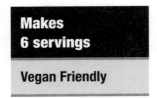

**Makes
6 servings**

Vegan Friendly

¼ cup	amaranth grains, thoroughly rinsed	60 mL
4	tomatoes, peeled and coarsely chopped	4
½ cup	chopped onion	125 mL
½ cup	chopped green bell pepper	125 mL
2	cloves garlic, minced	2
2 cups	vegetable stock	500 mL
1 cup	dried green or red lentils	250 mL
1	potato, peeled and coarsely chopped	1
1 cup	chopped carrot	250 mL
2 cups	cooked chickpeas or 1 can (19 oz/540 mL) chickpeas, drained and rinsed	500 mL
2 tbsp	chili powder	30 mL
2 tsp	ground cumin	10 mL
1 tsp	salt	5 mL

1. In a skillet, toast amaranth over medium-high heat, stirring constantly for about 10 or 15 seconds, until the seeds pop. Transfer to a small bowl and set aside.

2. In a large saucepan, combine tomatoes, onion, bell pepper and garlic. Simmer over medium heat for 5 minutes. Add stock. Increase heat to high and bring to a boil. Add lentils. Cover, reduce heat to low and simmer gently for 15 minutes, until lentils are tender.

3. Add amaranth, potato and carrot. Reduce heat and simmer for 15 minutes or until tender. Stir in chickpeas, chili powder, cumin and salt. Cook for 1 minute or until chickpeas are heated through. Serve immediately.

Variation

Use ¼ cup (60 mL) couscous instead of amaranth grains.

Black Bean Chili

Tips

Serve this robust chili over baked sweet or regular potatoes for a main dish or with whole-grain nachos for an appetizer or party dish.

Because many of the water-soluble nutrients are in the canning liquid, try to use both the beans and the liquid from the tin. When cooking fresh beans, however, do not use the cooking liquid.

2 tbsp	olive oil	30 mL
1 cup	chopped onions	250 mL
3	cloves garlic, minced	3
1½ cups	chopped red bell peppers	375 mL
2	whole chiles, crushed	2
2 tsp	ground cumin	10 mL
1	can (28 oz/796 mL) tomatoes with juice	1
1	can (19 oz/540 mL) black beans, with liquid	1
1	can (19 oz/540 mL) chickpeas, with liquid	1
2 tbsp	dried thyme leaves	30 mL
1 tbsp	dried savory leaves	15 mL
2 tbsp	fresh chopped parsley	30 mL

1. In a large skillet, heat oil over medium heat. Add onions, garlic, peppers and chiles; cook for 5 minutes or until soft.
2. Stir in cumin, tomatoes, black beans, chickpeas, thyme and savory. Bring to a boil; simmer for 5 minutes. Stir in parsley and serve.

Variations

Substitute 2 cups (500 mL) of any cooked beans.

Bean and Sweet Potato Chili on Garlic Polenta

Tip

Use any cooked beans that you have on hand.

Try fresh fennel instead of leeks.

Polenta is delicious, nutritious and takes minutes to make.

This dish is a great source of fiber.

Make Ahead

Prepare chili up to 2 days in advance. Cook polenta just before serving.

Chili

2 tsp	vegetable oil	10 mL
1½ tsp	minced garlic	7 mL
1½ cups	chopped leeks	375 mL
1 cup	chopped red bell peppers	250 mL
1	can (19 oz/540 mL) tomatoes, puréed	1
1½ cups	canned red kidney beans, rinsed and drained	375 mL
1¼ cups	chopped peeled sweet potatoes	300 mL
1 tbsp	fennel seeds	15 mL
2 tsp	chili powder	10 mL
1 tsp	dried basil	5 mL

Polenta

3¼ cups	vegetable stock	800 mL
1 cup	cornmeal	250 mL
1 tsp	minced garlic	5 mL

1. In a large nonstick saucepan, heat oil over medium-high heat. Add garlic, leeks and red peppers; cook 4 minutes or until softened. Stir in tomatoes, beans, sweet potatoes, fennel seeds, chili powder and basil; bring to a boil. Reduce heat to medium-low and cook, covered, for 20 to 25 minutes or until sweet potatoes are tender.

2. Meanwhile, in a deep saucepan, bring vegetable stock to a boil. Reduce heat to low and gradually whisk in cornmeal and garlic. Cook 5 minutes, stirring frequently.

3. Pour polenta into a serving dish. Spoon chili over top. Serve immediately.

Curry and Dal

Caribbean Curried Beef and
    Chickpeas 150

Thai Red Curry Tofu with
    Sweet Mango and Basil. 151

Lamb with Lentils. 152

Chicken Curry Baked with Lentils 153

Parsi Chicken Stew with Lentils and
    Vegetables 154

Thai Dry Vegetable Curry 156

Paneer with Chickpeas in
    Creamy Tomato Curry 157

Tofu and Snow Peas in Tamarind
    Ginger Curry. 158

Saffron Curry Mushrooms and Tofu 159

Pyaza Paneer and Navy Bean Curry. . . . 160

Caribbean Chickpea Curry
    with Potatoes 161

Caribbean Red Bean, Spinach
    and Potato Curry. 162

Curried Couscous with Tomatoes
    and Chickpeas 163

Tofu with Lime, Lemongrass and
    Coconut Curry 164

Punjabi Creamy Yellow Mung Beans . . . 165

Split Yellow Peas with Zucchini 166

Rajasthani Mixed Dal 167

Red Lentil Curry with Coconut
    and Cilantro 168

Bengali Red Lentils 169

Andhra Yellow Lentils with Tomatoes . . . 170

Brown Lentils with Peanuts. 171

Tomato Dal with Spinach 172

Caribbean Curried Beef and Chickpeas

This is a beef version of the famous Jamaican goat curry, just as meaty and zesty as its cousin and further fortified with the goodness and substance of chickpeas. It simmers for a long time, more or less unattended, while you perform other kitchen duties, filling the air with its aromatic promise.

Serves 8

Tips

Half of a Scotch bonnet pepper will give a pleasant but detectable heat. A whole one will provide a definite kick.

Garam masala from Guyana is a blend of roasted spices. If you have unroasted garam masala, toast in a dry small skillet over medium heat, stirring constantly, until the color darkens and spices smell toasted, about 2 minutes.

Reduced-sodium stock is best for this recipe. If using regular stock, use 1 cup (250 mL) stock and ½ cup (125 mL) water.

2 lbs	boneless beef for stew, cut into 1-inch (2.5 cm) pieces	1 kg
1	onion, finely chopped	1
½ to 1	Scotch bonnet pepper, minced	½ to 1
3 tbsp	curry powder, preferably Caribbean-style, divided	45 mL
2 tbsp	freshly squeezed lime juice	30 mL
2 tbsp	vegetable oil	30 mL
3	cloves garlic, minced	3
1 tbsp	minced gingerroot	15 mL
1 tbsp	garam masala, preferably Guyanese-style	15 mL
1	large ripe tomato, chopped	1
1½ cups	beef stock	375 mL
2	cans (14 to 19 oz/398 to 540 mL) chickpeas, drained and rinsed	2
2 tsp	chopped fresh thyme	10 mL
	Salt	
4	green onions, sliced	4

1. In a large bowl, combine beef, onion, Scotch bonnet pepper, 2 tbsp (30 mL) of the curry powder and the lime juice. Toss to coat evenly. Cover and marinate at room temperature for 30 minutes or refrigerate overnight.

2. In a large pot, heat oil over medium-high heat. Add remaining curry powder, garlic, ginger and garam masala; cook, stirring, until softened and fragrant, about 30 seconds. Add beef mixture with marinade and stir until coated with spices and beef starts to turn white, about 2 minutes.

3. Stir in tomato and stock; bring to a simmer. Reduce heat to medium-low, cover and simmer, stirring occasionally, for 45 minutes. Stir in chickpeas and simmer, covered, until beef is fork-tender, 45 to 60 minutes.

4. Stir in thyme. Increase heat to medium and simmer, uncovered, until sauce is slightly thickened, about 10 minutes. Season to taste with salt and serve sprinkled with green onions.

Thai Red Curry Tofu with Sweet Mango and Basil

Mango and tofu combine their charms in this Thai-inspired recipe. The sauce complements them without overpowering. It would make a lovely introduction to curry for uninitiated palates.

Serves 4

Vegan Friendly

Tip

This is flavorful and spicy, but not fiery hot. For more heat and spice, increase the curry paste to 4 tsp (20 mL).

1 tbsp	vegetable oil	15 mL
1	onion, sliced lengthwise	1
1	red bell pepper, thinly sliced	1
2 tbsp	minced gingerroot	30 mL
1/2 tsp	salt	2 mL
1 tbsp	Thai red curry paste	15 mL
12 oz	extra-firm or firm tofu, drained and cut into 1/2-inch (1 cm) cubes	375 g
2 tsp	packed brown or palm sugar	10 mL
1 cup	coconut milk	250 mL
3/4 cup	water	175 mL
1	firm ripe sweet mango, peeled and sliced	1
2 tbsp	freshly squeezed lime juice	30 mL
1/4 cup	shredded fresh Thai or sweet basil	60 mL

1. In a large skillet, heat oil over medium heat. Add onion and cook, stirring, until softened and starting to turn golden, about 3 minutes. Stir in red pepper, ginger salt and curry paste; cook, stirring, until spices are fragrant, about 1 minute.

2. Stir in tofu until coated with spices. Stir in brown sugar, coconut milk and water; bring to a simmer, scraping up bits stuck to pan. Reduce heat and simmer, stirring occasionally, until tofu is flavorful and sauce is slightly thickened, about 10 minutes.

3. Stir in mango. Increase heat to medium and cook, stirring gently, just until starting to soften, about 3 minutes. Stir in lime juice and season to taste with salt. Serve sprinkled with basil.

Masoor ma Gosht

Lamb with Lentils

This substantial dish is a classic of the Parsi community and is both delicious and nutritious. Rice and a vegetable side dish or salad complete the meal.

Serves 8

Tip

Sambhar powder is a South Indian blend used extensively in southern food. Its laundry list of ingredients includes fenugreek, peppercorns, red chiles, coriander, cumin, mustard seeds, tumeric, curry leaves and asafetida, among others. There are several good brands on the market that will remain fresh for one year if stored tightly closed and refrigerated.

1½ cups	brown lentils (sabat masoor)	375 mL
2 tbsp	oil	30 mL
5 cups	thinly sliced onions (lengthwise slices)	1.25 L
2 tbsp	minced garlic	30 mL
1½ tbsp	sambhar powder (see Tip, left) or garam masala	22 mL
1 tbsp	cumin seeds	15 mL
1 tbsp	coriander seeds	15 mL
1 tsp	cayenne pepper	5 mL
1 tsp	turmeric	5 mL
3 to 4 tbsp	freshly squeezed lime or lemon juice	45 to 60 mL
1 lb	boneless lamb, preferably leg or shoulder, cut into 1½-inch (4 cm) cubes	500 g
1 cup	cilantro, chopped	250 mL
3 cups	chopped tomatoes	750 mL
1½ tbsp	minced green chiles, preferably serranos	22 mL
2 tsp	salt or to taste	10 mL

1. Clean and pick through lentils for any small stones and grit. Rinse several times in cold water. Soak in 6 cups (1.5 L) water in a bowl at room temperature for 1 hour.

2. In a large saucepan, heat oil over medium-high heat. Add onions and garlic and sauté until golden brown, 10 to 12 minutes.

3. Add sambhar powder, cumin, coriander, cayenne, turmeric and lime juice. Reduce heat to medium-low and sauté for 4 minutes.

4. Increase heat to medium. Add lamb and cook until meat is brown, 10 to 15 minutes.

5. Drain lentils and add to meat. Add cilantro, tomatoes, chiles and salt. Add 2 cups (500 mL) water and mix well. Bring to a boil. Cover, reduce heat and simmer, stirring periodically, until meat is tender and lentils are cooked, 45 minutes to 1 hour. If mixture becomes too dry, add additional hot water to make a thick, creamy consistency.

Chicken Curry Baked with Lentils

Serves 4 to 6

- **Preheat oven to 375°F (190°C)**
- **10-cup (2.5 L) casserole dish**

2 lbs	boneless skinless chicken thighs, cut into bite-size pieces	1 kg
	Salt and freshly ground black pepper	
¼ cup	vegetable oil, divided	60 mL
2 tsp	black mustard seeds	10 mL
1½ cups	finely chopped onions	375 mL
2	cloves garlic, minced	2
1 tbsp	finely chopped gingerroot	15 mL
1 cup	dried lentils	250 mL
2 tsp	ground coriander	10 mL
2 tsp	curry powder	10 mL
Pinch	hot pepper flakes	Pinch
3 cups	chicken broth	750 mL
¾ cup	plain yogurt (not non-fat)	175 mL
2 tbsp	finely chopped fresh cilantro	30 mL

1. Season chicken with salt and pepper, to taste. In a large, deep skillet, heat half the oil over medium-high heat. Sauté chicken until browned on all sides; using a slotted spoon, remove to a plate.

2. Add the remaining oil to the pan. Sauté mustard seeds until they turn gray. Add onions and sauté until translucent. Add garlic and ginger; sauté for 1 minute. Stir in lentils, coriander, curry powder and hot pepper flakes. Add broth and bring to a boil.

3. Remove from heat and stir in chicken. Transfer to casserole dish and bake for 45 minutes, until heated through.

4. Meanwhile, combine yogurt and cilantro; serve with the casserole.

Variation

Indian Lamb and Rice: Follow preceding recipe, but substitute boneless leg of lamb for the chicken, 1½ cups (375 mL) long-grain white rice for the lentils, and beef broth for the chicken broth. Add 1 tbsp (15 mL) tomato paste with the broth. Serves 6.

Dhansak

Parsi Chicken Stew with Lentils and Vegetables

This is the signature dish of the Parsi community and is served with Parsi brown rice (dhansak na Chawal), Parsi meatballs (dhansak na kabab) and kachumbar, a fresh salad of tomatoes, cucumber and cilantro. It is somewhat laborious to make, but well worth the effort.

Serves 6 to 8

Tip

Dhansak is best served the next day. It can be frozen in an airtight container for up to 6 months. Reheat over low heat.

1/3 cup	red lentils (masoor dal)	75 mL
1/3 cup	yellow mung beans (yellow mung dal)	75 mL
1/4 cup	yellow lentils (toor dal)	60 mL
2 tbsp	Indian split white beans (val dal), optional	30 mL
12	bone-in skinless chicken thighs, rinsed (3 to 4 lbs/1.5 to 2 kg)	12
1 1/2 cups	chopped butternut squash	375 mL
1 1/2 cups	chopped eggplant	375 mL
1/4 cup	dried fenugreek leaves (kasuri methi)	60 mL
1 cup	chopped onion	250 mL
1	carrot, peeled and chopped	1
2 tsp	salt or to taste	10 mL
6 to 8	dried Indian red chiles	6 to 8
1/2 tsp	toasted coriander seeds	2 mL
1/2 tsp	toasted cumin seeds	2 mL
1	piece (1 inch/2.5 cm) cinnamon	1
6	whole cloves	6
6	black peppercorns	6
1 tbsp	sambhar powder (see Tip, page 152)	15 mL
1/2 tsp	turmeric	2 mL
1	cube (1 inch/2.5 cm) peeled gingerroot	1
8	cloves garlic	8
3 tbsp	oil	45 mL
3 cups	thinly sliced onions (lengthwise slices)	750 mL
3 cups	chopped tomatoes	750 mL
1 tbsp	jaggery (gur)	15 mL
3 tbsp	cilantro, chopped	45 mL
	Lemon wedges	

1. Clean and pick through masoor, mung, toor and val dals for any small stones and grit. Rinse several times in cold water until water is fairly clear. Add water to cover by 3 inches (7.5 cm) and soak at room temperature for 1 hour.

2. Drain dal. In a large pot, combine dal, chicken, squash, eggplant, fenugreek, onion, carrot, salt and 3 cups (750 mL) water. Bring to a boil over high heat. Reduce heat to medium-low and boil gently, partially covered, until vegetables are soft and mushy, about 45 minutes. Remove chicken and set aside.

3. Meanwhile, in a spice grinder, grind together red chiles, coriander, cumin, cinnamon, cloves, peppercorns, sambhar powder and turmeric to a powder.

4. In a blender, purée ginger, garlic, spice powder and 1/4 cup (60 mL) water to a smooth paste. Transfer to a bowl. In the same blender, purée dal mixture in 2 batches. Transfer to a separate bowl.

5. In a large saucepan, heat oil over medium-high heat. Add onions and sauté until dark brown, about 10 minutes. Reduce heat to medium. Add spice paste and sauté, stirring constantly, until mixture darkens and is aromatic, about 5 minutes. (Deglaze pan with 1 tbsp/15 mL water periodically if masala begins to stick.)

6. Add tomatoes, jaggery and cilantro. Cover, reduce heat to medium-low and cook until tomatoes are soft enough to be mashed with back of spoon, 5 to 6 minutes.

7. Add puréed dal mixture and chicken and mix well. Cover and simmer to allow flavors to combine, 15 to 20 minutes. Pass lemon wedges to squeeze over top.

Variation

You can use lamb here instead of chicken. Use 4 lbs (2 kg) lamb, preferably with bone, cut into bite-size pieces.

Thai Dry Vegetable Curry

This is a peculiarly Thai cooking method, where crisp, separately fried ingredients are cooked together with curry paste, sugar and fish sauce to make a dry curry. The dish incorporates a bit of oil, but the end result should not be greasy. In Thailand, fish is sometimes added to this type of preparation, as are fried lotus seeds and/or salted duck-egg yolks.

Tips

These vegetables complement each other well and are readily available at regular grocery stores. Cut each vegetable into a different shape to keep them distinct; all should be cut fairly thin but not less than $1/8$ inch (5 mm).

For stronger basil flavor, fry half the basil leaves for garnish and add the remaining leaves to the curry with the red chile rings.

1	small onion, thinly sliced	1
$1/2$ tsp	salt	2 mL
2 cups	vegetable oil	500 mL
2	carrots, cut crosswise into thirds and thinly sliced lengthwise	2
1	kohlrabi, cut in half and sliced into half-rounds	1
1	large baking or frying potato or taro root, cut into round slices	1
$1\frac{1}{2}$ cups	canned bamboo shoots, rinsed, drained and sliced	375 mL
1 cup	Chinese bean curd or firm tofu, cut into rectangles or square slices	250 mL
$2/3$ cup	loosely packed Thai or holy basil	150 mL
2 tbsp	Thai red curry paste	30 mL
2 tbsp	granulated sugar	30 mL
4 tsp	fish sauce	20 mL
1 or 2	red finger chiles, sliced into rings	1 or 2

1. In a bowl, combine onion and salt; set aside for 30 minutes. Drain, discarding liquid. Pat onion slices dry with paper towel.

2. In a wok or deep saucepan, heat oil to 350°F (180°C). Cook onion until golden and crisp; remove with slotted spoon and drain on paper towel. Cook separately the carrot, kohlrabi, potato, bamboo shoots and tofu in the hot oil until golden and crisp; drain on paper towels. Remove all but $1/3$ cup (75 mL) of the oil. Fry basil leaves until crispy but not browned; remove immediately from hot oil and drain on paper towel.

3. Add curry paste to oil; cook until fragrant. Stir in sugar and fish sauce; mix well. Add vegetables (except onion and basil); cook, stirring constantly, until curry paste adheres to all the vegetables. Add chile rings; mix. Serve garnished with fried onions and basil.

Paneer with Chickpeas in Creamy Tomato Curry

Cheese and chickpeas, a double dose of vegetarian proteins, are coddled in a rich tomato curry sauce and finished with cream. It's luxuriously suitable for a festive table.

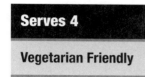

Serves 4

Vegetarian Friendly

Tip

Whipping cream adds a delightfully rich taste and texture; however, a lower-fat cream with a minimum of 10% milk fat can be used instead.

1 tbsp	vegetable oil	15 mL
3	green onions, sliced	3
½ tsp	ground cumin	2 mL
2 tbsp	Indian yellow curry paste or masala blend	30 mL
1 cup	canned crushed (ground) tomatoes	250 mL
½ cup	water	125 mL
5 oz	paneer, cut into ½-inch (1 cm) cubes (about 1 cup/250 mL)	150 g
1 cup	cooked or canned chickpeas, drained and rinsed	250 mL
⅓ cup	whipping (35%) cream	75 mL
	Chopped fresh cilantro	

1. In a skillet, heat oil over medium heat. Add green onions, cumin and curry paste; cook, stirring, until onions are softened and spices are fragrant, about 2 minutes. Stir in tomatoes and water; bring to a boil, scraping up bits stuck to pan.

2. Stir in paneer and chickpeas. Reduce heat and simmer, stirring often, until hot and flavorful, about 10 minutes. Stir in cream until heated through. Serve sprinkled with cilantro.

Tofu and Snow Peas in Tamarind Ginger Curry

Here's a springtime dish for when snow peas are in season and winter's heavy meat-eating can give way to far gentler, though equally nutritious, tofu. The combination of tangy Thai and Indian spices is an added bonus.

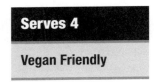

Serves 4

Vegan Friendly

Tips

To julienne ginger, cut a 3-inch (7.5 cm) piece of gingerroot into thin slices. Working with 3 slices at a time, stack and cut across into thin strips.

To make tamarind water, break a 2-oz (60 g) piece of block tamarind into small pieces and place in a heatproof bowl. Pour in 1 cup (250 mL) boiling water and let stand until very soft, about 30 minutes, or for up to 8 hours. Press through a fine mesh sieve, discarding seeds and skins.

Thai and Indian curry pastes will give very different flavors, but either works nicely in this recipe.

1 tbsp	vegetable oil	15 mL
1/4 cup	julienned gingerroot (see Tips, left)	60 mL
1	onion, sliced lengthwise	1
1/4 tsp	ground cinnamon	1 mL
Pinch	ground cardamom	Pinch
1 tbsp	Thai or Indian yellow curry paste or masala blend	15 mL
12 oz	firm or extra-firm tofu, drained and cut into 1/2-inch (1 cm) cubes	375 g
2 tsp	packed brown or palm sugar	10 mL
1 cup	coconut milk	250 mL
1/2 cup	tamarind water (see Tips, left)	125 mL
1/4 cup	water	60 mL
1 tbsp	fish sauce (nam pla) or 1/2 tsp (2 mL) salt	15 mL
1 1/2 cups	trimmed snow peas, halved diagonally	375 mL
	Salt, optional	
	Chopped fresh mint	

1. In a large skillet, heat oil over medium heat until hot but not smoking. Add ginger and cook, stirring, until softened and fragrant, about 1 minute. Using a slotted spoon, transfer half to a bowl and set aside.

2. Add onion, cinnamon, cardamom and curry paste to pan; cook, stirring, until onion is softened and starting to brown, about 5 minutes.

3. Stir in tofu until coated with spices. Stir in brown sugar, coconut milk, tamarind water, water and fish sauce; bring to a simmer, scraping up bits stuck to pan. Reduce heat and simmer, stirring occasionally, until sauce is slightly thickened, about 10 minutes.

4. Stir in snow peas, cover and simmer until snow peas are tender-crisp, about 5 minutes. Season to taste with salt, if using, and serve sprinkled with reserved ginger and mint.

Saffron Curry Mushrooms and Tofu

Saffron, exotic mushrooms and calorific cream turn this recipe into a luxury, yet an affordable and relatively sinless one, as tofu itself is inexpensive and easy on the calories. This one is for a special occasion or an elegant dinner party.

Serves 4 to 6

Vegetarian Friendly

Tips

Avoid very dark mushrooms, such as portobello, as they will discolor the sauce.

The whipping cream is essential to accent the flavor of the saffron and create a velvety texture. Don't be tempted to substitute a lower-fat cream in this one.

Medium tofu lends a soft texture to this dish that matches the mushrooms. For a contrasting texture, use firm tofu. If using medium, pat it dry after draining and avoid stirring too much, as this will cause it to break up.

1/8 tsp	saffron threads	0.5 mL
3/4 cup	vegetable stock, heated	175 mL
1 tsp	cumin seeds	5 mL
1/2 tsp	fennel seeds	2 mL
2 tbsp	butter or vegetable oil	30 mL
2	cloves garlic, minced	2
1	onion, chopped	1
1 tsp	garam masala	5 mL
1/2 tsp	ground coriander	2 mL
1/4 tsp	salt	1 mL
1/4 tsp	hot pepper flakes	1 mL
12 oz	exotic mushrooms (shiitake, cremini, oyster, king, etc.), trimmed and sliced	375 g
1/4 cup	dry white wine	60 mL
1/2 cup	whipping (35%) cream	125 mL
12 oz	medium or firm tofu, drained and cut into 1/2-inch (1 cm) cubes	375 g
	Chopped fresh cilantro	

1. In a measuring cup or bowl, combine saffron and stock; let stand for 15 minutes.
2. In a dry large skillet over medium-high heat, toast cumin seeds and fennel seeds, stirring constantly, until slightly darker and fragrant, about 30 seconds.
3. Add butter and swirl to coat pan. Add garlic, onion, garam masala, coriander, salt and hot pepper flakes; cook, stirring, until onion starts to soften, about 2 minutes. Add mushrooms and cook, stirring often, until liquid is released and mushrooms are browned, about 8 minutes.
4. Add wine and bring to a boil, scraping up bits stuck to pan. Stir in stock mixture and cream; bring to a boil. Boil for 2 minutes.
5. Gently stir in tofu. Reduce heat and simmer gently, stirring occasionally, until tofu is flavorful and sauce is slightly thickened, about 10 minutes. Season to taste with salt. Serve sprinkled with cilantro.

Pyaza Paneer and Navy Bean Curry

Beans, cheese and lots of onion combine for a hearty and versatile dish. Served with rice, it provides a satisfying lunch or light supper.

Serves 4

Vegetarian Friendly

2 tbsp	vegetable oil	30 mL
1 cup	diced onion	250 mL
1 cup	diced tomatoes	250 mL
1 tbsp	minced garlic	15 mL
1 tbsp	minced gingerroot	15 mL
1 tsp	ground cumin	5 mL
1 tsp	ground coriander	5 mL
1/2 tsp	salt	2 mL
1/4 tsp	ground turmeric	1 mL
1 cup	cooked or canned navy (cannellini) beans, drained and rinsed	250 mL
1 cup	boiled cubed peeled potato (1/2-inch/1 cm cubes)	250 mL
1 cup	water	250 mL
5 oz	paneer, cut into 1/2-inch (1 cm) cubes (about 1 cup/250 mL)	150 g
1/2 cup	chopped fresh cilantro	125 mL

1. In a skillet, heat oil over medium-high heat. Add onion and cook, stirring, until starting to soften, about 2 minutes. Add tomatoes and cook, stirring, until starting to soften, about 2 minutes.

2. Reduce heat to medium. Add garlic, ginger, cumin, coriander, salt and turmeric; cook, stirring, until softened and fragrant, 1 to 2 minutes. Stir in navy beans, potato and water; cook, stirring gently, until piping hot and bubbling, 2 to 3 minutes.

3. Gently fold in paneer and cilantro. Reduce heat to low and simmer, stirring gently, until paneer is heated through, about 3 minutes. Season to taste with salt.

Variation

If paneer is not available, substitute an equal amount of firm tofu or pressed dry-curd cottage cheese. If using dry-curd cottage cheese, break into pieces and be very careful when stirring to prevent it from breaking up too much.

Caribbean Chickpea Curry with Potatoes

This is the official stuffing of meatless Caribbean roti. It is filling and tasty, and has nourished generations of Jamaicans in search of a satisfying snack. The recipe also works well as a side dish for meat or chicken.

Serves 4 to 6

Vegan Friendly

Tips

If Scotch bonnet peppers are not available, substitute 1 tbsp (15 mL) minced jalapeño pepper (or to taste).

For the most authentic flavor, look for a Caribbean curry powder. Any Indian curry powder will work, but they tend to be hotter, so reduce the amount to 2 tsp (10 mL).

2 tbsp	vegetable oil	30 mL
1 tsp	cumin seeds	5 mL
1	onion, chopped	1
1	hot chile pepper, preferably Scotch bonnet, minced	1
1 tbsp	curry powder, preferably Caribbean-style (see Tips, left)	15 mL
½ tsp	salt	2 mL
¼ tsp	dried thyme (or 1 tsp/5 mL chopped fresh)	1 mL
Pinch	ground allspice	Pinch
2	boiling or all-purpose potatoes, cut into ½-inch (1 cm) cubes	2
1	can (14 to 19 oz/398 to 540 mL) chickpeas, drained and rinsed	1
½ cup	water or vegetable stock	125 mL
1 tbsp	chopped fresh cilantro or green onion	15 mL

1. In a large skillet, heat oil over medium heat until hot but not smoking. Add cumin seeds and cook, stirring, until starting to pop, about 1 minute. Add onion and cook, stirring, until starting to soften, about 2 minutes. Add chile pepper, curry powder, salt, thyme and allspice; cook, stirring, until onion is softened and starting to brown, about 3 minutes.

2. Stir in potatoes and chickpeas until coated with spices. Pour in water and cover pan quickly. Reduce heat to medium-low and boil gently, stirring occasionally, until potatoes are tender, about 20 minutes. Season to taste with salt. Serve sprinkled with cilantro.

Variation

To use for roti, spoon inside warmed roti skins or whole wheat flour tortillas.

Caribbean Red Bean, Spinach and Potato Curry

To combine the Caribbean staples of beans, potato and greens is to invite the sunshine of the islands to dinner or lunch. This dish works hot as a vegetarian main course or cold as a salad alongside seafood or fish. Bring on the reggae!

Serves 4 to 6

Vegan Friendly

Tip

There are several varieties of curry powder from the Caribbean that vary in spices from island to island. Any will work nicely in this recipe. If using a stronger, Indian curry powder, reduce the amount to 1½ to 2 tsp (7 to 10 mL) or according to taste.

2 lbs	baby new potatoes, halved (or quartered if large)	1 kg
	Cold water	
1 tsp	salt, divided	5 mL
2 tbsp	vegetable oil	30 mL
1	onion, sliced lengthwise	1
½	hot chile pepper, preferably Scotch bonnet, minced	½
1 tbsp	minced gingerroot	15 mL
1 tbsp	curry powder, preferably Caribbean-style (see Tip, left)	15 mL
1 tsp	ground coriander	5 mL
¼ tsp	ground allspice	1 mL
1	can (14 to 19 oz/398 to 540 mL) red kidney beans, drained and rinsed	1
½ cup	water or vegetable stock	125 mL
2 tbsp	freshly squeezed lemon juice	30 mL
2 cups	shredded fresh spinach	500 mL

1. In a pot, cover potatoes with cold water. Add ½ tsp (2 mL) of the salt and bring to a boil over high heat. Reduce heat and boil gently until potatoes are fork-tender, about 15 minutes. Drain well and transfer to a large bowl; set aside.

2. Meanwhile, in a skillet, heat oil over medium heat. Add onion, chile pepper, ginger, curry powder, coriander, allspice and remaining salt; cook, stirring, until onion is softened, about 3 minutes.

3. Stir in beans until coated with spices. Pour in water and bring to a boil, scraping up bits stuck to pan. Reduce heat and boil gently, stirring occasionally, until liquid is almost evaporated, about 5 minutes. Remove from heat and stir in lemon juice. Season to taste with salt. Pour over potatoes in bowl and stir in spinach just until wilted. Serve hot or let cool.

Variation

Replace spinach with Swiss chard, callaloo or another hearty green. Add with beans in Step 3, increasing time as necessary to make sure greens are tender.

Curried Couscous with Tomatoes and Chickpeas

Serves 4 to 6

Vegan Friendly

Tips

A great source of nutrition for vegetarians.

Cilantro can be replaced with basil, dill or parsley.

Couscous is available in the rice section of grocery stores.

Try quinoa in this recipe.

Make Ahead

Prepare up to 2 days in advance. Reheat gently.

2 cups	vegetable stock	500 mL
1½ cups	couscous	375 mL
1 tsp	vegetable oil	5 mL
3 cups	chopped plum tomatoes	750 mL
½ cup	vegetable stock	125 mL
2 tsp	curry powder	10 mL
2 tsp	minced garlic	10 mL
2 cups	canned chickpeas, rinsed and drained	500 mL
¾ cup	chopped fresh cilantro	175 mL
½ cup	chopped green onions	125 mL

1. In a saucepan, bring stock to a boil; stir in couscous, cover and remove from heat. Let stand 5 minutes; transfer to a serving bowl.

2. Meanwhile, in a large nonstick saucepan, heat oil over medium-high heat. Add tomatoes, stock, curry and garlic; cook, stirring, for 5 minutes or until tomatoes begin to break up. Stir in chickpeas; cook for 2 minutes or until heated through. Add to couscous along with cilantro and green onions; toss to combine. Serve immediately.

Tofu with Lime, Lemongrass and Coconut Curry

Vietnamese cuisine blends the flavors and textures of Thai and Chinese cookery in this sublimely aromatic tofu and eggplant dish that allows each ingredient to assert its own flavor while linking to the other in the lovely sauce.

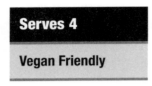

Serves 4

Vegan Friendly

Tips

To prepare lemongrass, trim off tough outer layers. Cut remaining stalk into 2-inch (5 cm) sections. Smash each piece with the broad side of a knife to bruise. This will help release the flavor when the lemongrass is cooked.

If lime leaves are not available, add ½ tsp (2 mL) finely grated lime zest with the lime juice in Step 3.

1 tbsp	vegetable oil	15 mL
1	onion, sliced lengthwise	1
3	cloves garlic, minced	3
2	stalks lemongrass, chopped and bruised (see Tips, left)	2
2	wild lime leaves (see Tips, left)	2
½ tsp	salt	2 mL
1 tbsp	Indian yellow curry paste or masala blend	15 mL
2 cups	cubed eggplant (½-inch/1 cm cubes)	500 mL
1 cup	coconut milk	250 mL
½ cup	vegetable stock or water	125 mL
12 oz	firm or extra-firm tofu, drained and cut into ¾-inch (2 cm) cubes	375 g
2 tbsp	freshly squeezed lime juice	30 mL
2	green onions, thinly sliced	2
¼ cup	thin strips red bell pepper	60 mL

1. In a large skillet, heat oil over medium heat. Add onion and cook, stirring, until softened and starting to turn golden, about 3 minutes. Stir in garlic, lemongrass, lime leaves, salt and curry paste; cook, stirring, until softened and fragrant, about 1 minute.

2. Stir in eggplant until coated with spices. Add coconut milk and stock; bring to a simmer, scraping up bits stuck to pan.

3. Stir in tofu. Reduce heat and simmer, stirring often, until eggplant is tender and sauce is slightly thickened, about 10 minutes. Discard lemongrass and lime leaves, if desired. Stir in lime juice and season to taste with salt. Serve sprinkled with green onions and red pepper.

Punjabi Malai Palak

Punjabi Creamy Yellow Mung Beans

The creamy dal gives this lightly spiced spinach dish a sensually silky texture.

Serves 8

Vegetarian Friendly

Tip

Beans and lentils, simply called "dal" in India, are unquestionably the basic food of all Indians. The variety of dals used throughout the country is astonishing, and they vary enormously in flavor, texture and starch content. With some exceptions, dal is usually cooked with plenty of water, which is seldom drained. A layer of water will be present on top of the cooked lentils. Instead of draining this off, when the dal is soft, it is mashed or blended with the remaining water, allowing the starch in the dal to break down and act as a thickener. The mashed dal is more often than not the consistency of cream soup. The cooked dal is then finished with flash-fried spices and seasonings.

1 cup	yellow mung beans (mung dal)	250 mL
3 cups	chopped fresh spinach	750 mL
2 tbsp	minced green chiles, preferably serranos	30 mL
1½ tbsp	minced peeled gingerroot	22 mL
½ tsp	turmeric	2 mL
2 tbsp	oil	30 mL
1 cup	finely chopped onion	250 mL
1½ tsp	salt or to taste	7 mL
½ tsp	cayenne pepper	2 mL
¼ cup	plain nonfat yogurt, divided	60 mL

1. Clean and pick through dal for any small stones and grit. Rinse several times in cold water until water is fairly clear. Soak in 3 cups (750 mL) water in a large pot for 10 minutes.

2. Add spinach, green chiles, ginger and turmeric to dal and bring to a boil over medium heat. Reduce heat to medium-low and boil gently, partially covered, until dal is very soft, about 30 minutes. Remove from heat. Using a blender, in batches if necessary, purée dal mixture until smooth. Set aside.

3. In a saucepan, heat oil over medium-high heat. Add onion and sauté until golden, 8 to 10 minutes. Stir in salt and cayenne and sauté for 1 minute. Add dal mixture and mix well.

4. Stir yogurt until creamy. Stir 2 tbsp (30 mL) into dal. If mixture is too thick, add ½ cup (125 mL) hot water. Cover and simmer for 5 minutes. Serve hot. Swirl remaining yogurt over top.

Channa Dal with Zucchini

Split Yellow Peas with Zucchini

Sindhis love channa dal and traditionally this dish would be made with turai, a long vegetable with a thick ridged skin but mild like zucchini on the inside. It is often available in Asian markets and is known as Chinese okra, although it bears no resemblance to okra. Unlike zucchini, the skin is peeled before cooking.

Serves 8

Vegan Friendly

Tips

When adding dry spices, it is important to sauté for 3 to 4 minutes to remove the "raw" taste of the spices. The spices will neither soften nor be recognizably fragrant. If anything, they may turn slightly darker.

This dish freezes well. To freeze, transfer to an airtight container and freeze for up to 3 months. Reheat in microwave or on stove top over low heat.

1 cup	split yellow peas (channa dal)	250 mL
2 tbsp	oil	30 mL
1½ tbsp	minced peeled gingerroot	22 mL
2 tsp	minced green chiles, preferably serranos	10 mL
1 cup	finely chopped onion	250 mL
3 cups	chopped zucchini (½-inch/1 cm pieces)	750 mL
1 tsp	ground coriander	5 mL
1 tsp	salt or to taste	5 mL
½ tsp	turmeric	2 mL
½ tsp	cayenne pepper	2 mL
1	can (14 oz/398 mL) tomatoes, including juice, chopped	1

1. Clean and pick through dal for any small stones and grit. Rinse several times in cold water until water is fairly clear. Soak in 2 cups (500 mL) water for 20 to 30 minutes.

2. In a saucepan, heat oil over medium-high heat. Add ginger and chiles and sauté for 1 minute. Add onion and sauté until soft and translucent, 6 to 7 minutes.

3. Add zucchini and mix well. Cover and cook for 5 minutes. Add coriander, salt, turmeric and cayenne. Mix well and cook, stirring, 3 to 4 minutes (see Tips, left).

4. Add tomatoes with juice and dal with soaking liquid, plus enough additional water to cover. Stir to mix well. Cover, reduce heat to low and simmer, stirring every 10 minutes, until dal is soft and a little liquid remains, resulting in a thin gravy (sauce), 20 to 25 minutes.

Rajasthani Mixed Dal

This is the dal cooked almost daily in many homes in Rajasthan. It is served with a baked whole wheat ball that is semihard and dry, called bati. *When cooked, the balls are soaked in warm ghee to soften. Serve it with steamed rice.*

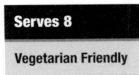

Serves 8

Vegetarian Friendly

Tip

If curry leaves have dried naturally in the refrigerator over several weeks, they are most likely still aromatic. The dried ones sold in Indian markets have no aroma or flavor and I would advise against those.

1 cup	split white lentils (urad dal)	250 mL
½ cup	yellow mung beans (mung dal)	125 mL
¼ cup	split yellow peas (channa dal)	60 mL
½ tsp	turmeric	2 mL
1½ tsp	salt	7 mL
2 tbsp	ghee	30 mL
1 tsp	cumin seeds	5 mL
¼ tsp	asafetida (hing)	1 mL
4	bay leaves	4
3	whole cloves	3
3	green cardamom pods, crushed	3
1	sprig fresh curry leaves, stripped (12 to 15 leaves) (see Tip, left), optional	1
1½ cups	chopped tomatoes	375 mL
2 tbsp	minced green chiles, preferably serranos	30 mL
1 tbsp	minced peeled gingerroot	15 mL
1 tsp	cayenne pepper	5 mL
1 cup	loosely packed cilantro	250 mL

1. Clean and pick through urad, mung and channa dals for any small stones and grit. Rinse several times in cold water until water is fairly clear. Soak in 7 cups (1.75 L) water in a saucepan for 1 hour.

2. Bring dals to a boil over medium-high heat. Stir in turmeric and boil gently, partially covered, until dals are soft but not mushy and water does not appear to be separated (see Tip, page 165), about 30 minutes. Stir in salt. Set aside.

3. In another saucepan, heat ghee over medium heat. Add cumin, asafetida, bay leaves, cloves, cardamom and curry leaves and sauté for 20 seconds. Add tomatoes, chiles, ginger and cayenne and sauté for 2 minutes.

4. Pour dal into tomato mixture and mix well. If there is excess water, cook, uncovered, over medium-low heat until water looks absorbed but without drying dal too much. (It should be thick but liquidy enough to pour over rice.) Adjust consistency with a little additional warm water if too thick. Sprinkle cilantro over dal before serving.

Red Lentil Curry with Coconut and Cilantro

Easy to make, these red lentils have a luxurious coconut finish and a lovely, bright yellow color. They partner any curry of your choice — vegetable or meat — as well as rice, for a complete and satisfying meal.

Tips

Traditionally, Indian lentil dishes such as this one are served very loose and almost soupy. You can adjust the texture to your taste by adding more water or simmering longer to thicken in Step 2.

Leftovers will thicken considerably upon cooling. If reheating in the microwave or a saucepan, add boiling water before heating to return to desired consistency.

2 tbsp	vegetable oil	30 mL
1	small onion, finely chopped	1
2	cloves garlic, minced	2
1 tbsp	minced gingerroot	15 mL
1 tsp	salt	5 mL
1 tsp	ground coriander	5 mL
1 tsp	ground cumin	5 mL
1/4 tsp	ground turmeric	1 mL
1 cup	red lentils (masoor dal), rinsed	250 mL
1	can (14 oz/400 mL) coconut milk	1
1 cup	water	250 mL
1/4 cup	torn cilantro leaves	60 mL
	Garam masala	

1. In a saucepan, heat oil over medium heat. Add onion and cook, stirring, until softened and starting to brown, about 5 minutes. Add garlic, ginger, salt, coriander, cumin and turmeric; cook, stirring, until softened and fragrant, about 2 minutes.

2. Stir in lentils until coated with spices. Stir in coconut milk and water; bring to a boil, scraping up bits stuck to pan and stirring to prevent lumps. Reduce heat to low, partially cover and simmer, stirring often, until lentils are very soft and mixture is thick, about 15 minutes.

3. Remove from heat, cover and let stand for 5 minutes. Season to taste with salt. Stir in all but a few leaves of cilantro. Serve sprinkled with remaining cilantro and garam masala.

Variation

To add some heat to this dish, add 1 or 2 hot red or green chile peppers, minced, with the garlic.

Bengali Red Lentils

This everyday dal can be seasoned in different ways to change the flavor profile. Cook the lentils and purée. Refrigerate for up to a week. Before serving, you can take a portion of the dal, bring it back to a boil and finish with a seasoning mix of your choice. The remainder of the unseasoned dal can be saved for another meal, when it can be seasoned differently.

Serves 6 to 8

Vegan Friendly

2 cups	red lentils (masoor dal)	500 mL
1 tsp	turmeric	5 mL
2 tsp	salt or to taste	10 mL

Tempering

1½ tbsp	oil	22 mL
1½ tsp	nigella seeds (kalaunji)	7 mL
2	green chiles, preferably serranos, slit	2

1. Clean and pick through dal for any small stones and grit. Rinse several times in cold water until water is fairly clear. Soak in 6 cups (1.5 L) water in a saucepan for 10 minutes.

2. Bring dal to a boil over medium-high heat. Reduce heat to low. Stir in turmeric and boil gently, partially covered, until dal is soft, about 20 minutes. Using an immersion blender or in a blender, in batches as necessary, purée until smooth. Return to saucepan. Add salt and cook over medium-low heat, stirring often, until consistency of pea soup, about 10 minutes.

3. *Tempering:* In a small saucepan, heat oil over medium heat. Add nigella and chiles and sauté, about 1 minute. Add to dal. Serve with rice.

Variations

Omit nigella and add 1 cup (250 mL) thinly sliced onions with the chiles in Step 3 and sauté until onions are light golden, 6 to 7 minutes. Add to dal.

Omit nigella and chiles and add 2 cups (500 mL) chopped tomatoes in Step 3 and sauté until soft and mushy, 6 to 7 minutes. Add ½ cup (125 mL) chopped cilantro and 1 tsp (5 mL) granulated sugar and cook for 1 minute. Add to dal.

Tomato Pappu

Andhra Yellow Lentils with Tomatoes

A delicious home-style dal without the fire of many Andhra dishes. This recipe comes from the chef at the Taj Banjara hotel in Hyderabad.

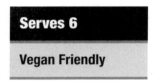

Serves 6

Vegan Friendly

1 cup	yellow lentils (toor dal)	250 mL
2	plum (Roma) tomatoes, cut into 1-inch (2.5 cm) pieces	2
1 tbsp	thinly sliced green chiles, preferably serranos	15 mL
½ tsp	turmeric	2 mL
1½ tbsp	oil	22 mL
1 tsp	dark mustard seeds	5 mL
1 tsp	cumin seeds	5 mL
2	dried Indian red chiles	2
1 tbsp	sliced garlic	15 mL
3	sprigs fresh curry leaves, stripped (30 to 40), divided	3
1 cup	chopped onion	250 mL
1 tsp	minced peeled gingerroot	5 mL
1 tsp	minced garlic	5 mL
1 tsp	salt or to taste	5 mL

1. Clean and pick through dal for any small stones and grit. Rinse several times in cold water until water is fairly clear. Soak in 4 cups (1 L) water in a saucepan for 10 minutes.

2. Bring dal to a boil over medium-high heat. Skim any foam off top. Reduce heat to medium-low. Add tomatoes, chiles and turmeric and boil gently, partially covered, until dal is soft and most of the water has been absorbed, 20 to 25 minutes.

3. In another large saucepan, heat oil over high heat until a couple of mustard seeds thrown in start to sputter. Add all the mustard seeds and cover quickly. When the seeds stop popping, in a few seconds, uncover, reduce heat to medium and add cumin seeds, red chiles, sliced garlic and about three-quarters of the curry leaves and sauté for 1 minute. Add onion and sauté until soft and just beginning to color, 3 to 4 minutes.

4. Pour dal over onion masala. Add ginger, minced garlic and salt and stir to mix. Cover and reduce heat to low. Simmer until dal is well mixed and mixture is thickened (see Tip, page 165), about 10 minutes. Sprinkle remaining curry leaves over top before serving over rice.

Masoor ani Shing

Brown Lentils with Peanuts

Peanuts are widely grown and extensively used in the cooking of Maharashtra. This simple home-style dal is typical of the area.

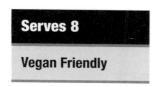

Serves 8

Vegan Friendly

Tip

Roasted peanuts in a jar can be used instead. Omit Step 3 if substituting them.

2 cups	brown lentils (sabat masoor)	500 mL
2/3 cup	raw peanuts, skinned (see Tip, left)	150 mL
1/4 cup	unsalted Thai tamarind purée	60 mL
4 tsp	jaggery (gur)	20 mL
2 tsp	salt or to taste	10 mL
1 tsp	cayenne pepper	5 mL
1 tbsp	oil	15 mL
1/2 tsp	ground cloves	2 mL
1/2 tsp	ground cinnamon	2 mL
3 tbsp	cilantro, chopped	45 mL

1. Clean and pick through dal for any small stones and grit. Rinse several times in cold water until water is fairly clear. Soak in 6 cups (1.5 L) water in a saucepan for 10 minutes.

2. Bring dal to a boil over high heat. Skim any froth off the top. Reduce heat to medium-low and boil gently, partially covered, until soft and dal can be mashed with back of spoon, about 30 minutes.

3. Meanwhile, in a heavy skillet over medium heat, toast peanuts, shaking pan often to brown evenly, 3 to 4 minutes.

4. Stir peanuts, tamarind, jaggery, salt and cayenne pepper into dal and simmer for 5 minutes.

5. In a small saucepan, heat oil over medium heat. Add cloves and cinnamon and immediately remove from heat. Pour infused oil over top of dal. Cover and simmer for 2 minutes. Garnish with cilantro. Serve hot with rice or any Indian bread.

Tomato Dal with Spinach

This mildly spiced but tasty dal is delicious over hot cooked rice or as a substantial side dish. Add the yogurt if you prefer a creamy finish.

Tips

Split yellow peas take a long time to cook and, despite what many say, need to be soaked before cooking. Soak this quantity in 8 cups (2 L) of water overnight or for 4 hours at room temperature. Drain and rinse before using in this recipe.

If you have leftover baby spinach for salad you can substitute it for the regular spinach in this recipe. About half of a 10-oz/300 g bag is an appropriate quantity as, unlike regular spinach, there is no waste.

If you prefer, substitute 2 parsnips for 2 of the carrots.

Make Ahead

This dish can be partially prepared the night before it is cooked. Complete Steps 1, 2 and 3. Cover and refrigerate overnight. The next day continue cooking as directed.

- **Medium (approx. 4 quart) slow cooker**

2 cups	yellow split peas (see Tips, left)	500 mL
2 tsp	cumin seeds	10 mL
1 tsp	whole coriander seeds	5 mL
1 tbsp	vegetable oil	15 mL
1	medium onion, finely chopped	1
6	carrots, peeled and diced	6
6	cloves garlic, finely chopped	6
1 tbsp	minced gingerroot	15 mL
1 tsp	salt	5 mL
½ tsp	cracked black peppercorns	2 mL
1	can (28 oz/796 mL) tomatoes, including juice, coarsely chopped	1
2 cups	vegetable stock	500 mL
8 oz	fresh spinach leaves, washed, or 1 package (10 oz/300 g) frozen spinach, thawed (see Tips, left)	250 g
1 tbsp	freshly squeezed lemon juice	15 mL
	Plain yogurt (optional)	

1. Soak peas in 8 cups (2 L) water overnight or for 4 hours at room temperature. Drain and rinse and set aside.

2. In a dry skillet, toast cumin and coriander seeds until they release their aroma. Transfer to a spice grinder or mortar, or use the bottom of a measuring cup or wine bottle, to coarsely grind. Set aside.

3. In same skillet, heat oil over medium heat. Add onion and carrots and cook, stirring, until softened, about 7 minutes. Add garlic, gingerroot, salt and peppercorns and cook, stirring, for 1 minute. Add tomatoes with juice and bring to a boil, breaking up with a spoon. Transfer to slow cooker stoneware. Add vegetable stock and yellow split peas and stir to combine.

4. Cover and cook on Low for 10 to 12 hours or on High for 4 to 5 hours, until peas are soft. Add spinach and lemon juice. Cover and cook on High for 20 minutes, until spinach is cooked and mixture is bubbling. Ladle into bowls and drizzle with yogurt, if using.

Mains with Meat, Poultry, Fish and Seafood

Southwestern Shepherd's Pie 174

Beans, Beef and Biscuits 175

Best-Ever Cholent 176

Kim's Mexican Casserole 177

Stuffed Veal Rolls with White Beans. . . .178

Prairie Fire Beans. 179

Braised Stuffed Bean Curd 180

Braised Roasted Pork with Tofu
   and Green Onions. 182

Make-Ahead Southwestern
   Pork Stew. .183

Pork and Black Bean Stew
   with Sweet Potatoes 184

Maple Baked Pork and Beans
   with Caramelized Apples 185

Mediterranean Pork and Beans. 186

Home-Style Pork and Beans 187

Molasses Baked Beans 188

The Best Pork 'n' Beans. 189

Bistro Lentils with Smoked Sausage . . .190

Sausage-Spiked Peas 'n' Rice 191

Baked Beans 'n' Barley 192

Quick Cassoulet. 193

Cheater's Cassoulet 194

Potato and Chickpea Stew
   with Spicy Sausage. 196

Quince-Laced Lamb Shanks
   with Yellow Split Peas 198

Country-Style Salted Pork
   with Lentils. 199

Lamb with Flageolet Gratin 200

Spicy Lamb with Chickpeas 202

Cheesy Beans and Hot Dogs. 203

Braised Lamb with Beans and Dates . . .204

Chicken Baked with Black Beans
   and Lime 205

Brunswick-Style Chicken Pot Pie. 206

Manicotti Stuffed with Chickpeas
   and Cheese 207

Rice and Red Lentil Pilaf
   with Fried Zucchini 208

Linguine with Tuna, White Beans
   and Dill 209

Saucy Halibut on a Bed of Lentils 210

Salmon over White-and-Black Bean
   Salsa 211

Baked Shrimp Enchiladas 212

Tuscan Shrimp and Beans 213

Steamed Shrimp-Stuffed Tofu
   with Broccoli. 214

Southwestern Shepherd's Pie

Traditional shepherd's pie is great, but shepherd's pie with a little kick of the Southwest? Terrific!

Makes 6 servings

Tips

Yukon gold potatoes add extra flavor, but the butter and cilantro will enhance 2½ cups (375 mL) of your favorite instant mashed potatoes.

If you want to use canned corn, use a 14- or 15-oz (398 or 425 mL) can and drain first.

- **Preheat oven to 350°F (180°C)**
- **11- by 7-inch (28 by 18 cm) glass baking dish**

1½ lbs	Yukon gold potatoes, cut into 1-inch (2.5 cm) cubes	750 g
½ cup	milk	125 mL
2 tbsp	butter	30 mL
2 tbsp	chopped fresh cilantro	30 mL
1 tsp	salt, divided	5 mL
1 tsp	freshly ground black pepper, divided	5 mL
1 lb	lean ground beef	500 g
2	cloves garlic, minced	2
½ cup	chopped onion	125 mL
1	can (14 to 19 oz/398 to 540 mL) black beans, drained and rinsed	1
1	can (14 oz/398 mL) diced tomatoes	1
1½ cups	corn kernels (thawed if frozen)	375 mL
½ cup	shredded Cheddar cheese	125 mL

1. Place potatoes in a large saucepan and add enough water to cover. Cover and bring to a boil over high heat. Reduce heat and simmer for about 15 minutes or until potatoes are just tender. Drain, return to the pot and add milk, butter, cilantro, half the salt and half the pepper; mash until smooth.

2. Meanwhile, in a large nonstick skillet, over medium-high heat, cook beef, garlic and onion, breaking beef up with the back of a spoon, for 8 to 10 minutes or until beef is no longer pink. Drain off fat.

3. Stir in beans, tomatoes and the remaining salt and pepper; bring to a boil. Reduce heat and simmer, stirring often, for 5 to 7 minutes or until heated through.

4. Spread beef mixture in baking dish. Spread corn evenly over meat. Spread mashed potatoes over corn. Sprinkle with cheese.

5. Bake in preheated oven for 20 minutes or until top is golden.

Beans, Beef and Biscuits

Topped with hot biscuits, this hearty mix looks as good as it tastes. Serve with a tossed green salad for a great family meal.

Tips

Placing the biscuits on a hot filling prevents them from becoming mushy on the bottom during baking.

Arrabbiata is a popular spicy tomato sauce.

- **Preheat oven to 375°F (190°C)**
- **8-cup (2 L) baking dish, lightly greased**

1 tbsp	vegetable oil	15 mL
1 lb	lean ground beef, thawed if frozen	500 g
1 cup	diced onion	250 mL
½ cup	finely chopped celery	125 mL
2 cups	spicy tomato sauce	500 mL
2	cans (each 14 oz/398 mL) baked beans in tomato sauce	2
1 tbsp	Worcestershire sauce	15 mL
1	can (8 oz/250 g) country-style biscuit dough	1

1. In a skillet, heat oil over medium heat. Add beef, onion and celery and cook, breaking up meat with a spoon, until beef is no longer pink and vegetables are softened, about 7 minutes. Add tomato sauce, baked beans and Worcestershire sauce and bring to a boil. Reduce heat to low and simmer for 2 minutes. Pour into prepared dish.

2. Separate dough into individual biscuits. Arrange evenly over top of bean mixture (there will be spaces in between). Bake in preheated oven until biscuits are puffed and brown, 10 to 12 minutes. Serve immediately.

> **Celery:** Celery is one of nature's convenience foods. Available year-round, it is very versatile and if stored in a vented plastic bag will keep for about a week in the crisper. Its slightly salty flavor complements a wide variety of foods and makes celery a useful crudité. It adds crunch to salads and flavor to soups and stews. If you run out of parsley, use celery leaves as a garnish instead. When purchasing celery, choose heads that are firm and tight, with ribs that snap easily, and avoid any that seem woody. When it begins to pass its peak, break off the ribs and refresh in a bowl of ice water for 30 minutes.

Best-Ever Cholent

This version of a Sabbath dish traditionally made by observant Jews has been adapted from a number of one family's treasured recipes. It is more liquidy than many. Serve it with the conventional condiments: horseradish, dill pickles and good mustard.

Serves 10 to 12

Tips

If the whole piece of brisket won't fit in your slow cooker, cut it in half and lay the two pieces on top of each other.

If you are halving this recipe, be sure to use a small (2½ to 3½ quart) slow cooker.

Celery root is actually a type of celery with crispy white flesh and a pleasing peppery flavor. Since it oxidizes quickly on contact with air, be sure to use it as soon as it is shredded or toss with 1 tbsp (15 mL) lemon juice and water to prevent discoloration. It is usually available in fall and winter. If you can't find it, substitute 6 stalks of diced celery instead. If using celery, soften it in oil along with the carrots and onions.

Use pearled, pot or whole barley in this recipe — whichever you prefer.

- **Large (minimum 5 quart) slow cooker**

½ cup	dried red kidney beans, soaked and drained	125 mL
½ cup	dried white navy or kidney beans, soaked and drained	125 mL
4 to 5 lbs	double beef brisket, trimmed (see Tips, left)	2 to 2.5 kg
2	bone-in English-style short ribs (about 8 oz/250 g)	2
1 tbsp	olive oil	15 mL
2	large potatoes, peeled and cut into ½-inch (1 cm) cubes	2
3	onions, finely chopped	3
4	carrots, peeled and diced	4
6	cloves garlic, minced	6
2 tsp	dried thyme leaves	10 mL
2 tsp	each salt and cracked black peppercorns	10 mL
2 cups	shredded peeled celery root (see Tips, left)	500 mL
½ cup	barley (see Tips, left)	125 mL
4 cups	beef stock, divided	1 L
	Horseradish	
	Dill pickles	
	Dijon or grainy mustard	

1. Pat brisket and short ribs dry. In a large skillet, heat oil over medium-high heat. Add brisket, fat side down, and brown, turning once, about 6 minutes. Transfer to slow cooker stoneware. Add short ribs and cook, turning, until well browned, about 6 minutes. Transfer to stoneware. Add potatoes to skillet, in batches, and cook, stirring, until lightly browned, about 4 minutes. Transfer to stoneware as completed. Drain off all but 2 tbsp (30 mL) of fat.

Complete Step 2, adding 1 tbsp (15 mL) oil to pan before softening vegetables. Cover and refrigerate mixture for up to 2 days. When you're ready to cook, complete the recipe.

2. Reduce heat to medium. Add onions and carrots and cook, stirring, until softened, about 7 minutes. Add garlic, thyme, salt and peppercorns and cook, stirring and scraping up brown bits from bottom of pan, for 1 minute. Add celery root and barley and toss to coat. Add beans and 2 cups (500 mL) of the stock and bring to a boil, stirring and scraping up brown bits from pan. Boil for 1 minute.

3. Transfer to stoneware. Add remaining stock and water barely to cover. Cover and cook on Low for 8 to 10 hours or on High for 4 to 5 hours, until meat and beans are very tender. Serve with horseradish, pickles and mustard.

Kim's Mexican Casserole

This dish would be great for a Mexican-themed party. Serve with dollops of sour cream and salsa, garnished with minced seeded jalapeños or finely chopped bell peppers for added crunch and color. On the side, serve a mixed green salad with orange sections.

Makes 8 servings

Tip

Use a nonstick skillet when browning ground turkey, chicken or beef, as it eliminates the need for oil or butter.

- **Preheat oven to 350°F (180°C)**
- **13- by 9-inch (33 by 23 cm) glass baking dish, greased**

1 lb	lean ground beef	500 g
1	envelope (1¼ oz/37 g) taco seasoning mix	1
6	6- or 7-inch (15 or 18 cm) flour tortillas	6
1	can (16 oz/454 mL) refried beans	1
8 oz	shredded Mexican-blend cheese (2 cups/500 mL)	250 g

1. In a large nonstick skillet, over medium-high heat, cook beef and taco seasoning, breaking beef up with the back of a spoon, for 8 to 10 minutes or until beef is no longer pink. Drain off fat.

2. Arrange tortillas in prepared baking dish, overlapping as necessary. Spread half the beans over tortillas, then half the beef mixture. Sprinkle with half the cheese. Repeat layers with the remaining beans, beef mixture and cheese.

3. Cover and bake in preheated oven for 45 minutes or until bubbling.

Involtini con Fagioloni Bianchi
Stuffed Veal Rolls with White Beans

Make sure the veal you use here is as thin as possible. To achieve this, place veal slices between sheets of waxed paper and gently pound with a kitchen mallet or rolling pin, being careful not to tear the meat.

Serves 6

Sauce

1/4 cup	olive oil	60 mL
2 oz	pancetta, chopped	60 g
3	cloves garlic, finely chopped	3
1	medium onion, finely chopped	1
1/4 cup	finely chopped flat-leaf parsley	60 mL
4	large plum tomatoes, peeled and chopped, or canned Italian plum tomatoes, drained	4
3 cups	cooked white beans	750 mL

Filling

8 oz	mushrooms, minced	250 g
1/3 cup	dry red wine	75 mL
4 oz	Italian salami, finely chopped	125 g
1/3 cup	grated Parmigiano-Reggiano	75 mL
1	egg	1
1/2 tsp	salt	2 mL
1/4 tsp	freshly ground black pepper	1 mL
	Dry bread crumbs, as needed	
2 lbs	veal (about 12 slices)	1 kg
1/4 cup	butter	60 mL

1. In a skillet, heat half of the olive oil over medium heat. Add pancetta, 2 of the chopped garlic cloves, the onion and half of the parsley; cook until onion is softened. Add tomatoes and beans; cook for 15 minutes or until slightly thickened. Season with salt and pepper to taste. Transfer beans/sauce mixture to a bowl; set aside.

2. Wipe the skillet clean and sauté remaining garlic in remaining olive oil. Add mushrooms and cook, stirring, for 1 minute. Add wine and cook until it is absorbed by mushrooms. Allow mushroom mixture to cool, then mix with the salami, Parmigiano-Reggiano, egg, salt and pepper. (Add a small amount of dry bread crumbs if too wet.)

3. Spread some of this mixture on each of the veal scallops. Roll slices up firmly and secure each with a toothpick. Wipe skillet clean.

4. Over medium heat, heat butter in the skillet; cook the veal rolls, turning once or twice, for 8 to 10 minutes or until golden brown. (Do not overcook, or they will toughen.) Add beans and their sauce and simmer gently for 15 minutes or until heated through. Serve immediately.

Prairie Fire Beans

Dried beans keep indefinitely and, when eaten with rice or other grains, are a complete protein — high in fiber and complex carbohydrates, as well as low in fat.

In Texas and Mexico, red beans or mottled pinto beans are most common and are the basis for most chili dishes. Further north, the Great Northern bean is grown. This large white bean is the North American version of the haricot bean or Italian cannellini bean. Navy or pea beans are smaller white beans, used for pots of molasses-spiked baked beans or in soups. Heirloom beans like tongues of fire, Anasazi, flageolets and rattlesnakes have taken on a new cachet as today's Western cooks search for healthier ways to cut down on fat and protein in their traditionally meat-based diets.

Serves 10

2 lbs	dried pinto beans (about 5 cups/1.25 L), soaked overnight in water to cover	1 kg
1	large ham hock or ham bone	1
1	small whole onion, peeled	1
Pinch	salt	Pinch
2 tbsp	butter	30 mL
1 lb	sharp Cheddar cheese, shredded	500 g
1 tsp	Prairie Fire hot sauce or other hot sauce	5 mL
1 cup	finely chopped onions	250 mL
2	cloves garlic, minced	2
	Additional hot sauce to taste	
	Salt and pepper to taste	

1. In a large saucepan, combine drained beans, ham hock, whole onion and a pinch of salt. Add cold water to cover beans by 2 inches (5 cm). Bring to a boil, reduce heat to low and simmer, covered, for 1 hour or until beans are tender.

2. Discard ham hock and onion. Drain beans; return to saucepan. Stir in butter, cheese, hot sauce, onions and garlic. Cook, covered, over low heat for 20 minutes or until cheese melts and everything is tender.

3. Season to taste with additional hot sauce, salt and pepper.

Braised Stuffed Bean Curd

In this Chinese dish, the bean curd is stuffed with either a meat or vegetarian filling, then braised; the vegetarian filling is given on page 181 (see Variation). Served with a green vegetable and rice, this constitutes a rich and tasty main course.

the vegetarian filling is given on page 181 (see Variation).

Serves 4 to 5

Tip

Bean curd (*dofu* in Chinese or *tofu* in Japanese) is a cooked, solid form of soybean milk that has been used in Chinese cookery for at least 2,000 years and has spread throughout East and Southeast Asia. It is bland by nature and therefore acts as a good background for tasty sauces. Although it is very important as a protein source for vegetarians — in North America it is almost synonymous with vegetarian food — Asians often cook bean curd with meat or fish. It helps a small amount of meat go a long way.

2 lbs	bean curd or firm tofu, cut into 6 pieces about 2½ inches (7 cm) square	1 kg
¼ cup	cornstarch	60 mL
1 cup	vegetable oil	250 mL
2 tbsp	finely chopped green onion, white part only	30 mL
6 oz	ground pork	175 g
¼ tsp	white pepper	1 mL
1 cup	finely chopped mushrooms	250 mL
2 tsp	Chinese rice wine or dry sherry or sake	10 mL
¼ tsp	salt	1 mL
1	beaten egg	1
2 tbsp	finely chopped green onion, green part only	30 mL
2 tbsp	finely chopped Chinese celery, cilantro or parsley	30 mL
1 tbsp	cornstarch	15 mL
½ tsp	sesame oil	2 mL
2 tbsp	grated gingerroot	30 mL
1 cup	chicken stock	250 mL
2 tbsp	soy sauce	30 mL

1. Drain and rinse bean curd; weigh down with a plate for at least 30 minutes to remove excess water. Pat dry with paper towels. Dip all sides in cornstarch, shaking off extra. In a nonstick frying pan, heat oil over medium-high heat; when oil is hot, cook bean curd for 5 minutes per side or until golden. Drain on paper towels. Cool.

2. Remove all but 1 tbsp (15 mL) oil from the frying pan; cook white part of green onion until softened. Stir in pork and pepper; cook, stirring, until no longer pink. Stir in mushrooms; cook for 30 seconds. Stir in rice wine and salt; cook until liquid evaporates. Remove from heat; cool. Drain off any liquid, adding it to the stock. Mix meat with egg, green part of green onion, celery, cornstarch and sesame oil.

3. Cut each cooked bean curd cake in half horizontally. Scoop 2 tsp (10 mL) of bean curd from center of each half; fill indentation in each bottom half with meat filling, mounding it up, and cover with a top half.

4. Wrap ginger in a piece of cheesecloth and squeeze out juice over a bowl. Mix ginger pulp with 2 tbsp (30 mL) of the stock and squeeze out juice through cheesecloth again. In a large shallow saucepan, combine ginger juice, remaining stock and soy sauce; bring to a simmer over medium heat. Carefully add stuffed bean curd cakes, cover and simmer for 12 minutes. Transfer cakes to warm serving platter; cut in half diagonally with a sharp knife. Bring sauce to a boil; cook until slightly thickened and pour over bean curd.

Variation

For a vegetarian dish, replace the meat with 7 oz (210 g) finely diced eggplant. Mix eggplant with 1 tsp (5 mL) salt and let sit 20 minutes. Wrap eggplant in cloth or paper towels and squeeze out as much liquid as you can. Proceed with recipe as above, reducing added salt to $1/8$ tsp (0.5 mL) and replacing chicken stock with vegetable stock.

Braised Roasted Pork with Tofu and Green Onions

Crispy-skinned and succulent roasted pork, sold by the pound, is one of our favorite treats from the Chinese barbecue shop. It's hard not to eat it right away, but if there's anything left, this is a great way to use it up.

4	dried Chinese black mushrooms	4
1 tbsp	vegetable oil	15 mL
5	thin slices gingerroot	5
1 tsp	minced garlic	5 mL
1 lb	crispy-skin roasted pork or barbecued pork or leftover roast pork, cut into 1/2-inch (1 cm) slices	500 g
2 tbsp	oyster sauce	30 mL
1 tbsp	soy sauce	15 mL
1 tbsp	dark soy sauce	15 mL
1/2 cup	chicken stock or water	125 mL
	Salt and freshly ground black pepper to taste	
1 tbsp	cornstarch, dissolved in 2 tbsp (30 mL) chicken stock or water	15 mL
2	packages (10 oz/300 g) soft tofu, cut into pieces 1 inch (2.5 cm) by 1/2 inch (1 cm)	2
3	green onions, cut into 1-inch (2.5 cm) lengths	3

1. In a heatproof bowl, soak mushrooms in boiling water for 15 minutes. Remove stems, slice caps thinly and set aside.

2. In a wok or deep skillet, heat oil over medium-high heat. Add gingerroot, garlic and mushrooms and sauté until fragrant (about 1 minute). Add pork and stir-fry for 1 minute. Add oyster sauce, soy sauce, dark soy sauce and stock; mix well. Reduce heat to medium and cook for 3 minutes. Season to taste with salt and pepper. Add dissolved cornstarch and cook until sauce is thickened.

3. Gently fold tofu and green onions into mixture; cover and allow to absorb flavors for 2 minutes. Transfer to a deep platter and serve immediately.

Make-Ahead Southwestern Pork Stew

Here's a soothing dish to serve for casual get-togethers. This stew requires no more preparation time than a stir-fry or one-pot dish. Cutting the meat into smaller pieces also shortens the cooking time.

Serves 6

Tip

Lean stewing beef can be substituted for the pork. For a vegetarian dish, replace meat with cubes of firm tofu. Add along with kidney beans.

4 tsp	olive oil	20 mL
1 lb	lean stewing pork, cut into $\frac{3}{4}$-inch (2 cm) cubes	500 g
2	medium onions, chopped	2
3	cloves garlic, finely chopped	3
4 tsp	chili powder	20 mL
$1\frac{1}{2}$ tsp	dried oregano	7 mL
1 tsp	ground cumin	5 mL
$\frac{3}{4}$ tsp	salt	3 mL
$\frac{1}{2}$ tsp	red pepper flakes	2 mL
3 tbsp	all-purpose flour	45 mL
2 cups	beef stock or chicken stock	500 mL
1	can (28 oz/796 mL) tomatoes, chopped	1
2	bell peppers (assorted colors), cubed	2
2 cups	frozen corn kernels	500 mL
1	can (19 oz/540 mL) kidney beans or black beans, rinsed and drained	1
	Chopped cilantro (optional)	

1. In a large Dutch oven, heat half the oil over high heat; brown pork in batches. Transfer to a plate. Add remaining oil to pan; reduce heat to medium. Add onions, garlic, chili powder, oregano, cumin, salt and red pepper flakes; cook, stirring, for 2 minutes or until softened.

2. Sprinkle with flour; stir in stock and tomatoes. Bring to a boil, stirring until thickened. Return pork and accumulated juices to pan; reduce heat, cover and simmer for 1 hour or until meat is tender.

3. Add bell peppers, corn and kidney beans; simmer, covered, for 15 minutes or until vegetables are tender. Garnish with chopped cilantro, if desired.

Pork and Black Bean Stew with Sweet Potatoes

This is a gorgeous stew — tender pieces of boneless pork, highlighted by shiny black beans and cubes of deep orange sweet potatoes. A sprinkling of chopped cilantro just before serving adds real Western flavor and even more bright color to the mix. I like this healthy combination served with a mound of creamy mashed potatoes or cornbread.

Serves 6

Tip

To save time, use canned black beans, rinsed and drained.

- **Preheat oven to 350°F (180°C)**
- **12-cup (3 L) casserole dish with lid**

2 tbsp	olive oil	30 mL
4 lbs	boneless pork shoulder, cut into 1-inch (2.5 cm) cubes	2 kg
2 tbsp	all-purpose flour	30 mL
2	sweet potatoes (about 1 lb/500 g), peeled and cubed	2
1½ cups	chicken stock	375 mL
1½ cups	chopped onions	375 mL
1 cup	dry white wine	250 mL
½ cup	chopped fresh parsley	125 mL
¼ cup	red wine vinegar	60 mL
6	cloves garlic, minced	6
1 tbsp	ground cumin	15 mL
2 cups	cooked black beans	500 mL
1 tsp	ground cumin	5 mL
½ tsp	freshly ground black pepper	2 mL
½ cup	chopped cilantro	125 mL

1. In a large frying pan, heat oil over medium-high heat. In batches, cook pork, turning occasionally, for 5 minutes or until browned. Transfer pork to casserole dish as it is browned.

2. Sprinkle flour over the pork and toss. Add the sweet potatoes, chicken stock, onions, wine, parsley, vinegar, half of the garlic and 1 tbsp (15 mL) cumin; mix well. Cover and bake for 1 hour.

3. Stir in beans, 1 tsp (5 mL) cumin, pepper and remaining garlic. Bake, uncovered, for 15 minutes or until slightly thickened. Just before serving, stir in the cilantro.

Maple Baked Pork and Beans with Caramelized Apples

This recipe makes a delicious old-fashioned bean dish, good alongside your barbecue beef on a bun — or even with pancakes — for a Stampede breakfast. It's a variation of a recipe Calgarian Rick Gauthier entered in a bean contest and for which he won second place.

Serves 8

- **12-cup (3 L) bean pot or casserole dish**

2 cups	dried navy beans, rinsed	500 mL
1 tbsp	molasses	15 mL
8 oz	back bacon, preferably double-smoked	250 g
4	Granny Smith apples	4
1	large onion, chopped	1
½ cup	maple syrup	125 mL
1 tbsp	dry mustard	15 mL
1 tsp	coarse salt	5 mL
¼ cup	butter	60 mL
¼ cup	packed brown sugar	60 mL
½ cup	rum	125 mL

1. In a saucepan combine beans, molasses and 8 cups (2 L) water; bring to a boil. Remove from heat; let stand, covered, for 1 hour. Uncover. Bring to a boil, reduce heat to low and simmer, covered, for 45 minutes to 1 hour or until beans are starting to get tender. Drain.

2. Preheat oven to 325°F (160°C). Chop bacon into thin slivers. Peel and chop 2 of the apples. In a bean pot, combine drained beans, bacon, chopped apples, onion, maple syrup, mustard and salt. Cover and bake for 3 hours. Stir; if beans seem dry, add a little hot water. Cover and bake 1 to 2 hours longer.

3. Meanwhile, core remaining apples and slice into ½-inch (1 cm) rings. In a frying pan, melt butter over medium heat. Stir in brown sugar; cook for 2 minutes, stirring occasionally. Add apple rings, stirring to coat with sugar. Add half of the rum; increase heat to medium-high and cook, turning rings occasionally, for 8 minutes or until the liquid evaporates and apples are tender. Set aside.

4. Remove cover from bean pot and arrange caramelized apple slices on top of the beans. Bake, uncovered, for 30 minutes. Just before serving, pour the remaining rum slowly over the beans.

Mediterranean Pork and Beans

This dish is loaded with flavor. To complement the Mediterranean ingredients, accompany this with a platter of marinated roasted peppers. Add warm crusty bread, such as ciabatta.

Tips

To purée garlic, use a fine, sharp-toothed grater, such as those made by Microplane.

Use 2 cups (250 mL) dried white kidney or navy beans, soaked, cooked and drained (see Basic Beans in the Slow Cooker, page 277), or 2 cans (each 14 to 19 oz/398 to 540 mL), drained and rinsed.

This makes a large quantity but reheats well.

Make Ahead

Complete Step 1. Heat 1 tbsp (15 mL) of the oil and complete Step 3. Cover and refrigerate meat and onion mixtures separately for up to 2 days. When you're ready to cook, complete the recipe.

- **Large (minimum 4 quart) slow cooker**

1 tbsp	puréed garlic (see Tips, left)	15 mL
1 tsp	salt	5 mL
½ tsp	cracked black pepper	2 mL
2 lbs	boneless pork shoulder blade (butt), trimmed and cut into bite-size pieces	1 kg
2 tbsp	olive oil (approx.), divided	30 mL
6	anchovy fillets, minced	6
3	onions, thinly sliced	3
2 tsp	dried thyme	10 mL
1 cup	dry white wine	250 mL
1 tsp	white wine vinegar	5 mL
1	can (14 oz/398 mL) diced tomatoes, with juice	1
4 cups	cooked white beans, drained and rinsed	1 L
1 cup	finely chopped fresh parsley	250 mL
1 cup	chopped pitted kalamata olives (about 48)	250 mL
1 tsp	paprika (preferably smoked), dissolved in 1 tbsp (15 mL) white wine or water	5 mL

1. In a bowl large enough to accommodate the pork, combine garlic, salt and pepper. Add pork and toss to coat. Cover and refrigerate overnight. Pat pork dry.

2. In a skillet, heat 1 tbsp (15 mL) of the oil over medium-high heat for 30 seconds. Add pork to pan, in batches; cook, stirring, until lightly browned, about 5 minutes per batch, adding oil between batches if necessary. Using a slotted spoon, transfer to slow cooker stoneware as completed.

3. Reduce heat to medium and add more oil to the pan if necessary. Add anchovies and onions; cook, stirring, until onions are softened, about 3 minutes. Add thyme and cook, stirring, for 1 minute. Add wine and vinegar; cook for 2 minutes, stirring and scraping up any brown bits on the bottom of the pan. Add tomatoes with juice and bring to a boil. Transfer to stoneware and stir well.

4. Stir in beans. Cover and cook on Low for 8 hours or on High for 4 hours, until pork is very tender (it should be falling apart). Stir in parsley, olives and paprika solution. Cover and cook on High for 15 minutes, until heated through.

Home-Style Pork and Beans

There is nothing fancy about this dish — it's real down-home cooking that is simply delicious. Serve it with thick slices of hearty bread, a big salad and cold beer or robust red wine. This is a great recipe for a tailgate or Super Bowl party.

Serves 6

Tips

If you are halving this recipe, be sure to use a small (approx. 1 1/2 to 3 quart) slow cooker.

If you prefer, cook the beans in your slow cooker (see Basic Beans in the Slow Cooker, page 277) and skip Step 2, reserving 1 1/2 cups (375 mL) of the cooking liquid.

If you are using pork belly, cut it into two equal pieces. If bacon, slice it thinly.

Make Ahead

Complete Step 1, retaining enough cooking liquid to cover the cooked beans. Cover and refrigerate for up to 2 days. When you're ready to cook, drain the beans, reserving 1 1/2 cups (375 mL) of the cooking liquid, and continue with the recipe.

• **Medium to large (3 1/2 to 6 quart) slow cooker**

2 cups	dried white beans such as Great Northern or navy, soaked, drained and rinsed (see Tips, left)	500 mL
1/2 cup	pure maple syrup	125 mL
1/2 cup	grainy mustard	125 mL
1/2 cup	ketchup	125 mL
1/2 cup	tomato paste	125 mL
1 tsp	salt	5 mL
1 tsp	cracked black peppercorns	5 mL
8 oz	chunk pork belly or bacon (see Tips, left)	250 g
3	onions, finely chopped	3
4	cloves garlic, minced	4

1. In a saucepan, combine rinsed beans with 6 cups (1.5 L) fresh cold water (see Tips, left). Bring to a boil over medium heat. Reduce heat and simmer until beans are just tender to the bite but not fully cooked, about 30 minutes. Scoop out 1 1/2 cups (375 mL) of the cooking liquid and set aside. Drain beans and set aside, discarding remaining liquid.

2. In a large measuring cup, combine maple syrup, mustard, ketchup, tomato paste, salt, peppercorns and 1/2 cup (125 mL) of the bean cooking liquid. Stir well and set aside.

3. In slow cooker stoneware, place half the pork. Add half the onions and garlic, sprinkling evenly over bottom of stoneware. Add half of the beans and remaining pork. Repeat with remaining onion, garlic and beans. Pour tomato mixture evenly over top.

4. Cover and cook on Low for 8 hours or on High for 4 hours, adding more bean cooking liquid, if necessary to keep beans moist, until beans are tender and mixture is hot and bubbly.

Molasses Baked Beans

Here's an old-time favorite that stirs memories of the pioneer spirit. This rustic dish is a winter standby and wonderful when served with home-baked bread.

Serves 8

Tip

For a vegetarian version, omit bacon and cook onions and garlic in 2 tbsp (30 mL) vegetable oil.

- **Preheat oven to 300°F (150°C)**
- **12-cup (3 L) casserole dish or bean pot**

1 lb	dried Great Northern or white pea beans (about 2¼ cups/560 mL), rinsed and picked over	500 g
6	slices lean smoky bacon, chopped	6
1	large onion, chopped	1
3	cloves garlic, finely chopped	3
1	can (7½ oz/213 mL) tomato sauce	1
⅓ cup	molasses	75 mL
¼ cup	packed brown sugar	60 mL
2 tbsp	balsamic vinegar	30 mL
2 tsp	dry mustard	10 mL
1 tsp	salt	5 mL
¼ tsp	pepper	1 mL

1. In a Dutch oven, combine beans with 6 cups (1.5 L) cold water. Bring to a boil over high heat; boil for 2 minutes. Remove from heat, cover and let stand for 1 hour.

2. Drain beans and cover with 8 cups (2 L) cold water; bring to a boil. Reduce heat and simmer, covered, for 30 to 40 minutes or until beans are just tender but still hold their shape. Drain, reserving 2 cups (500 mL) cooking liquid. Place beans in casserole dish or bean pot.

3. Meanwhile, in a saucepan, cook bacon over medium heat, stirring often, for 5 minutes or until crisp. Drain all but 2 tbsp (30 mL) fat in pan. Add onion and garlic; cook, stirring, for 3 minutes or until softened.

4. Add 2 cups (500 mL) reserved bean-cooking liquid, tomato sauce, molasses, brown sugar, balsamic vinegar, mustard, salt and pepper. Stir into beans.

5. Cover and bake in preheated oven for 2½ to 3 hours or until most of liquid has been absorbed.

The Best Pork 'n' Beans

A great make-ahead meal and a favorite side dish for family cookouts and barbecues at all times of year. Serve with lots of freshly baked cornbread. The beans taste even better when gently reheated in the oven the following day.

Serves 4 to 6

• **Large casserole with lid**

2 cups	dried navy beans	500 mL
1	bay leaf	1
	Salt and freshly ground black pepper	
2 tbsp	vegetable oil	30 mL
1	onion, coarsely chopped	1
2	cloves garlic, minced	2
1 cup	ketchup	250 mL
¼ cup	light (fancy) molasses	60 mL
¼ cup	packed brown sugar	60 mL
2 tbsp	Worcestershire sauce	30 mL
12 oz	smoked pork hock	375 g

1. Soak beans in water to cover overnight in the refrigerator.

2. Drain beans. In a saucepan, cover beans with 8 cups (2 L) fresh water and add bay leaf. Bring to a boil over medium-high heat. Reduce heat and simmer, partially covered, until beans are tender, 35 to 45 minutes. Remove from heat and add 1 tsp (5 mL) salt. Let stand for 5 minutes. Drain and set aside.

3. Meanwhile, preheat oven to 325°F (160°C).

4. In a large skillet, heat oil over medium heat. Add onion and sauté until soft, 4 to 5 minutes. Add garlic and sauté for 1 to 2 minutes. Set aside.

5. In a bowl, combine ketchup, ½ cup (125 mL) water, molasses, brown sugar, Worcestershire sauce, 1 tsp (5 mL) salt and ¼ tsp (1 mL) pepper. Set aside.

6. In casserole, combine beans, onion mixture, molasses mixture and pork hock. Stir to mix everything together well. Cover casserole and bake in preheated oven until beans are very tender, 1¾ to 2 hours. Remove pork hock and, when cool enough to handle, pull off pieces of lean meat, discarding fat, trim and bone, and return meat to the pot. Taste and adjust seasoning.

Variation

Vegetarian Baked Beans: Omit pork hock. Add 1 tbsp (15 mL) ground coffee to molasses mixture.

Bistro Lentils with Smoked Sausage

It's Friday night. You've worked hard all week. Don't even bother setting the table. Here's a supper dish that's easy to balance on your lap while you relax in front of the TV set. As an added bonus, this dish goes great with a cold beer.

Serves 6

Tip

Any kind of smoked sausage or ham works well. The smaller-sized green Laird lentils hold their shape in cooking and are preferred for this recipe.

3½ cups	chicken stock or vegetable stock (approximate)	875 mL
1½ cups	lentils, picked over and rinsed	375 mL
½ tsp	dried thyme	2 mL
2 tbsp	olive oil	30 mL
1 cup	diced red onions	250 mL
3	cloves garlic, finely chopped	3
2	carrots, peeled and diced	2
1 cup	diced fennel or celery	250 mL
1	red bell pepper, diced	1
2 tbsp	balsamic vinegar	30 mL
8 oz	smoked sausage, such as kielbasa, cut into ½-inch (1 cm) chunks	250 g
	Black pepper	
¼ cup	chopped fresh parsley	60 mL

1. In a large saucepan, bring stock to a boil over high heat; add lentils and thyme. Reduce heat to medium-low and simmer, covered, for 25 to 30 minutes or until lentils are just tender but still hold their shape.

2. Meanwhile, heat oil in a large nonstick skillet over medium heat. Add onions, garlic, carrots and fennel; cook, stirring often, for 8 minutes. Add red pepper; cook, stirring, for 2 minutes or until vegetables are just tender. Stir in vinegar; remove from heat.

3. Add vegetables and smoked sausage to lentils in saucepan; season to taste with pepper. Cover and cook for 5 to 8 minutes or until sausage is heated through. (Add more stock or water, if necessary, to prevent lentils from sticking.) Stir in parsley. Serve warm or at room temperature.

Sausage-Spiked Peas 'n' Rice

What could be easier than this combination of brown and wild rice and split peas, seasoned with sausage and fennel? The flavors are fantastic and the way the split peas dissolve into the sauce creates a luscious texture that is extremely satisfying. Add a simple green salad or some steamed green beans and enjoy.

Makes 6 servings

Tips

You can cook the split peas yourself, reserving 1/4 cup (60 mL) of the cooking liquid, or you can use a can (14 to 19 oz/398 to 540 mL) yellow split peas, rinsed and drained, plus 1/4 cup (60 mL) water, instead. Be aware that the canned peas will be much higher in sodium than those you cook yourself.

If you have fresh thyme on hand, substitute 2 whole sprigs, stem and all, for the dried. Remove and discard before serving.

2 cups	cooked yellow split peas, with 1/4 cup (60 mL) cooking liquid (see Tips, left)	500 mL
1 tbsp	olive oil	15 mL
12 oz	hot or mild Italian sausage, removed from casings	375 g
1	bulb fennel, cored and chopped	1
1	onion, finely chopped	1
4	cloves garlic, minced	4
1 tsp	dried thyme leaves (see Tips, left)	5 mL
	Freshly ground black pepper	
1 cup	brown and wild rice mixture, rinsed and drained	250 mL
2 cups	reduced-sodium chicken stock	500 mL

1. In a large saucepan with a tight-fitting lid or Dutch oven, heat oil over medium heat for 30 seconds. Add sausage, fennel and onion and cook, stirring and breaking sausage up with a spoon, until meat is cooked through, about 6 minutes. Add garlic, thyme, pepper to taste and rice and cook, stirring, for 1 minute. Stir in peas with reserved liquid and stock and bring to a boil.

2. Reduce heat to low. Cover tightly and simmer until grains of wild rice begin to split, about 50 minutes. Ladle into soup plates.

Slow Cooker Method

Complete Step 1. Transfer mixture to slow cooker stoneware. Cover and cook on Low for 8 hours or on High for 4 hours, until wild rice is tender and grains begin to split.

Baked Beans 'n' Barley

If you're a fan of Boston baked beans, this dish is for you. It's every bit as delicious as the best versions of the original. This is the perfect choice for a chilly day or a potluck or tailgate party. If you're serving it for dinner, complete the meal with warm whole-grain rolls and a tossed green salad.

Serves 6

Tips

Although any kind of maple syrup works well in this recipe, the dark amber or grade B versions, which are more strongly flavored are preferable. They are also more economical than the lighter kinds.

Use pearled, pot or whole barley in this recipe — whichever you prefer. Whole (also known as hulled) barley is the most nutritious form of the grain.

If you like heat, the chile peppers add a pleasant note, but they are not essential.

- **Large (minimum 4 quart) slow cooker**

¾ cup	ketchup	175 mL
⅔ cup	pure maple syrup (see Tips, left)	150 mL
4	cloves garlic, minced	4
1 tbsp	minced gingerroot	15 mL
1 tsp	dry mustard	5 mL
1 tsp	salt	5 mL
1 tsp	cracked black peppercorns	5 mL
4 oz	chunk pancetta or salt pork, diced	125 g
2	onions, halved and thinly sliced on the vertical	2
1 cup	barley (see Tips, left), rinsed and drained	250 mL
1 cup	dried navy beans, soaked, cooked and drained, cooking liquid reserved (see pages 6 to 10)	250 mL
2	dried red chile peppers (optional)	2

1. In a bowl, combine ketchup, maple syrup, garlic, ginger, dry mustard, salt and peppercorns. Set aside.

2. In slow cooker stoneware, combine pancetta, onions, barley, beans and ketchup mixture. Stir well. Add reserved bean liquid barely to cover. Cover and cook on Low for 8 hours or on High for 4 hours. Stir in chile peppers, if using. Cover and cook on High for 30 minutes to meld flavors.

Variations

Baked Beans 'n' Wheat Berries: Substitute an equal quantity of wheat, spelt or Kamut berries for the barley.

Crusty Baked Beans 'n' Barley: Forty-five minutes before you're ready to serve, preheat oven to 325°F (160°C). Stir in chile peppers, if using, as per Step 2, but do not cook to meld flavors. If your stoneware insert isn't ovenproof, transfer mixture to a baking dish or individual ramekins. Bake until top is crusty, about 30 minutes. Remove and discard chile peppers, if using.

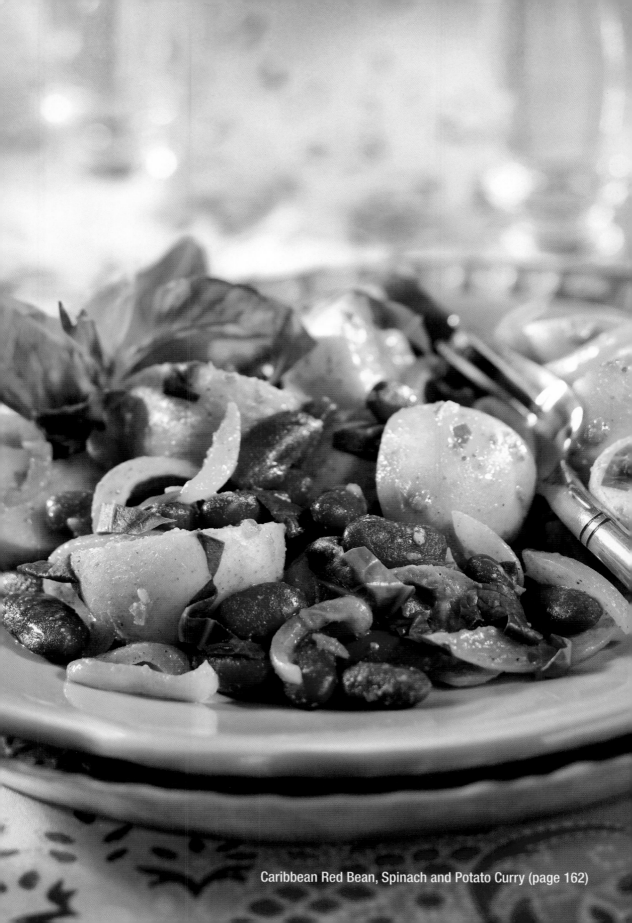

Caribbean Red Bean, Spinach and Potato Curry (page 162)

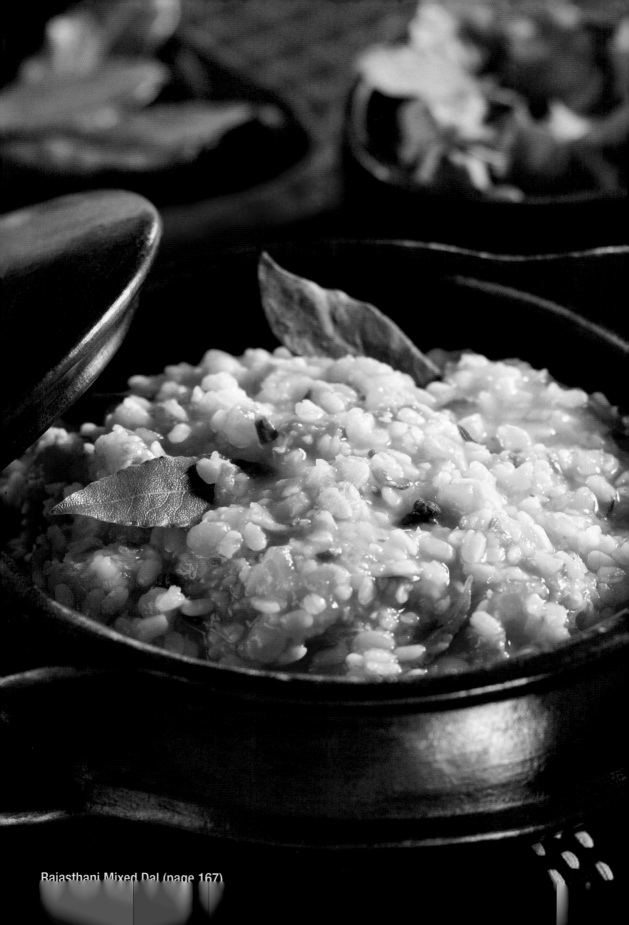

Rajasthani Mixed Dal (page 167)

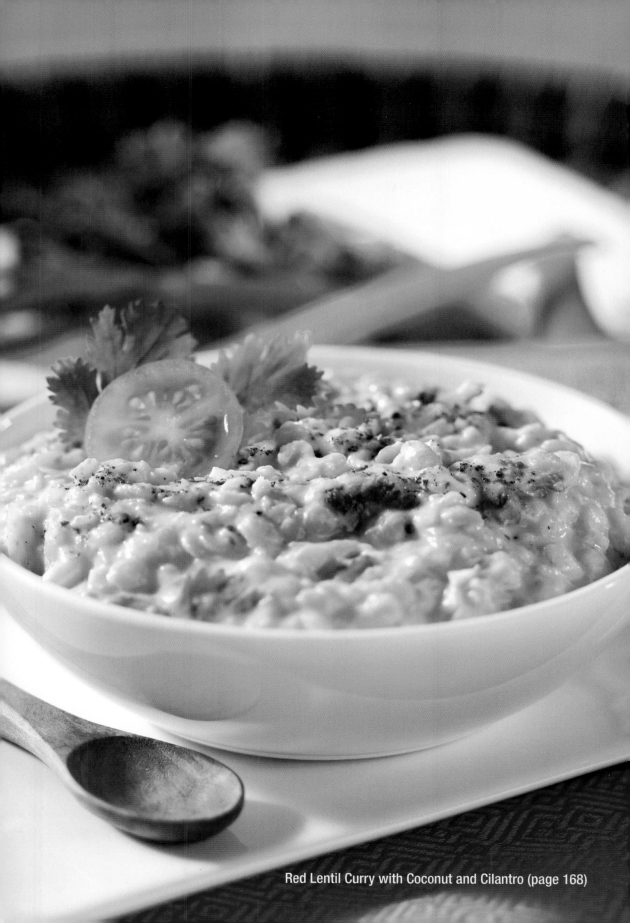

Red Lentil Curry with Coconut and Cilantro (page 168)

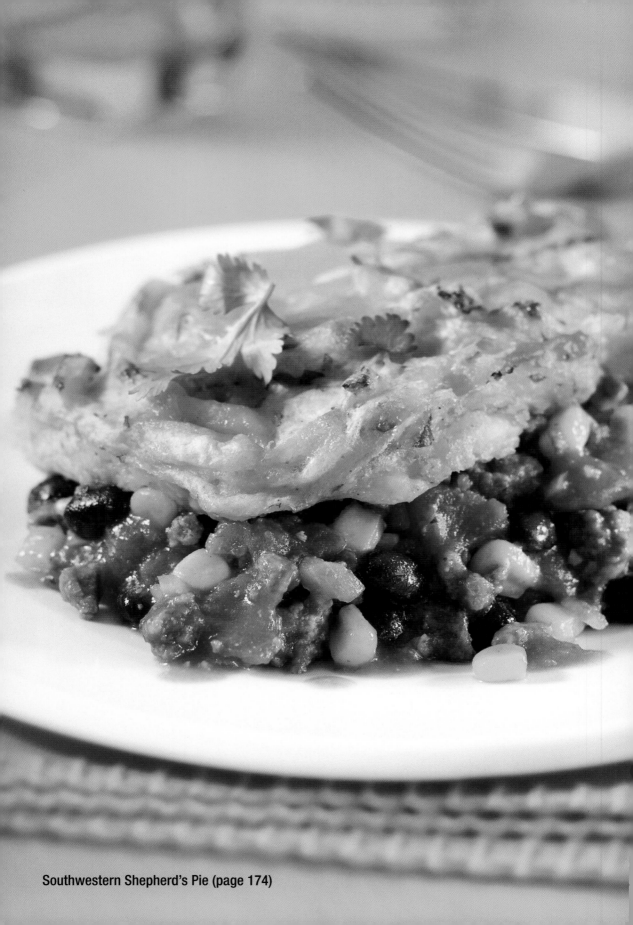

Southwestern Shepherd's Pie (page 174)

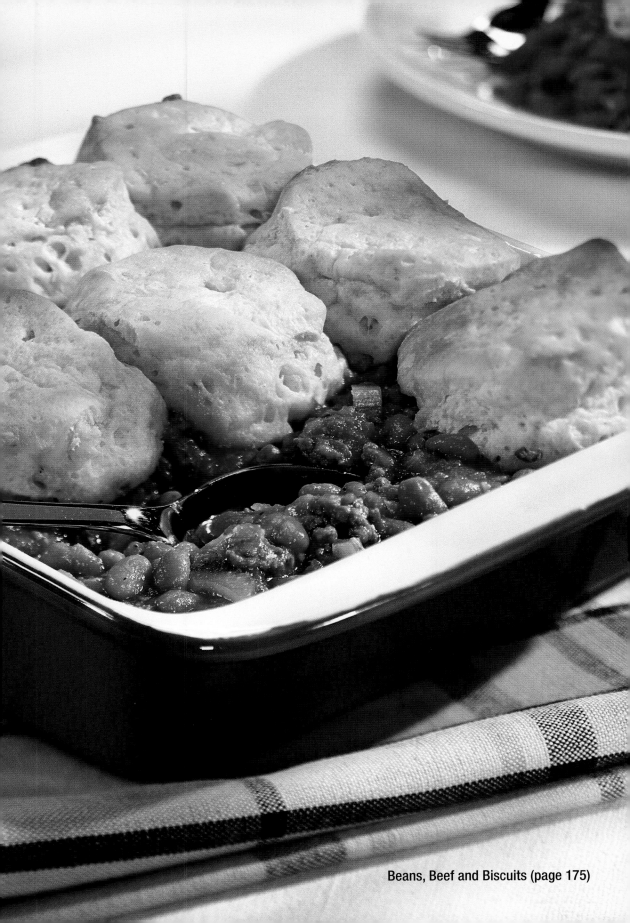

Beans, Beef and Biscuits (page 175)

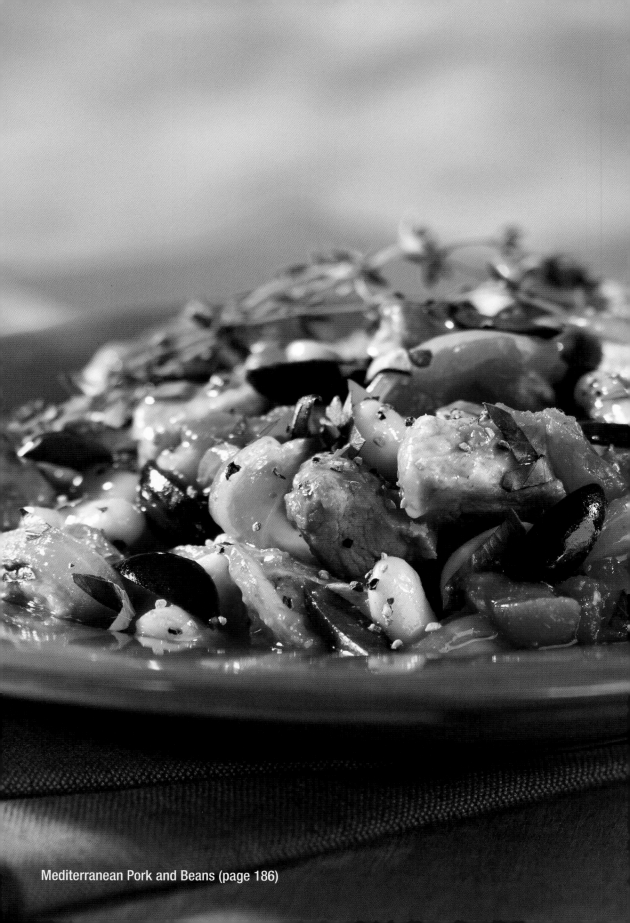

Mediterranean Pork and Beans (page 186)

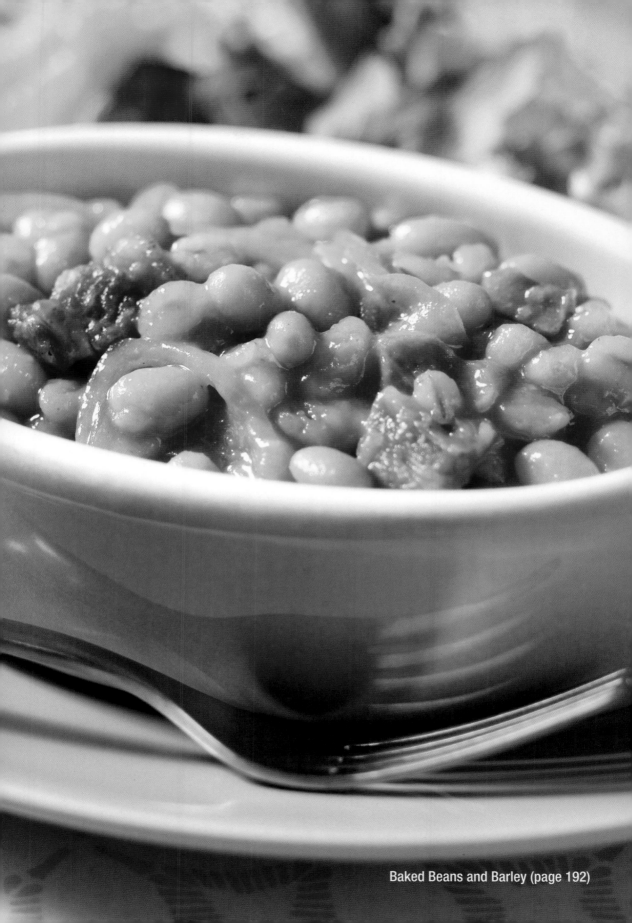

Baked Beans and Barley (page 192)

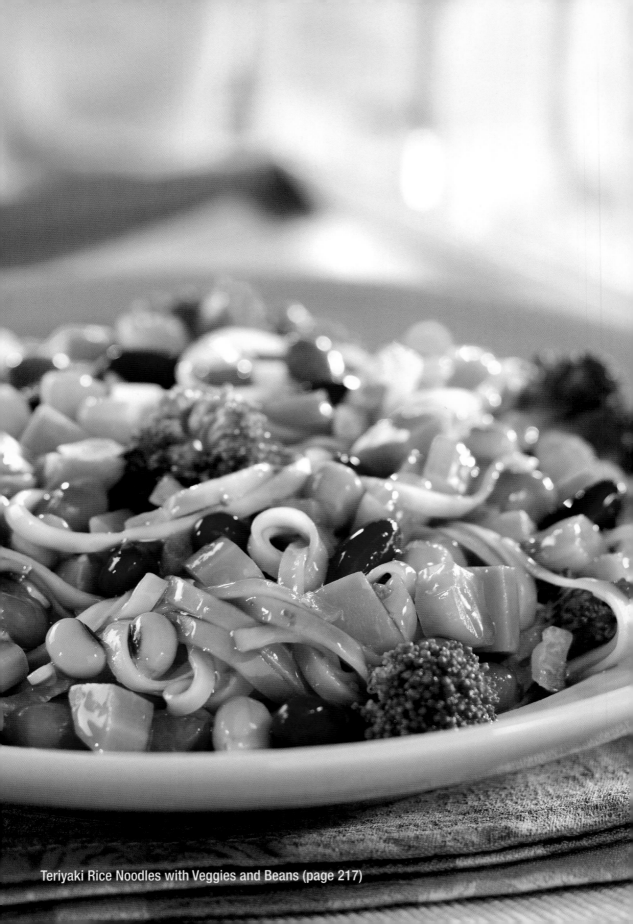

Teriyaki Rice Noodles with Veggies and Beans (page 217)

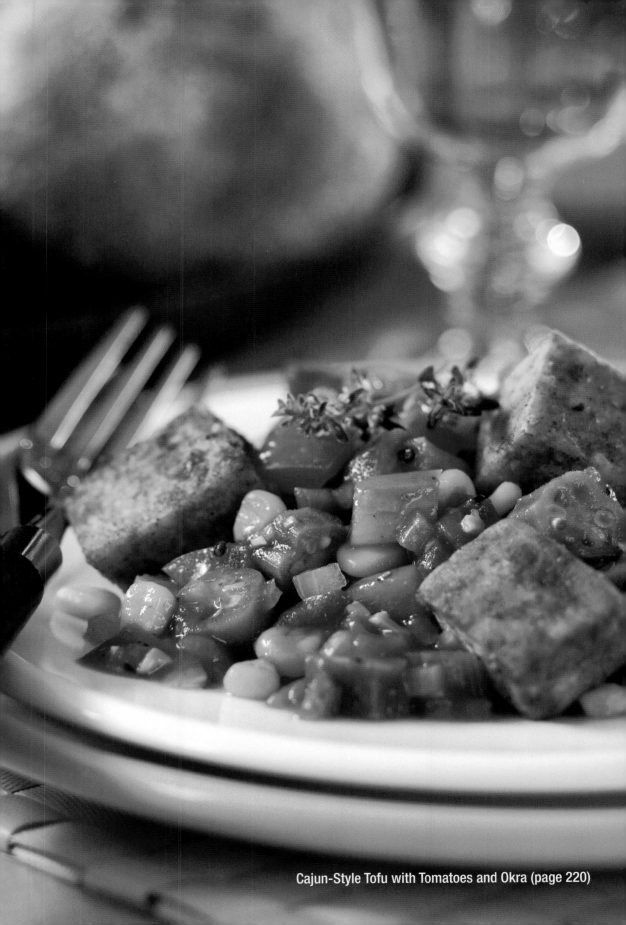

Cajun-Style Tofu with Tomatoes and Okra (page 220)

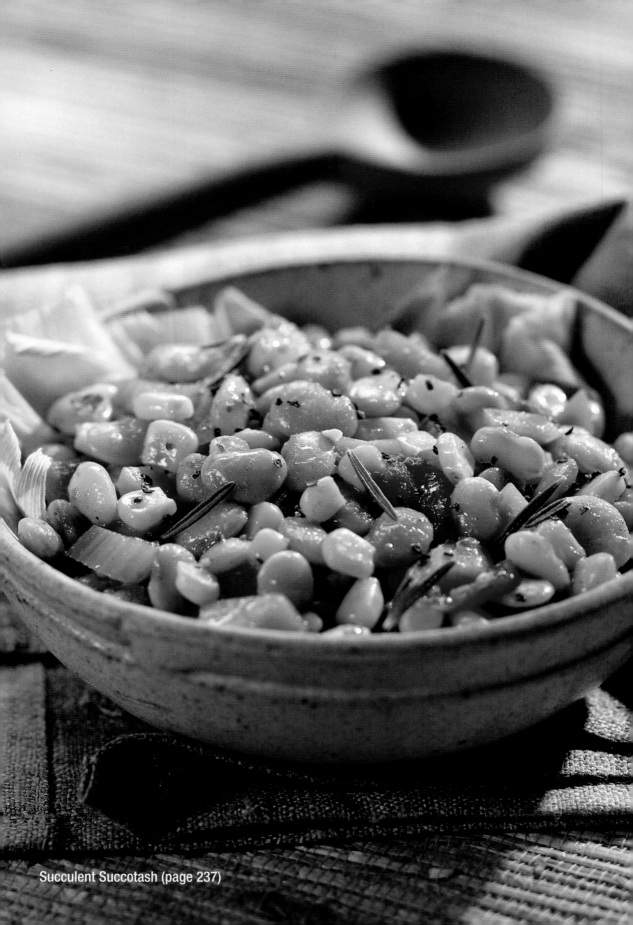

Succulent Succotash (page 237)

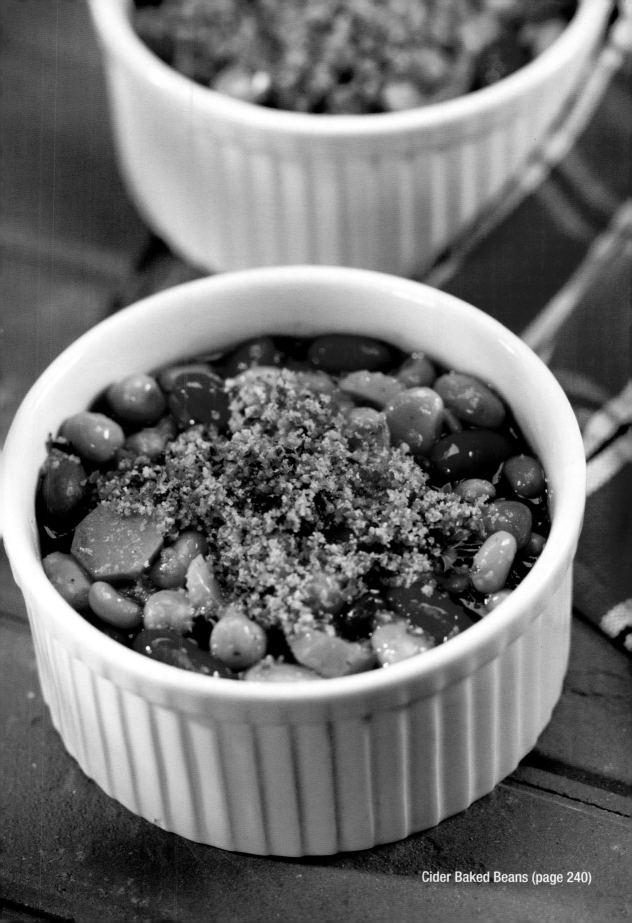

Cider Baked Beans (page 240)

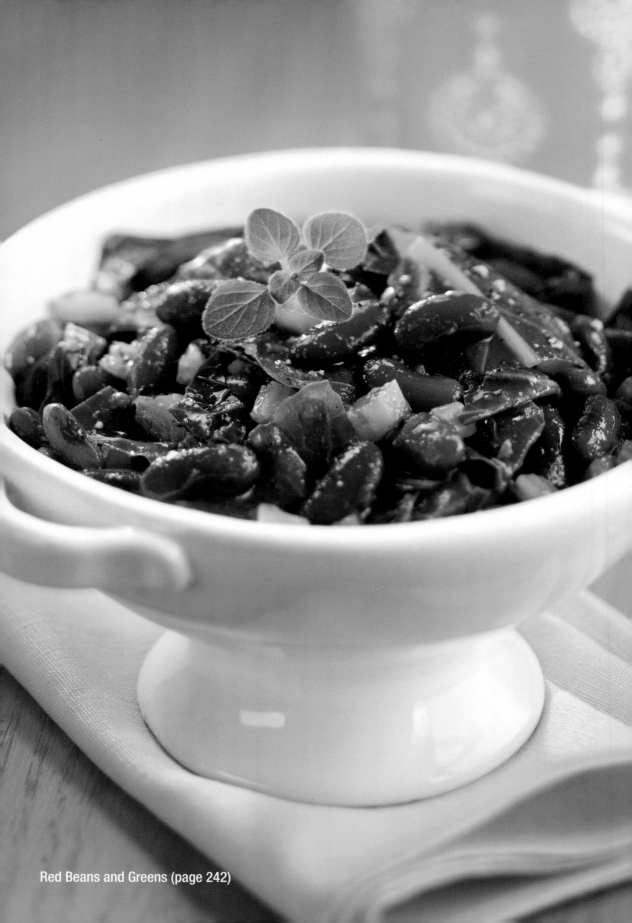

Red Beans and Greens (page 242)

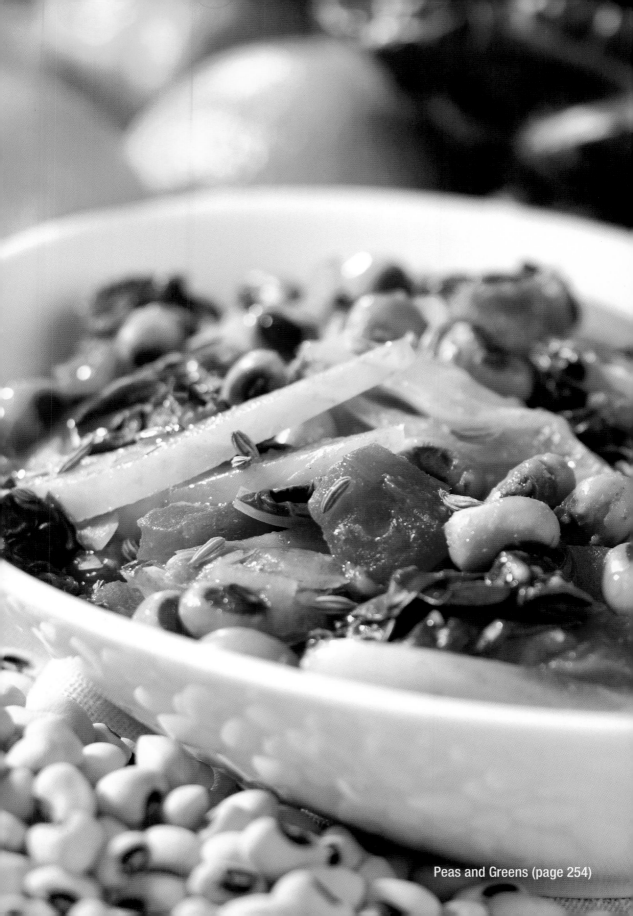

Peas and Greens (page 254)

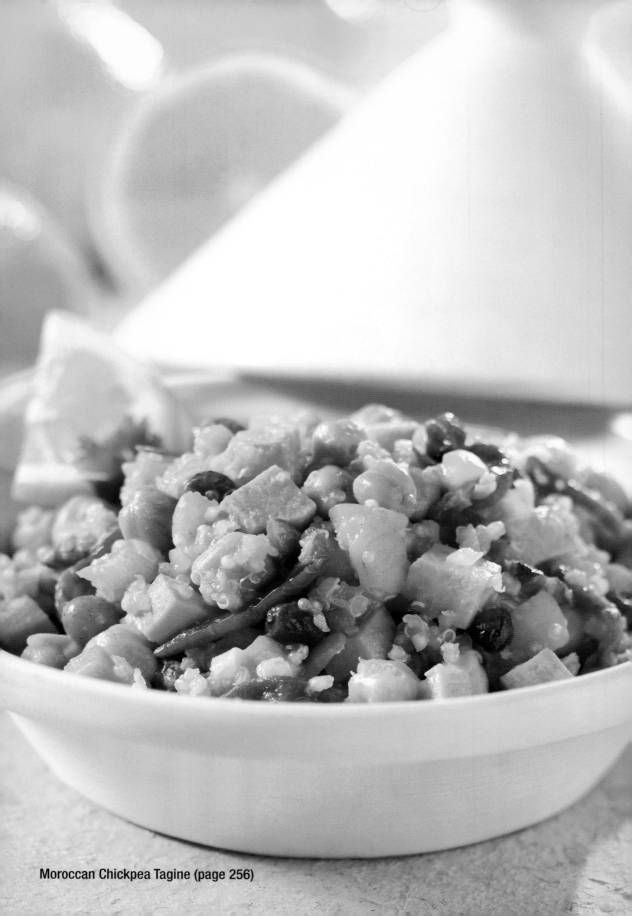

Moroccan Chickpea Tagine (page 256)

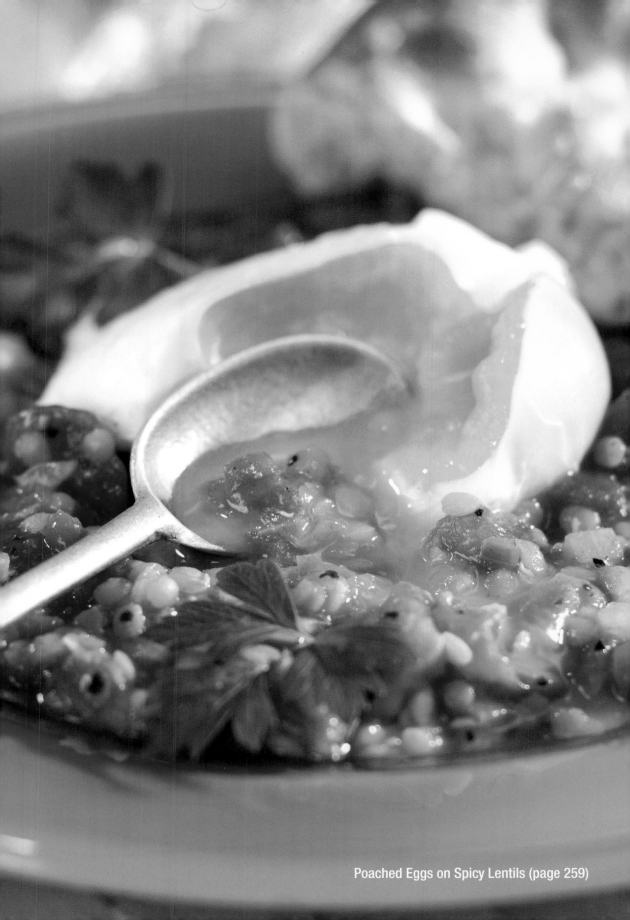

Poached Eggs on Spicy Lentils (page 259)

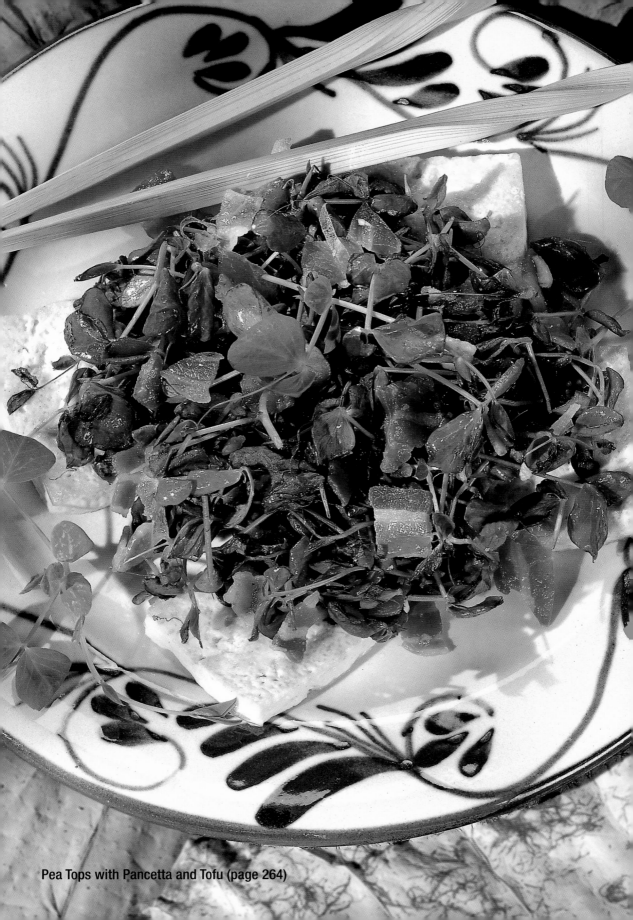

Pea Tops with Pancetta and Tofu (page 264)

Quick Cassoulet

- **Preheat oven to 350°F (180°C)**
- **10-cup (2.5 L) casserole dish**

4	slices bacon, coarsely chopped	4
1 lb	smoked sausage (such as kielbasa), sliced	500 g
1 cup	chopped onion	250 mL
4	cloves garlic, minced	4
1 tbsp	ground coriander	15 mL
1 tsp	ground cumin	5 mL
1 tsp	ground ginger	5 mL
1 tsp	dry mustard	5 mL
Pinch	ground cloves	Pinch
1/2 cup	dry white wine	125 mL
2	cans (each 14 to 19 oz/398 to 540 mL) Great Northern beans, drained and rinsed	2
2 tbsp	chopped fresh Italian (flat-leaf) parsley	30 mL
2 tsp	chopped fresh dill	10 mL
	Salt and freshly ground black pepper to taste	
1/2 cup	seasoned dry bread crumbs	125 mL

1. In a skillet, over medium heat, sauté bacon until crisp. Add sausage and onion; sauté until onion is tender and sausage is lightly browned. Add garlic, coriander, cumin, ginger, mustard and cloves; sauté until aromatic. Add wine, increase heat to high and boil until wine has evaporated.

2. Stir in beans, parsley, dill, salt and pepper. Pack into casserole dish and smooth top. Sprinkle with bread crumbs. Bake in preheated oven for 1 hour, until browned and bubbling.

Cheater's Cassoulet

While it is still a fair bit of work to make this version of the classic French dish, it is not nearly as onerous as the traditional approach, which first roasts the pork and braises the lamb, then combines them with the beans and sausage to simmer. Cassoulet has a real mystique, perhaps because it usually takes several days to make, but it is actually a country dish — rich, delicious and substantial.

Serves 12

Tips

Be sure to use sausage that is seasoned with "traditional French spices." Those containing chile pepper, such as chorizo, will disrupt the flavors of the dish.

Many butchers sell cut-up pork stewing meat, which is fine to use in this recipe.

If you prefer, substitute 1 1/2 cups (375 mL) chicken stock plus 2 tbsp (30 mL) lemon juice for the white wine.

Make Ahead

Complete Step 2. Cover and refrigerate mixture for up to 2 days. When you're ready to cook, complete the recipe.

• **Large (minimum 6 quart) slow cooker**

4 cups	cooked white beans, such as navy or Great Northern, drained and rinsed (see pages 6 to 10)	1 L
2 tbsp	olive oil, divided	30 mL
1 lb	pork sausage, removed from casings (see Tips, left)	500 g
2 lbs	trimmed boneless pork shoulder or blade (butt), cut into 1-inch (2.5 cm) cubes, and patted dry (see Tips, left)	1 kg
1 lb	trimmed lamb shoulder, cut into 1-inch (2.5 cm) cubes, and patted dry	500 g
4	onions, chopped	4
6	cloves garlic, minced	6
2 tsp	dried thyme leaves	10
2	bay leaves	2
1 tsp	salt	5 mL
1 tsp	cracked black peppercorns	5 mL
1	can (5 1/2 oz/156 mL) tomato paste	1
1 1/2 cups	dry white wine (see Tips, left)	375 mL
3 cups	chicken stock	750 mL
8 oz	pork belly, thinly sliced	250 g

Topping

2 cups	bread crumbs	500 mL
1/2 cup	finely chopped parsley	125 mL
2	cloves garlic, minced	2
	Freshly ground black pepper	
1/4 cup	melted butter	60 mL

1. In a skillet, heat 1 tbsp (15 mL) of the oil over medium-high heat. Add sausage and cook, stirring, until no hint of pink remains, about 5 minutes. Transfer to slow cooker stoneware. Add pork shoulder, in batches, and cook, stirring, until browned, about 4 minutes per batch.

2. Transfer to slow cooker stoneware. Add lamb, in batches, and cook, stirring, until browned, about 4 minutes per batch. Transfer to stoneware.

3. Reduce heat to medium. Add remaining 1 tbsp (15 mL) of oil to pan. Add onions and cook, stirring, until softened, about 5 minutes. Add garlic, thyme, bay leaves, salt and peppercorns and cook, stirring, for 1 minute. Stir in tomato paste. Add wine, bring to a boil and boil for 2 minutes, scraping up brown bits from bottom of pan.

4. Transfer to slow cooker stoneware. Add chicken stock, pork belly and cooked beans. Stir well. Cover and cook on Low for 8 to 10 hours or on High for 4 to 5 hours, until hot and bubbly.

5. *Topping:* Preheat oven to 350°F (180°C). In a bowl, combine bread crumbs, parsley, garlic and pepper to taste. Mix well. Spread evenly over bean mixture. Drizzle with butter. Bake in preheated oven until top has formed a crust, about 30 minutes.

Variation

If you are serving this to guests, you can easily bump it up a notch if you have access to prepared duck confit (many butchers are selling it these days). Just cut it into bite-size pieces and add to the cooked cassoulet before adding the topping. Don't use more than 8 oz (250 g).

Potato and Chickpea Stew with Spicy Sausage

During the long winter months, this is the kind of hearty, legume-based stew with which southern Europeans bring the sunshine back into their homes. The version we present here is virtually foolproof, requiring just a minimum of attention — and little effort if one uses canned chickpeas (washed with cold running water and strained).

Serves 4

Tip

Leftovers are wonderful, since the flavors will intensify upon reheating the next day. It can be enjoyed as a vegetarian main course (just omit the sausages) or you can experiment with substitutes for the sausage; any stewing meat (pork, lamb or chicken) will work well. In all cases, the stew is wonderful if served with a salad and crusty bread.

$1/2$ cup	red lentils (masoor dal)	125 mL
1 cup	diced peeled potatoes	250 mL
$1/2$ cup	scraped carrots, cut into $1/4$-inch (5 mm) cubes	125 mL
	Boiling water	
$1/4$ cup	olive oil	60 mL
1 tsp	sweet paprika	5 mL
$3/4$ tsp	salt	3 mL
$1/4$ tsp	freshly ground black pepper	1 mL
$1/4$ tsp	turmeric	1 mL
2 cups	chopped onions	500 mL
$1/4$ tsp	chile flakes	1 mL
2 tbsp	finely chopped garlic	30 mL
2	medium tomatoes, cut into $1/2$-inch (1 cm) wedges	2
2	bay leaves	2
1 tsp	red wine vinegar	5 mL
$1/2$ tsp	dried oregano	2 mL
$1/2$ tsp	dried thyme	2 mL
2 cups	cooked chickpeas or 1 can (19 oz/540 mL) chickpeas, rinsed and drained	500 mL
2	dried figs, cut into $1/4$-inch (5 mm) cubes	2
1 lb	spicy sausage (such as merguez, chorizo or spicy Italian)	500 g
2 tbsp	finely minced red onions	30 mL
	Few sprigs fresh parsley, chopped	

1. Soak lentils in boiling water to cover for 20 minutes; drain. Bring 5 cups (1.25 L) water to a boil; stir in lentils and cook for 5 minutes. Add potatoes and carrots; return to a boil. Reduce heat to medium; cook, stirring very occasionally, for 10 minutes or until the potatoes are tender, but not quite crumbling. Drain, reserving cooking liquid. Set lentils and vegetables aside. Measure out $1\frac{1}{2}$ cups (375 mL) of the cooking liquid and set aside. (If there isn't enough liquid, make up the difference with water.)

2. In a large deep saucepan, heat olive oil over medium-high heat. Add paprika, salt, pepper and turmeric; cook, stirring, for 1 minute, being careful not to let the spices burn. Add onions and chile flakes; cook, stirring, 4 minutes or until the onions are soft and beginning to catch on the bottom of the pan. Add garlic and cook, stirring, for 1 minute. Add tomatoes, bay leaves, vinegar, oregano and thyme; cook, stirring, for 2 to 3 minutes or until tomatoes are starting to break up and a sauce forms.

3. Stir in lentil-vegetable mixture, chickpeas, figs and reserved cooking liquid; bring to a boil. Reduce heat to medium-low and cook for 20 minutes, uncovered, stirring occasionally from the bottom up to avoid scorching. Take off heat, cover and let rest for 10 minutes.

4. While stew rests, grill, broil or fry the sausages. Serve stew garnished with sausages, red onions and parsley.

Quince-Laced Lamb Shanks with Yellow Split Peas

This is a version of a traditional Middle Eastern dish. Fragrant quince, which is very fibrous in its raw state, cooks up beautifully in the slow cooker and pairs with the hint of pomegranate to add luscious fruitiness. Serve this over couscous, preferably a whole wheat version.

Serves 4 to 8

Tips

If you are halving this recipe, be sure to use a small (2 to 3½ quart) slow cooker.

Whether you cook the lamb shanks whole or halved or have them cut into pieces is a matter of preference. However, if the shanks are left whole, you will be able to serve only four people — each will receive one large shank.

If you can't find quinces, substitute 4 Granny Smith apples, peeled, cored and thinly sliced, and add them to the stew 2 hours before it is finished, if you're cooking on Low, or 1 hour, if you're cooking on High.

Make Ahead

Complete Steps 1 and 3. Cover and refrigerate mixture for up to 2 days. When you're ready to cook, complete the recipe.

- **Large (approx. 5 quart) slow cooker**

2 tsp	each cumin seeds and coriander seeds	10 mL
2 tbsp	olive oil, divided	30 mL
4	large lamb shanks, halved (about 4 lbs/2 kg) (see Tips, left)	4
2	onions, finely chopped	2
4	cloves garlic, minced	4
2 tbsp	minced gingerroot	30 mL
½ tsp	salt	2 mL
½ tsp	cracked black peppercorns	2 mL
3	quinces (about 1½ lbs/750 g), peeled, cored and sliced (see Tips, left)	3
¼ cup	yellow split peas	60 mL
2 cups	chicken stock	500 mL
2 tbsp	pomegranate molasses	30 mL

1. In a large dry skillet over medium heat, toast cumin and coriander seeds, stirring constantly, until fragrant, about 3 minutes. Using a mortar and pestle or a spice grinder, pound or grind as finely as you can. Set aside.

2. Return skillet to element and heat 1 tbsp (15 mL) oil. Add lamb, in batches, and brown on all sides, about 4 minutes per batch. Transfer to slow cooker stoneware. Drain off fat from pan.

3. Reduce heat to medium. Add remaining 1 tbsp (15 mL) of oil to pan. Add onions and cook, stirring, until softened, about 3 minutes. Add garlic, ginger, salt, peppercorns and reserved cumin and coriander and cook, stirring, for 1 minute. Add quinces and toss to coat. Add split peas and toss to coat. Stir in chicken stock and pomegranate molasses and bring to a boil, scraping up brown bits from bottom of pan.

4. Transfer to slow cooker stoneware. Cover and cook on Low for 10 hours or on High for 5 hours, until meat is falling off the bone.

Country-Style Salted Pork with Lentils

This is a variation of a classic French country dish — dry-brined pork simmered with lentils and aromatics. It makes a sumptuous winter meal. Steamed baby turnips along with sliced green beans are the perfect accompaniment.

Serves 6 to 8

Tips

For best results, use Puy lentils, a French green lentil with robust flavor that holds its shape during cooking. Red lentils, which are very soft and dissolve during cooking, would not work well in this recipe.

If you prefer, substitute 1 cup (250 mL) chicken stock plus 1 tbsp (15 mL) lemon juice for the wine.

Make Ahead

Complete Steps 1 and 3, refrigerating meat and vegetable mixtures separately for up to 2 days. When you're ready to cook, brown the pork and continue with the recipe. Or, if you prefer, add the unbrowned pork to the stoneware along with the vegetable mixture; the result will not be as flavorful as that produced using browned meat.

• **Medium (approx. 4 quart) slow cooker**

1 tbsp	fennel seeds, toasted and ground	15 mL
1 tbsp	puréed garlic	15 mL
2 tsp	coarse salt	10 mL
1 tsp	cracked black peppercorns	5 mL
2 lbs	trimmed boneless pork shoulder or blade (butt), patted dry	1 kg
2 tbsp	olive oil, divided	30 mL
2	onions, finely chopped	2
2	stalks celery, diced	2
2	carrots, peeled and diced	2
4	cloves garlic, minced	4
2	whole cloves	2
2	bay leaves	2
1½ cups	green or brown lentils (see Tips, left)	375 mL
1 cup	dry white wine (see Tips, left)	250 mL
4 cups	chicken stock	1 L

1. In a small bowl, combine fennel seeds, garlic, salt and peppercorns. Mix well. Pat meat dry and rub all over with mixture. Cover and refrigerate overnight. Set any juices aside.

2. In a skillet, heat 1 tbsp (15 mL) of the oil over medium-high heat. Add pork and brown, about 4 minutes per side. Transfer to slow cooker stoneware.

3. Reduce heat to medium. Add remaining 1 tbsp (15 mL) of oil to pan. Add onions, celery and carrots and cook, stirring, until vegetables are softened, about 7 minutes. Add garlic, cloves and bay leaves and cook, stirring, for 1 minute. Add lentils and toss until coated. Stir in any reserved meat juices. Add wine, bring to a boil and boil for 2 minutes, scraping up brown bits from bottom of pan. Transfer to slow cooker stoneware. Pour in chicken stock.

4. Cover and cook on Low for 8 hours or on High for 4 hours, until pork is very tender.

Lamb with Flageolet Gratin

This ambrosial concoction of highly seasoned lamb, fennel and flageolets (small dried beans that traditionally accompany lamb in France) is a superb dish for entertaining. For an elegant presentation, transfer the mixture to individual gratin dishes, and place under the broiler. If your slow cooker stoneware is ovenproof you can do it directly in the stoneware and serve from that.

Serves 6 to 8

Tips

Use a fine-tooth grater to purée the garlic.

To toast fennel seeds: Place seeds in a dry skillet over medium heat, stirring until fragrant, about 3 minutes. Using a mortar and pestle or a clean spice grinder, pound or grind as finely as you can.

Flageolets are available in well-stocked supermarkets or specialty stores. Although they usually do not need to be soaked before using, I find they cook better in the slow cooker if they receive a quick soak as directed in Step 2.

- **Large (approx. 5 quart) slow cooker**

Marinade

2 tbsp	olive oil	30 mL
1 tbsp	puréed garlic (3 to 4 cloves) (see Tips, left)	15 mL
1 tsp	dried thyme leaves	5 mL
1 tsp	dried rosemary leaves	5 mL
1 tsp	fennel seeds, toasted and ground (see Tips, left)	5 mL
1 tsp	cracked black peppercorns	5 mL
2 lbs	trimmed stewing lamb, cut into 1-inch (2.5 cm) cubes, and patted dry	1 kg
1½ cups	dried flageolets (see Tips, left)	375 mL
2 cups	chicken stock	500 mL
2 cups	water	500 mL
2 tbsp	olive oil, divided	30 mL
2	onions, thinly sliced on the vertical	2
1	bulb fennel, cored and diced	1
4	cloves garlic, minced	4
1 tsp	dried thyme leaves or 1 sprig fresh thyme	5 mL
1 tsp	dried rosemary or 1 sprig fresh rosemary	5 mL
2	bay leaves	2
1 tsp	salt	5 mL

Topping

2 cups	dry bread crumbs	500 mL
½ cup	finely chopped parsley	125 mL
1 tsp	Aleppo pepper, optional (see Tip, right)	5 mL
¼ tsp	salt	1 mL
¼ cup	melted butter	60 mL

1. *Marinade:* In a bowl, combine olive oil, garlic, thyme, rosemary, fennel and peppercorns. Mix well. Add lamb and toss until well coated. Cover and refrigerate overnight or up to 2 days.

Aleppo pepper is a
mild chile pepper from
Syria. It is available
in specialty stores or
supermarkets with
a well-stocked spice
section. If you want a
bit of heat and don't
have it, substitute
$\frac{1}{4}$ tsp (1 mL) cayenne
pepper.

Make Ahead

Complete Steps
1 and 4, adding
1 cup (250 mL) of
the chicken stock
called for in Step 2
to the onion mixture
after sautéing the
garlic, etc. Cover
and refrigerate for
up to 2 days. When
you're ready to cook,
complete the recipe.

2. In a saucepan, combine flageolets, stock and water. Bring to a boil and boil rapidly for 2 minutes. Set aside for 20 minutes.

3. In a skillet, heat 1 tbsp (15 mL) of the oil over medium-high heat. Add lamb, in batches, and cook, stirring, until browned, about 4 minutes per batch, transferring to slow cooker stoneware as completed.

4. Reduce heat to medium. Add remaining 1 tbsp (15 mL) oil to pan. Add onions and fennel and cook, stirring, until softened, about 5 minutes. Add garlic, thyme, rosemary, bay leaves and salt and cook, stirring, for 1 minute, scraping up brown bits from bottom of pan.

5. Transfer to slow cooker stoneware. Add flageolets with liquid. Stir well. Cover and cook on Low for 8 hours or on High for 4 hours, until flageolets are tender.

6. *Topping:* Preheat broiler. After lamb has cooked, ladle it into individual heatproof tureens. (If your stoneware is ovenproof, you may prefer to leave it in that.) In a bowl, combine bread crumbs, parsley, Aleppo pepper, if using, and salt and mix well. Sprinkle over lamb mixture and drizzle with butter. Place under broiler until topping is lightly browned and mixture is bubbly, about 3 minutes.

Spicy Lamb with Chickpeas

Here's a dish with robust flavor that will delight even your most discriminating guests. Serve over whole-grain couscous or, for a New World spin, hot quinoa, and open a good Rioja for a perfect accompaniment.

Serves 6

Tips

If you are halving this recipe, be sure to use a small (2 to 3½ quart) slow cooker.

For the best flavor, toast and grind the cumin and coriander yourself. Place seeds in a dry skillet over medium heat, stirring until fragrant, about 3 minutes. Using a mortar and pestle or a spice grinder, pound or grind as finely as you can.

You can soak and cook your own chickpeas (see pages 6 to 10) or use canned chickpeas, thoroughly rinsed and drained.

Aleppo pepper is a mild Syrian chile pepper. It is increasingly available in specialty shops or well-stocked supermarkets. If you don't have it, substitute another mild chile powder such as ancho or New Mexico, or add another ¼ tsp (1 mL) cayenne.

- **Medium to large (4 to 6 quart) slow cooker**

1 tbsp	ground cumin (see Tips, left)	15 mL
2 tsp	ground coriander	10 mL
1 tsp	ground turmeric	5 mL
1 tsp	salt	5 mL
1 tsp	cracked black peppercorns	5 mL
1 tsp	finely grated lime zest	5 mL
2 tbsp	freshly squeezed lime juice	30 mL
2 lbs	trimmed stewing lamb, cut into 1-inch (2.5 cm) cubes	1 kg
2 tbsp	olive oil, divided	30 mL
2	onions, finely chopped	2
2	carrots, diced	2
2	parsnips, peeled and diced	2
4	cloves garlic, minced	4
2 tbsp	minced gingerroot	30 mL
4	black cardamom pods, crushed	4
1	piece (2 inches/5 cm) cinnamon stick	1
6	whole cloves	6
½ tsp	salt	2 mL
½ tsp	cracked black peppercorns	2 mL
1	can (28 oz/796 mL) tomatoes with juice, coarsely chopped	1
1 cup	chicken or vegetable stock	250 mL
3 cups	cooked chickpeas, mashed (see Tips, left)	750 mL
1 tsp	Aleppo pepper (see Tips, left)	5 mL
¼ tsp	cayenne pepper	1 mL

1. In a bowl, combine cumin, coriander, turmeric, salt, peppercorns and lime zest and juice. Stir well. Add lamb and toss to coat. Cover and set aside in refrigerator for 4 hours or overnight.

2. Pat lamb dry. In a skillet, heat 1 tbsp (15 mL) of the oil over medium heat. Add lamb, in batches, and cook, stirring, until lightly browned, about 4 minutes per batch. Transfer to slow cooker as completed.

Complete Steps 1
and 3. Cover and
refrigerate overnight.
When you're ready
to cook, complete
the recipe.

3. Add remaining 1 tbsp (15 mL) oil to pan. Add onions, carrots and parsnips and cook, stirring and scraping up brown bits from the bottom of the pan, until carrots are softened, about 7 minutes. Add garlic, ginger, cardamom, cinnamon stick, cloves, salt and peppercorns and cook, stirring, for 1 minute. Add tomatoes with juice and chicken stock and bring to a boil, scraping up brown bits from bottom of pan.

4. Transfer to slow cooker stoneware. Stir in chickpeas. Cover and cook on Low for 8 hours or on High for 4 to 5 hours, until meat is very tender. Stir in Aleppo and cayenne peppers. Cover and cook on High for 10 minutes to meld flavors.

Cheesy Beans and Hot Dogs

Beans, cheese and hot dogs — if you're a kid, you have to love this one!

**Makes 4 to
6 servings**

Tip

When you're stirring
the cheese into the
sauce, if it looks
like the cheese
isn't incorporating
smoothly, just remove
the pan from the heat.
The residual heat
in the sauce will be
enough to melt the
cheese, and it's less
likely to split.

- **Preheat oven to 375°F (190°C)**
- **8-inch (20 cm) square glass baking dish**

1 tbsp	olive oil	15 mL
1	small onion, finely chopped	1
2$\frac{1}{2}$ tbsp	all-purpose flour	37 mL
1$\frac{3}{4}$ cups	milk	425 mL
3 cups	shredded Cheddar cheese	750 mL
2	cans (each 14 to 19 oz/398 to 540 mL) pinto beans, drained and rinsed	2
8 oz	all-beef frankfurters, halved lengthwise and cut crosswise into $\frac{1}{2}$-inch (1 cm) slices	250 g
$\frac{1}{2}$ tsp	salt	2 mL
$\frac{1}{4}$ tsp	freshly ground black pepper	1 mL
$\frac{1}{2}$ cup	dry bread crumbs	125 mL

1. In a skillet, heat oil over medium heat. Sauté onion for 5 to 7 minutes or until softened. Sprinkle with flour and cook, stirring constantly, for 2 minutes. Gradually whisk in milk and cook, whisking constantly, for 2 to 3 minutes or until slightly thickened. Add cheese, 1 cup (250 mL) at a time, stirring until melted after each addition.

2. Remove from heat and stir in beans, frankfurters, salt and pepper. Spoon into baking dish and sprinkle with bread crumbs.

3. Bake in preheated oven for 15 to 20 minutes or until top is golden. Let cool slightly before serving.

Braised Lamb with Beans and Dates

Choose a cold winter night and dazzle the loved ones with this sweet-hot stew and its soothing beans and carrots (ideal alongside rice). The sweetness comes from dates (pitted, please), while the heat from crushed chiles provides a necessary counterpoint to the ultimately cloying effect of a sweet-only sauce. If chiles absolutely don't agree with you (a real pity), substitute 1 tsp (5 mL) white wine vinegar (add along with the chicken stock) for a sweet-and-sour result.

Serves 4 or 5

2 tbsp	olive oil	30 mL
½ tsp	ground allspice	2 mL
½ tsp	ground cumin	2 mL
½ tsp	salt	2 mL
¼ tsp	freshly ground black pepper	1 mL
2 cups	finely diced onions	500 mL
¼ to ½ tsp	chile flakes, or to taste	1 to 2 mL
2½ lbs	lamb leg or shoulder cut into 1½-inch (4 cm) pieces (bone in, fat trimmed)	1.25 kg
1	large carrot, peeled and cut into ¼-inch (5 mm) rounds	1
2	stalks celery with leaves, finely chopped	2
1 cup	diced peeled tomatoes, with juice, or canned tomatoes	250 mL
3 cups	boiling chicken stock	750 mL
1 tsp	dried oregano	5 mL
1 tsp	dried thyme	5 mL
1 cup	pitted dates (about 4 oz/125 g)	250 mL
2 cups	cooked white kidney beans or 1 can (19 oz/540 mL), rinsed and drained	500 mL
¼ cup	packed chopped fresh parsley	60 mL
	Steamed rice as an accompaniment	

1. In a large saucepan, heat olive oil, allspice, cumin, salt and pepper over high heat, stirring, for 1 minute. Add onions and chile flakes; stir-fry for 4 minutes or until starting to brown. Add lamb and cook, stirring actively, for 5 to 7 minutes or until the lamb is thoroughly browned and everything is well mixed together. Add carrot, celery, tomatoes, chicken stock, oregano and thyme; mix together to settle everything in the liquid.

2. Bring to a boil and reduce heat to medium. Cook uncovered for 45 minutes or until the lamb is tender. Stir every 15 minutes and keep up a steady but not vigorous bubble.

3. Fold in dates, beans and parsley; wait for the steady-but-not-vigorous bubble to return. Cook for 20 minutes, folding from the bottom up every 5 minutes to avoid scorching. Remove from heat and cover. Let rest for 5 to 10 minutes.

4. Portion alongside steamed rice with plenty of sauce; serve immediately.

Chicken Baked with Black Beans and Lime

Serves 4 to 6

- **Preheat oven to 375°F (190°C)**
- **10-cup (2.5 L) casserole dish**

1½ lbs	boneless skinless chicken thighs, cut into bite-size pieces	750 g
	Salt and freshly ground black pepper	
2 tbsp	olive oil	30 mL
2	carrots, finely diced	2
1	onion, finely chopped	1
2	cloves garlic, minced	2
2 oz	chorizo or other spicy sausage, finely chopped	60 g
3 cups	drained rinsed canned black beans	750 mL
1 cup	chicken broth	250 mL
¼ cup	chopped fresh cilantro	60 mL
	Finely grated zest and juice of 4 limes	
2 cups	shredded Monterey Jack cheese	500 mL

1. Season chicken with salt and pepper, to taste. In a large skillet, heat oil over medium-high heat. Sauté carrots and onion until almost tender. Add chicken and sauté until browned on all sides. Stir in garlic, chorizo, beans and broth; bring to a boil. Stir in cilantro, lime zest and lime juice.

2. Pack half the chicken mixture into casserole dish and sprinkle with half the cheese. Repeat layers. Bake in preheated oven for 45 minutes, until bubbling.

Brunswick-Style Chicken Pot Pie

Brunswick stew, a traditional dish from the southeast United States, is usually tomato-based and includes lima beans, corn and other vegetables. Authentic recipes often include squirrel or rabbit, but chicken, pork and beef are common too.

Makes 6 servings

Tip

When draining tomatoes, freeze the liquid, then add it to soups, stews and sauces.

- **Preheat oven to 350°F (180°C)**
- **11- by 7-inch (28 by 18 cm) glass baking dish, greased**

½ cup	all-purpose flour	125 mL
½ tsp	freshly ground black pepper	2 mL
6	boneless skinless chicken breasts	6
¼ cup	butter	60 mL
1 cup	chopped onion	250 mL
1	can (10 oz/284 mL) condensed chicken broth	1
1	can (14 oz/398 mL) stewed tomatoes, drained	1
1	can (11 oz/312 mL) whole kernel corn, drained	1
1	package (10 oz/300 g) frozen baby lima beans, thawed	1
1½ tsp	dried thyme	7 mL
1	can (10 oz/300 g) refrigerated biscuit dough	1

1. In a shallow bowl, combine flour and pepper. Dredge chicken in seasoned flour, coating evenly and shaking off excess. Discard excess flour mixture.
2. In a large skillet, melt butter over medium-high heat. In batches as necessary, cook chicken, turning once, for 8 to 10 minutes or until no longer pink inside. Transfer to a plate and let cool slightly.
3. Add onion to fat remaining in skillet; sauté for 3 to 5 minutes or until softened. Stir in broth, tomatoes, corn, beans and thyme; bring to a boil. Reduce heat to low, cover and simmer for 15 to 20 minutes or until beans are tender.
4. Shred chicken with a fork and stir into onion mixture. Pour into prepared baking dish. Cut biscuit dough into quarters and arrange over chicken mixture.
5. Bake in preheated oven for 15 to 20 minutes or until biscuits are golden brown.

Manicotti Stuffed with Chickpeas and Cheese

Tips

As an alternative, use about 16 jumbo pasta shells, with 2 tbsp (30 mL) of stuffing per shell.

Substitute Swiss or mozzarella for Cheddar cheese.

Make Ahead

Stuff shells and make sauce up to a day ahead. Pour over just before baking. If sauce is too thick, add extra stock.

- Preheat oven to 350°F (180°C)
- Food processor
- 9- by 13-inch (3 L) baking dish, sprayed with vegetable spray

10	manicotti shells	10

Sauce

2 tsp	margarine or butter	10 mL
1 tbsp	all-purpose flour	15 mL
½ cup	2% milk	125 mL
½ cup	chicken stock	125 mL
2 tbsp	grated Parmesan cheese	30 mL
1½ cups	canned chickpeas, drained	375 mL
1 cup	5% ricotta cheese	250 mL
½ cup	chopped green onions (about 4 medium)	125 mL
⅓ cup	grated Cheddar cheese	75 mL
1	egg	1
3 tbsp	grated Parmesan cheese, divided	45 mL
1½ tsp	minced garlic	7 mL
1 tsp	dried basil	5 mL

1. In a large pot of boiling water, cook pasta according to package directions or until tender but firm; rinse under cold water and drain.

2. In a saucepan, melt margarine over medium heat; add flour and cook, stirring, for 1 minute. Gradually add milk and stock; stir constantly for 7 minutes or until sauce begins to simmer and thicken slightly. Stir in 2 tbsp (30 mL) Parmesan and remove from heat.

3. Put chickpeas, ricotta, green onions, Cheddar cheese, egg, 2 tbsp (30 mL) Parmesan, garlic and basil in food processor; pulse on and off until well mixed. Stuff 3 tbsp (45 mL) into each shell and put in prepared dish. Pour white sauce over and sprinkle with remaining 1 tbsp (15 mL) Parmesan. Bake, covered, for 15 minutes or until heated through.

Rice and Red Lentil Pilaf with Fried Zucchini

Most "modern" types of cuisine borrow from a number of cultures to create a brand-new dish. And this aromatic rice-and-red-lentil concoction is a perfect example. It could have come from India just as easily as from Turkey, while its fried zucchini garnish is strictly Greek. It entails several different procedures but they're all easy and can be performed at leisure — one by one, not simultaneously. The result is satisfyingly exotic and tasty, a most viable (and healthier) alternative to pasta for a light supper or lunch.

Serves 4

Tip

After soaking (Step 1) the lentils will absorb most of the water.

$1/2$ cup	red lentils (masoor dal)	125 mL
1 cup	water	250 mL
$1/2$ tsp	salt	2 mL
$1/4$ cup	olive oil	60 mL
$1/4$ tsp	ground cinnamon	1 mL
$1/4$ tsp	ground cumin	1 mL
$1/4$ tsp	turmeric	1 mL
$1/2$ tsp	salt	2 mL
$1/4$ tsp	freshly ground black pepper	1 mL
$3/4$ cup	finely diced onions	175 mL
$1/2$ cup	finely diced red bell peppers	125 mL
2 tbsp	finely chopped garlic	30 mL
2 tbsp	dried currants	30 mL
$1/2$ cup	short-grain rice	125 mL
2 cups	boiling chicken stock	500 mL
1	zucchini (about 8 oz/250 g)	1
3 tbsp	all-purpose flour	45 mL
Pinch	salt	Pinch

1. Rinse and drain lentils. Put in a saucepan with water and $1/2$ tsp (2 mL) salt. Bring to a boil. Remove from heat; pour into a bowl. Let soak for 10 to 15 minutes.

2. Meanwhile in a heavy-bottomed pot with a tight-fitting lid over high heat, combine 2 tbsp (30 mL) of the oil, cinnamon, cumin, turmeric, salt and pepper. Cook, stirring, for 1 minute. Add onions and red peppers; stir-fry for 2 minutes or until beginning to char. Add garlic and currants; stir-fry for 1 minute.

3. Immediately drain the leftover water from the lentils; add to pot along with rice. Cook, stirring, for 1 minute or until rice and lentils are coated with oil. Add chicken stock and stir. Reduce heat to low, cover tightly and cook undisturbed for 20 minutes. Remove from heat. Let rest, covered, for 10 minutes.

4. Meanwhile, cut the zucchini lengthwise into long, thin ($\frac{1}{8}$- to $\frac{1}{4}$-inch/3 to 5 mm) slices (you should get 8 slices). Dredge lightly in flour. In a large frying pan, heat 2 tbsp (30 mL) olive oil and pinch of salt over high heat for 1 minute. Add zucchini in a single layer and fry each side for 2 minutes or until golden brown. Transfer to a paper-towel-lined plate to drain excess oil.

5. Uncover rice/lentil mixture. Fluff, folding from the bottom up to distribute all ingredients throughout. Put portions onto 4 plates. Garnish with 2 slices of fried zucchini per portion and serve immediately.

Linguine with Tuna, White Beans and Dill

Serves 6

Tips

For color variation, try red kidney beans or black beans instead of white beans.

For a more sophisticated meal, replace canned tuna with cooked tuna or swordfish.

Make Ahead

Prepare sauce up to a day ahead. Reheat gently, adding more stock if too thick.

12 oz	linguine	375 g
1 tbsp	olive oil	15 mL
2 tsp	crushed garlic	10 mL
1	can (19 oz/540 mL) white kidney beans, drained	1
4 tbsp	lemon juice	60 mL
1$\frac{3}{4}$ cups	cold chicken stock	425 mL
4 tsp	all-purpose flour	20 mL
1	can (6.5 oz/185 g) flaked tuna packed in water, drained	1
$\frac{1}{2}$ cup	chopped fresh dill (or 1 tbsp/15 mL dried)	125 mL
$\frac{1}{3}$ cup	sliced black olives	75 mL
$\frac{1}{4}$ cup	chopped green onions	60 mL

1. Cook pasta in boiling water according to package instructions or until firm to the bite. Drain and place in a serving bowl.

2. In a large nonstick skillet, heat oil; add garlic, beans and lemon juice. Cook for 2 minutes or until hot.

3. Meanwhile, in a small bowl combine stock and flour until smooth. Add to bean mixture; simmer for 3 minutes or until sauce thickens slightly. Pour over pasta. Add tuna, dill, olives and green onions. Toss to combine.

Saucy Halibut on a Bed of Lentils

Thanks to English chef Simon Hopkinson, whose recipe we've adapted here. Hearty yet light and nutritious, this is a perfect dish for entertaining. (Double the quantity if you're serving more people.) It is so easy to make that you can also serve it for a family meal.

Tips

For best results (or if you're serving this to guests) use Puy lentils, a French green lentil with robust flavor that holds its shape during cooking.

We always use Italian flat-leaf parsley because it has so much more flavor than the curly-leaf variety. Unless the stems or sprigs are specifically called for, use only the tender leaves.

Lentils

1 tbsp	butter or olive oil	15 mL
1	onion, finely chopped	1
2	cloves garlic, minced	2
1	bay leaf	1
	Salt and freshly ground black pepper	
1 cup	dried brown or green lentils, rinsed and drained (see Tips, left)	250 mL
2½ cups	chicken or vegetable broth	625 mL

Parsley Sauce

4 cups	Italian flat-leaf parsley leaves	1 L
10	basil leaves	10
15	mint leaves	15
2	cloves garlic, coarsely chopped	2
1 tbsp	Dijon mustard	15 mL
4	anchovy fillets	4
1 tbsp	drained capers	15 mL
⅓ cup	extra virgin olive oil	75 mL
	Salt and freshly ground black pepper	

Halibut

3 tbsp	freshly squeezed lemon juice	45 mL
1 tsp	salt	5 mL
1½ lbs	Pacific halibut fillet, cut into 4 pieces	750 g

1. *Lentils:* In a large heavy saucepan over medium heat, melt butter. Add onion and cook, stirring, until softened, about 3 minutes. Add garlic, bay leaf, and salt and black pepper to taste, and cook, stirring, for 1 minute. Add lentils and toss until coated with mixture. Add broth and bring to a boil. Reduce heat and simmer until lentils are tender and liquid is absorbed, about 40 minutes.

Tip

You may need a bit more or less water, depending upon the configuration of the pan you are using to poach the fish. You want the fish to just be covered with the liquid.

2. *Parsley Sauce:* Meanwhile, in a food processor fitted with metal blade, pulse parsley, basil, mint, garlic, mustard, anchovies and capers to chop, about 15 times, stopping and scraping down sides of the bowl as necessary. With motor running, slowly add oil through feed tube until oil is well integrated. Season with salt and black pepper to taste, and set aside.

3. *Halibut:* Bring 8 cups (2 L) water (see Tip, left) to a boil in a large covered skillet or fish poacher. Add lemon juice and salt. Add fish and return to a boil. Cover and turn off heat. Set aside for 5 minutes, until fish is cooked through.

4. To serve, spread lentils on a serving dish or deep platter. Remove skin from fish, if necessary, and arrange on top of lentils. Spoon a good dollop of sauce over each piece of fish and pass the remainder in a sauceboat at the table. Serve immediately.

Salmon over White-and-Black Bean Salsa

Serves 4

Tips

Swordfish or tuna can be substituted for salmon.

Other varieties of beans can be substituted if black or white navy beans are unavailable.

If you're not using canned beans, 1 cup (250 mL) dry yields 3 cups (750 mL) cooked.

Make Ahead

Prepare bean mixture earlier in the day and keep refrigerated. Stir before serving.

• **Start barbecue or preheat oven to 425°F (220°C)**

1 cup	canned black beans, drained	250 mL
1 cup	canned white navy beans, drained	250 mL
3/4 cup	chopped tomatoes	175 mL
1/2 cup	chopped green bell peppers	125 mL
1/4 cup	chopped red onions	60 mL
1/4 cup	chopped fresh cilantro	60 mL
2 tbsp	balsamic vinegar	30 mL
2 tbsp	lemon juice	30 mL
1 tbsp	olive oil	15 mL
1 tsp	minced garlic	5 mL
1 lb	salmon steaks	500 g

1. In a bowl combine black beans, white beans, tomatoes, green peppers, red onions and cilantro. In a small bowl, whisk together vinegar, lemon juice, olive oil and garlic; pour over bean mixture and toss to combine.

2. Barbecue salmon or bake uncovered for approximately 10 minutes per 1 inch (2.5 cm) thickness or until fish flakes with a fork. Serve over bean salsa.

Baked Shrimp Enchiladas

This easy casserole makes an excellent weeknight meal. It's loaded with flavor and has much less fat than traditional shrimp enchiladas.

Makes 8 servings

Tip

Precooked shrimp are a great time-saver in this recipe.

- **Preheat oven to 425°F (220°C)**
- **13- by 9-inch (33 by 23 cm) glass baking dish, greased**

2	cans (each 4½ oz/127 mL) chopped mild green chiles	2
1 lb	cooked medium shrimp, diced	500 g
2 cups	enchilada sauce, divided	500 mL
1 cup	frozen corn kernels, thawed	250 mL
12	6-inch (15 cm) corn tortillas	12
1	can (15 oz/426 mL) fat-free refried beans	1
1 cup	shredded reduced-fat Mexican-blend cheese	250 mL
½ cup	chopped fresh cilantro	125 mL

1. In a medium bowl, combine chiles, shrimp, ½ cup (125 mL) of the enchilada sauce and corn. Set aside.

2. Spread ½ cup (125 mL) of the remaining enchilada sauce in prepared baking dish. Arrange 6 tortillas on top, overlapping as necessary. Spread refried beans evenly over tortillas. Top with shrimp mixture. Arrange the remaining 6 tortillas on top and pour the remaining sauce over tortillas.

3. Cover and bake in preheated oven for about 30 minutes or until bubbling. Sprinkle with cheese and bake for about 5 minutes or until cheese is melted. Serve garnished with cilantro.

Tuscan Shrimp and Beans

One taste of these spicy garlic shrimp, combined with fresh tomatoes and herbs and perfectly cooked white beans, and you are transported to sunny Italy. Serve with a green vegetable and a wedge of crusty Italian bread.

Serves 6

1½ cups	dried white beans	375 mL
2	bay leaves, divided	2
	Kosher or sea salt	
¼ cup	extra virgin olive oil	60 mL
4	cloves garlic, finely chopped	4
Pinch	hot pepper flakes	Pinch
6	ripe Roma (plum) tomatoes, seeded and diced	6
1 lb	large shrimp, peeled and deveined	500 g
2 tbsp	basil chiffonade	30 mL
2 tbsp	finely chopped flat-leaf parsley	30 mL
	Freshly ground black pepper	

1. Soak beans in water to cover overnight. Drain beans and place in a large saucepan with 6 cups (1.5 L) fresh water and 1 bay leaf. Bring to a boil. Reduce heat and simmer, partially covered, until beans are tender, 40 to 45 minutes. Remove from heat. Add a pinch of salt and let stand for 5 minutes. Drain and set aside.

2. In a large sauté pan, heat oil over medium heat. Add garlic and hot pepper flakes and sauté for 1 to 2 minutes. Add beans, tomatoes and remaining bay leaf and cook, stirring, 4 to 5 minutes. Add shrimp and stir diligently until pink and opaque, 4 to 5 minutes.

3. Remove from heat and stir in basil and parsley. Season with pepper to taste.

Variation

For speed and convenience, replace dried beans with 2 cans (14 to 19 oz/398 to 540 mL) white beans, rinsed and drained.

Steamed Shrimp-Stuffed Tofu with Broccoli

This is one of our favorite adaptations from classical Cantonese cooking. If you want to eat more tofu for its health benefits, this should convince you that it can also be delicious.

Tip

Before placing the tofu on the plate, make sure it will fit in your steamer.

• **Preheat steamer over medium-high heat**

Stuffing

8 oz	raw shrimp, coarsely chopped	250 g
1 tsp	minced gingerroot	5 mL
½ cup	water chestnuts, finely chopped	125 mL
2 tbsp	finely chopped green onions	30 mL
1	egg white, beaten	1
¼ tsp	salt	1 mL
1 tbsp	cornstarch	15 mL
1 lb	soft tofu, drained	500 g
2 cups	broccoli florets, cut into bite-sized pieces	500 mL

Sauce

2 tsp	sesame oil	10 mL
2 tbsp	soy sauce	30 mL
1 tbsp	chicken stock	15 mL
Pinch	granulated sugar	Pinch

1. In a mixing bowl, combine shrimp, gingerroot, water chestnuts, green onions, egg white, salt and cornstarch; mix well and set aside.

2. Gently cut tofu in half lengthwise, then slice each half into ½-inch (1 cm) thick slices. Pat dry with paper towel. Lay tofu in a flat layer in the center of a plate (see Tip, left) and line the outside with a ring of broccoli florets. Spoon a portion (about 1 tbsp/15 mL) of shrimp stuffing onto each slice of tofu, pressing gently with the back of the spoon so it sticks to the tofu. Place plate in preheated steamer, cover and steam for 5 minutes or until shrimp mixture is firm to the touch.

3. *Sauce:* In a small saucepan over medium-high heat, combine ingredients; heat just until boiling. Pour sauce evenly over cooked tofu and broccoli; serve immediately.

Meatless Mains

Hoisin Stir-Fried Vegetables and Tofu
over Rice Noodles 216

Teriyaki Rice Noodles with Veggies
and Beans 217

Tofu Ratatouille 218

Cantonese Noodles 219

Cajun-Style Tofu with Tomatoes
and Okra 220

Moussaka with Tofu Topping 222

Tofu in Indian-Spiced Tomato Sauce . . . 223

Soy-Braised Tofu 224

Mediterranean-Style Braised Tofu 224

Chickpea Tofu Stew 225

Baked Orzo and Beans 226

Penne with Creamy White Bean
Sauce 227

Three-Cheese Creamy Pasta Bean
Bake 228

All-in-One Pasta and Chickpea
Ragoût 229

Roasted Vegetable Lasagna 230

Spicy Rice, Bean and Lentil
Casserole 231

Rice and Black Bean Stuffed
Peppers 232

Assamese Khichri 234

Bengali Khichri 235

Khichri with Tomatoes and
Green Peppers 236

Succulent Succotash 237

Mushroom Cholent 238

Green Beans Gado Gado 239

Cider Baked Beans 240

Romano Bean Stew 241

Red Beans and Greens 242

Vegetable Tamale Pie 243

Leek-Potato-Lentil Pie 244

Olive Oil Crust 245

Vegetarian Shepherd's Pie
with Peppered Potato Topping 246

Lentil Shepherd's Pie 247

Zesty Black Bean Pie 248

Black Bean, Corn and Leek Frittata 249

Creamy Chipotle Black Bean
Burrito Bake 250

Southwest Butternut Squash
Tortilla Bake 251

Enchiladas in Salsa Verde 252

Southwest Bread Pudding 253

Peas and Greens 254

Potato and Adzuki Latkes 255

Moroccan Chickpea Tagine 256

Garlic Greens with Chickpeas
and Cumin 257

Lentil Sloppy Joes 258

Poached Eggs on Spicy Lentils 259

Cumin-Laced Lentils with Sun-Dried
Tomatoes and Roasted Peppers 260

Indian-Spiced Lentils with
Peppery Apricots 261

Eggplant Lentil Ragoût 262

Hoisin Stir-Fried Vegetables and Tofu over Rice Noodles

Tips

Tofu is sold in the produce section of supermarkets. Be sure to use a firm or extra-firm variety or it will fall apart in the stir-fry.

Tofu can be replaced with 6 oz (175 g) cooked beans of your choice.

If rice noodles are unavailable, use regular pasta. Cook according to package directions.

Make Ahead

Prepare sauce up to 2 days in advance. Stir-fry just before serving.

Sauce

1/3 cup	hoisin sauce	75 mL
1/3 cup	soy sauce	75 mL
1/4 cup	rice wine vinegar	60 mL
1/4 cup	packed brown sugar	60 mL
1 tsp	minced garlic	5 mL
1 tsp	minced gingerroot	5 mL

Stir-Fry

8 oz	thin rice vermicelli	250 g
2 tsp	vegetable oil	10 mL
2 1/4 cups	chopped red bell peppers	560 mL
2 1/4 cups	chopped leeks	560 mL
2 cups	sliced mushrooms	500 mL
1 1/4 cups	shredded carrots	300 mL
1 1/4 cups	chopped zucchini	300 mL
6 oz	firm tofu, cubed	175 g

1. In a small bowl, whisk together hoisin sauce, soy sauce, vinegar, brown sugar, garlic and ginger. Set aside.

2. Pour boiling water over noodles to cover; soak for 10 minutes or until soft. Drain well.

3. In a nonstick wok or large saucepan sprayed with vegetable spray, heat oil over high heat. Add red peppers and leeks; stir-fry for 4 minutes. Add mushrooms and stir-fry for 2 minutes. Add carrots and zucchini; stir-fry for 2 minutes or until vegetables are tender-crisp. Add noodles, tofu and sauce; stir-fry for 2 minutes or until bubbly and hot. Serve immediately.

Teriyaki Rice Noodles with Veggies and Beans

This is a variation on the noodle dish Pad Thai, but it uses beans as the protein instead of shrimp and chicken, which is the more usual combination. Teriyaki sauce is a favorite of children because of its sweet taste.

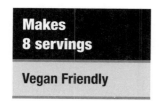

**Makes
8 servings**

Vegan Friendly

Preparation time:
8 minutes

Cooking time:
25 minutes

Tips

For a milder flavor, omit the hot pepper sauce.

This recipe reheats well, so it makes for a great packed lunch the next day.

2 cups	rice noodles	500 mL
1 tbsp	olive oil	15 mL
1	small onion, diced	1
1 cup	chopped carrots	250 mL
1 cup	chopped celery	250 mL
2	cloves garlic, chopped	2
2 cups	broccoli florets	500 mL
1/2 cup	reduced-sodium teriyaki sauce	125 mL
Dash	hot pepper sauce	Dash
1	can (19 oz/540 mL) mixed beans, drained and rinsed (about 2 cups/500 mL)	1

1. Prepare rice noodles according to package directions. Drain and set aside.
2. In a large skillet, heat oil over medium heat. Sauté onion, carrots and celery until onions are softened, about 5 minutes. Add garlic and broccoli; cover and cook for 5 minutes. Stir in teriyaki sauce, hot pepper sauce, beans and rice noodles; cover and cook for 5 minutes.

Variation

To change the texture of this recipe, substitute couscous for the rice noodles.

Tofu Ratatouille

Like any good ratatouille, this one involves quite a bit of preparation. Although it is time-consuming, sautéeing the vegetables individually ensures that their unique flavors aren't lost when the dish is complete. The results are worth the extra effort. Serve this to your most discriminating guests and expect requests for seconds.

Tip

If you are too busy to cook at the end of the day, fry the tofu when you cook the zucchini. Cover and refrigerate. Add to the slow cooker along with the zucchini and cook until heated through.

Make Ahead

This dish can be partially prepared the night before it is cooked. Complete Steps 1 through 3. Cover and refrigerate zucchini and eggplant mixtures separately, overnight. When you're ready to cook, complete the recipe.

- **Large (approx. 5 quart) slow cooker**

Ratatouille

1	large eggplant, peeled, cubed (1 inch/ 2.5 cm) and sweated (see Tips, page 222)	1
2 tbsp	oil, divided (approx.)	30 mL
8 oz	mushrooms, stems removed, quartered	250 g
2	small zucchini, thinly sliced	2
1	large onion, finely chopped	1
3	cloves garlic, minced	3
½ tsp	cracked black peppercorns	2 mL
½ tsp	dried thyme	2 mL
½ tsp	ground cinnamon	2 mL
1	can (28 oz/796 mL) tomatoes with juice, coarsely chopped	1
	Salt, to taste	

Tofu

8 oz	firm tofu with fine herbs, cut into 1-inch (2.5 cm) cubes	250 g
	Salt and freshly ground black pepper	
1 tbsp	oil	15 mL

1. *Ratatouille:* In a skillet, heat 1 tbsp (15 mL) of the oil over medium heat. Add mushrooms and cook, stirring, just until they begin to lose their liquid. Using a slotted spoon, transfer to slow cooker stoneware. Return pan to element and add more oil, if needed.

2. Add zucchini, in batches, and cook, stirring, until it softens and begins to brown. Using a slotted spoon, transfer to a bowl. Cover and refrigerate.

3. Add eggplant to pan, in batches, and sauté until lightly browned, adding more oil as needed. Transfer to slow cooker as completed. Add onion to pan and cook, stirring, until softened. Add garlic, peppercorns, thyme and cinnamon and cook, stirring, for 1 minute. Add tomatoes with juice and bring to a boil. Add salt, to taste. Pour over contents of slow cooker. Stir to blend.

4. Cover and cook on Low for 6 hours or High for 3 hours, until hot and bubbly. Add reserved zucchini and cook on High for 15 minutes, until heated through.

5. *Tofu:* Season tofu with salt and pepper, to taste. In a skillet, heat oil over medium heat. Add tofu and cook, stirring, until lightly browned, about 15 minutes. Spread tofu over top of eggplant mixture and serve immediately.

Cantonese Noodles

Tofu is now available in Tetra Paks so it can be kept in a cupboard to have readily on hand. All the other ingredients are easily available for this fast and easy dinner dish.

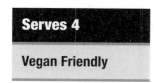

Serves 4

Vegan Friendly

Tip

If using store-bought Cajun spice, start with 1 1/2 tsp (7 mL) because it may be stronger than the homemade version. Taste and add more as required.

1 tbsp	Cajun Black Spice (page 98) or store-bought (see Tip, left)	15 mL
1 tbsp	Chinese black bean sauce	15 mL
1/2 cup	chopped onion	125 mL
4 cups	vegetable stock, divided	1 L
1 tbsp	tamari or soy sauce	15 mL
6 oz	dried somen (buckwheat) noodles	175 g
4	oyster mushrooms, sliced	4
4 oz	firm tofu, cut into small dice	125 g
2 cups	spinach, shredded	500 mL
1	sheet nori, shredded	1
	Salt and freshly ground pepper	
2	green onions, thinly sliced, optional	2

1. In a wok or large saucepan, combine Cajun spice and black bean sauce. Heat gently over medium-low heat for 1 minute. Stir in onion and 2 tbsp (30 mL) of the stock. Increase heat to medium and cook for 5 minutes or until onions are soft.

2. Stir in remaining stock and tamari. Increase heat to high and bring to a boil. Add noodles and mushrooms. Reduce heat and simmer for 8 minutes or until noodles are tender.

3. Add tofu, spinach and nori and simmer for 2 minutes. Taste and add more black bean sauce, tamari or salt, if required. Add salt and pepper, to taste. Ladle into soup bowls and garnish with green onions, if using.

Variations

Soy or rice milk can replace the vegetable stock.

Use frozen spinach or canned lima or green beans in place of the spinach.

Cajun-Style Tofu with Tomatoes and Okra

Here's a dish that is Cajun-inspired in its ingredients yet packs just a hint of heat and yields a great sense of freshness. Deliciously different, served over rice, it makes a great one-pot meal.

Serves 4 to 6

Vegan Friendly

Tips

If you're using Italian San Marzano tomatoes, which are very rich, omit the tomato paste.

Okra, a tropical vegetable, has a great flavor but it becomes unpleasantly sticky when overcooked. Choose young okra pods, 2 to 4 inches (5 to 10 cm) long, that don't feel sticky to the touch. (If sticky they are too ripe.) Gently scrub the pods and cut off the top and tail before slicing.

Whether you add cayenne depends upon how spicy your Cajun spice mix is and how much you like heat.

Make Ahead

Complete Step 1. Cover and refrigerate for up to 2 days. When you're ready to cook, complete the recipe.

- **Medium (approx. 3 quart) slow cooker**

2 tbsp	oil	30 mL
1	onion, finely chopped	1
4	stalks celery, diced	4
4	cloves garlic, minced	4
1 tsp	salt	5 mL
1 tsp	cracked black peppercorns	5 mL
1 tsp	dried thyme	5 mL
2	bay leaves	2
1 tbsp	tomato paste (see Tips, left)	15 mL
1	can (14 oz/398 mL) diced tomatoes with juice	1
2 cups	thinly sliced okra (see Tips, left)	500 mL
1 cup	corn kernels	250 mL
1	red or green bell pepper, seeded and diced	1

Tofu

¼ cup	all-purpose flour	60 mL
1 tbsp	Cajun spice mix	15 mL
¼ tsp	cayenne pepper, optional (see Tips, left)	1 mL
1 lb	firm tofu, cut into 1-inch (2.5 cm) squares	500 g
1 tbsp	oil	15 mL

1. In a skillet, heat oil over medium heat. Add onion and celery and cook, stirring, until softened, about 5 minutes. Add garlic, salt, peppercorns, thyme and bay leaves and cook, stirring, for 1 minute. Stir in tomato paste. Add tomatoes with juice and bring to a boil. Transfer to slow cooker stoneware.

2. Cover and cook on Low for 6 hours or on High for 3 hours. Stir in okra, corn and bell pepper. Cover and cook on High for 20 minutes, until pepper is tender. Discard bay leaves.

3. Meanwhile, on a plate, mix together flour, Cajun spice mix and cayenne pepper, if using. Roll tofu in mixture until lightly coated. Discard excess flour. In a skillet, heat oil over medium-high heat. Add dredged tofu and sauté, stirring, until nicely browned, about 4 minutes. Spoon tomato mixture into a serving dish. Layer tofu on top and serve.

Variation

Cajun-Style Tempeh with Tomatoes and Okra:
Substitute 1 lb (500 g) sliced tempeh for the tofu. Omit the flour. Combine Cajun spice and cayenne, if using, and sprinkle over the sliced tempeh. Before starting Step 1, heat the oil in a skillet over medium-high heat. Sauté tempeh, turning once, until browned on both sides, about 7 minutes. Cover and refrigerate. Reduce heat to medium and continue with Step 1, using the oil in the pan to soften the vegetables. Add tempeh to slow cooker along with the okra.

Moussaka with Tofu Topping

This delicious rendition of the classic Greek dish, with an unusual tofu topping, is every bit as good as the original.

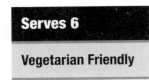
Tips

To sweat eggplant: Place cubed eggplant in a colander, sprinkle liberally with salt, toss well and set aside for 30 minutes to 1 hour. If time is short, blanch the pieces for a minute or two in heavily salted water. In either case, rinse thoroughly in fresh cold water and, using your hands, squeeze out excess moisture. Pat dry with paper towels.

Make Ahead

Complete Steps 1 through 3. Cover and refrigerate for up to 2 days. When you're ready to cook, complete the recipe.

- **Large (minimum 5 quart) oval slow cooker**
- **Food processor or blender**

2	medium eggplants (each about 1 lb/500 g), peeled, cubed (2 inches/5 cm) and sweated (see Tips, left)	2
2 tbsp	oil (approx.)	30 mL
2	onions, finely chopped	2
4	cloves garlic, minced	4
1 tsp	dried oregano	5 mL
1 tsp	ground cumin (see Tips, page 236)	5 mL
1/2 tsp	salt	2 mL
1/2 tsp	cracked black peppercorns	2 mL
2 cups	drained cooked chickpeas	500 mL
3 cups	tomato sauce	750 mL

Topping

1 lb	medium tofu	500 g
2	eggs	2
1/2 cup	freshly grated Parmesan cheese	125 mL
Pinch	ground nutmeg	Pinch
Pinch	ground cinnamon	Pinch

1. In a skillet, heat oil over medium-high heat. Add eggplant, in batches, and cook until browned, adding more oil, if necessary. Set aside.

2. Add onions to pan and cook, stirring, until softened, about 3 minutes. Add garlic, oregano, cumin, salt and peppercorns and cook, stirring, for 1 minute. Add chickpeas and stir well.

3. Spread 1 cup (250 mL) of the tomato sauce evenly over bottom of slow cooker stoneware. Spread one-third of the eggplant over sauce and half of the chickpea mixture over eggplant. Repeat. Finish with remaining eggplant and pour remaining tomato sauce over top.

4. *Topping:* In a food processor or blender, purée tofu, eggs, Parmesan, nutmeg and cinnamon. Spread over eggplant. Place a clean tea towel, folded in half (so you will have two layers), over top of stoneware to absorb moisture. Cover and cook on Low for 6 hours or on High for 3 hours.

Tofu in Indian-Spiced Tomato Sauce

This robust dish makes a lively and different meal. Serve it with fresh green beans and naan, an Indian bread, to soak up the sauce.

Serves 4 to 6

Vegan Friendly

Tip

If halving this recipe, be sure to use a small (approx. 2 quart) slow cooker.

Make Ahead

Complete Step 1. Cover and refrigerate for up to 2 days. When you're ready to cook, complete the recipe.

- **Medium (approx. 4 quart) slow cooker**

1 tbsp	oil	15 mL
2	onions, finely chopped	2
2	cloves garlic, minced	2
½ tsp	minced gingerroot	2 mL
6	whole cloves	6
4	white or green cardamom pods	4
1	piece (2 inches/5 cm) cinnamon stick	1
1 tsp	caraway seeds	5 mL
1 tsp	salt	5 mL
½ tsp	cracked black peppercorns	2 mL
1	can (28 oz/796 mL) tomatoes with juice	1
1	long green chile pepper, seeded and finely chopped	1

Tofu

¼ cup	all-purpose flour	60 mL
1 tsp	curry powder	5 mL
¼ tsp	cayenne pepper	1 mL
8 oz	firm tofu, cut into 1-inch (2.5 cm) cubes	250 g
1 tbsp	vegetable oil	15 mL

1. In a skillet, heat oil over medium heat. Add onions and cook, stirring, until softened, about 3 minutes. Add garlic, ginger, cloves, cardamom, cinnamon stick, caraway seeds, salt and peppercorns and cook, stirring, for 1 minute. Add tomatoes with juice and bring to a boil. Transfer to slow cooker stoneware.

2. Cover and cook on Low for 6 hours or on High for 3 hours, until hot and bubbly. Discard cloves, cardamom and cinnamon stick. Stir in chile pepper.

3. *Tofu:* On a plate, mix together flour, curry powder and cayenne. Roll tofu in mixture until lightly coated. Discard excess flour. In a skillet, heat oil over medium-high heat. Add dredged tofu and sauté, stirring, until nicely browned. Spoon tomato mixture into a serving dish. Lay tofu on top and serve.

Soy-Braised Tofu

Use this hot braised tofu as a centerpiece to a meal of vegetarian dishes that might include stir-fried bok choy or wilted greens garnished with toasted sesame seeds. You can also transform this flavorful tofu into a wrap. Place on lettuce leaves, garnish with shredded carrots and fold.

**Makes about
3 cups (750 mL)**

Vegan Friendly

Tip

To drain tofu: Place a layer of paper towels on a plate. Set tofu in the middle. Cover with another layer of paper towels and a heavy plate. Set aside for 30 minutes. Peel off paper and cut tofu into cubes.

- **Small to medium (1½ to 3½ quart) slow cooker**

1 lb	firm tofu, drained and cut into 1-inch (2.5 cm) cubes (see Tip, left)	500 g
¼ cup	light soy sauce	60 mL
1 tbsp	puréed gingerroot (see Tip, below left)	15 mL
1 tbsp	pure maple syrup	15 mL
1 tbsp	toasted sesame oil	15 mL
1 tbsp	freshly squeezed lemon juice	15 mL
1 tsp	puréed garlic	5 mL
½ tsp	cracked black peppercorns	2 mL

1. In slow cooker stoneware, combine soy sauce, ginger, maple syrup, toasted sesame oil, lemon juice, garlic and peppercorns. Add tofu and toss gently until coated on all sides. Cover and refrigerate for 1 hour.
2. Toss well. Cover and cook on Low for 5 hours or on High for 2½ hours, until tofu is hot and has absorbed the flavor.

Mediterranean-Style Braised Tofu

Serve this flavorful tofu as the centerpiece of a vegetarian meal, or use it as the main ingredient in a salade composée. It is particularly good as a substitute for tuna in a salade niçoise.

**Makes about
2 cups (500 mL)**

Vegan Friendly

Tip

Use a fine Microplane grater to purée the gingerroot or garlic for these recipes. It creates tiny particles that integrate into the mixture, enhancing the flavor.

- **Small to medium (1½ to 3½ quart) slow cooker**

1 lb	firm tofu, drained and cut into 1-inch (2.5 cm) cubes (see Tip, above)	500 g
¼ cup	extra virgin olive oil	60 mL
1 tbsp	balsamic or red wine vinegar	15 mL
1 tbsp	dried Italian seasoning	15 mL
4	cloves garlic, puréed (see Tip, left)	4
½ tsp	salt	2 mL
½ tsp	cracked black peppercorns	2 mL

1. In slow cooker stoneware, combine olive oil, vinegar, Italian seasoning, garlic, salt and peppercorns. Add tofu and toss gently until coated on all sides. Cover and refrigerate for 1 hour. Complete Step 2, above.

Chickpea Tofu Stew

A filling and flavorful winter dish, this stew is bolstered with the addition of super-nutritious tofu. It is imperative to use firm tofu (often called "pressed tofu"), since the soft variety will disintegrate.

Serves 4

Tips

For chickpeas, you can either cook your own or use the canned variety.

Excellent served with a salad, steamed rice and a yogurt-based sauce.

For a spicier flavor, substitute cayenne pepper for the chili powder.

- **Preheat oven to 375°F (190°C)**
- **6-cup (1.5 L) casserole dish**

1 lb	ripe tomatoes (about 4)	500 g
3 tbsp	olive oil	45 mL
½ tsp	salt	2 mL
½ tsp	paprika	2 mL
½ tsp	whole cumin seeds	2 mL
½ tsp	chili powder	2 mL
2½ cups	thinly sliced onions	625 mL
½	green bell pepper, thinly sliced	½
4	cloves garlic, thinly sliced	4
2	bay leaves	2
1 cup	hot water	250 mL
2 tsp	lime juice	10 mL
2 cups	cooked chickpeas	500 mL
8 oz	firm tofu, cut into ½-inch (1 cm) cubes	250 g
1 tsp	olive oil (optional)	5 mL
¼ cup	finely diced red onions	60 mL
	Few sprigs fresh cilantro, chopped	

1. Blanch tomatoes in boiling water for 30 seconds. Over a bowl, peel, core and deseed them. Chop tomatoes into chunks and set aside. Strain any accumulated tomato juices from bowl; add the juices to the tomatoes.

2. In a large frying pan, heat olive oil over high heat for 30 seconds. Add salt, paprika, cumin seeds and chili powder in quick succession. Stir-fry for 30 seconds. Add onions and stir-fry for 1 minute. Add green pepper and stir-fry for 2 to 3 minutes or until soft. Add garlic and stir-fry for 1 minute. Add the tomato flesh and juices. Cook, stirring, for 3 minutes, breaking up the tomato somewhat. Add the bay leaves, hot water and lime juice. Cook, stirring often, for 5 minutes.

3. Transfer sauce to casserole dish. Fold the chickpeas into the sauce. Distribute the tofu cubes evenly over the surface, and gently press them down into the sauce.

4. Bake the stew, uncovered, for 25 to 30 minutes, until bubbling and bright. Drizzle with olive oil (if using) and garnish with red onions and cilantro.

Baked Orzo and Beans

Orzo — a jumbo rice lookalike — may be the most versatile of all pastas. This recipe comes from a long line of similarly baked Greek dishes but borrows from Italian cuisine in its cheese topping. Use a plainer tomato sauce (mine may be too piquant) and omit the sautéed red onion, and you'll have a dish that delights young children, who seem to have a natural affinity to orzo (maybe because it's so much fun to pick up individual grains with tiny fingers).

Serves 4 to 6

Vegetarian Friendly

- **Preheat oven to 350°F (180°C)**
- **10-cup (2.5 L) casserole with lid**

2½ cups	orzo	625 mL
1 tbsp	olive oil	15 mL
½ cup	sliced red onions	125 mL
2	tomatoes, roughly chopped	2
2 cups	tomato sauce	500 mL
2 cups	cooked red kidney beans	500 mL
1 cup	tomato juice	250 mL
1 cup	shaved Parmesan cheese	250 mL
1 tbsp	extra virgin olive oil	15 mL
	Few sprigs fresh parsley, chopped	
	Grated Romano cheese (optional)	

1. In a large pot of boiling salted water, cook orzo for 10 minutes or until al dente.

2. Meanwhile, in a skillet, heat oil over high heat for 30 seconds; add onions and cook, stirring, for 1 or 2 minutes or until slightly charred. Remove from heat and set aside.

3. When the orzo is cooked, drain well and transfer to casserole. Add sautéed onions to orzo and stir to combine. Add tomatoes and tomato sauce; mix thoroughly. Add cooked beans; fold until evenly distributed.

4. Cover the orzo mixture and bake, covered, for 30 minutes. Remove from oven and mix in tomato juice. Top with Parmesan shavings and return to the oven, uncovered, for another 10 to 12 minutes or until the cheese is melted. Serve on pasta plates, making sure each portion is topped with some of the melted cheese. Drizzle a few drops of extra virgin olive oil on each portion and garnish with chopped parsley. Serve immediately, with Romano as an optional accompaniment.

Penne with Creamy White Bean Sauce

Serves 4 to 6

Vegetarian Friendly

Tips

Use any medium-sized pasta, such as rotini or medium shells.

Puréed kidney beans give this sauce a texture similar to canned tuna.

Add other vegetables to replace red peppers and peas. Snow peas, broccoli or sliced green beans are good choices.

Make Ahead

Prepare sauce early in the day. Sauté vegetables and cook pasta just before serving.

- **Food processor**

12 oz	penne	375 g
1	can (19 oz/540 mL) white kidney beans, rinsed and drained	1
1 cup	vegetable stock, heated	250 mL
2 tbsp	olive oil	30 mL
2 tbsp	light mayonnaise	30 mL
1 tbsp	freshly squeezed lemon juice	15 mL
1 tbsp	drained capers	15 mL
1½ tsp	minced garlic	7 mL
⅓ cup	chopped fresh dill (or 1 tbsp/15 mL dried)	75 mL
¼ tsp	freshly ground black pepper	1 mL
2 tsp	vegetable oil	10 mL
1 cup	chopped onions	250 mL
1 cup	chopped red bell peppers	250 mL
1 cup	fresh or frozen peas	250 mL

1. In a large pot of boiling water, cook penne for 8 to 10 minutes or until tender but firm. Meanwhile, prepare the sauce.

2. In a food processor, combine beans, stock, olive oil, mayonnaise, lemon juice, capers, garlic, dill and pepper; process until well mixed.

3. In a nonstick frying pan, heat vegetable oil over medium-high heat. Add onions and red peppers; cook for 4 minutes or until browned. Stir in peas; cook for 1 minute.

4. Toss drained pasta with bean mixture and vegetables. Serve immediately.

Three-Cheese Creamy Pasta Bean Bake

Tips

Fettuccine, spaghetti or small shell pasta can replace the linguine.

Try other bean combinations such as chickpeas, navy beans or black beans.

Replace the Italian seasoning with dried basil.

Make Ahead

Prepare all elements of recipe, except for pasta, up to 2 days in advance. Assemble early in the day, then bake.

- **Preheat oven to 350°F (180°C)**
- **8-cup (2 L) casserole dish sprayed with vegetable spray**

1 cup	shredded part-skim mozzarella cheese (about 4 oz/125 g)	250 mL
1 cup	5% ricotta cheese	250 mL
¾ cup	light sour cream	175 mL
¼ cup	2% milk	60 mL
2 tbsp	grated Parmesan cheese	30 mL
8 oz	linguine, broken into thirds	250 g
2 tsp	vegetable oil	10 mL
1½ tsp	minced garlic	7 mL
1 cup	chopped onions	250 mL
½ cup	chopped green bell peppers	125 mL
2 cups	prepared tomato pasta sauce	500 mL
¾ cup	canned red kidney beans, rinsed and drained	175 mL
¾ cup	canned white kidney beans, rinsed and drained	175 mL
2 tsp	Italian seasoning	10 mL

Topping

⅓ cup	dry seasoned bread crumbs	75 mL
4 tsp	grated Parmesan cheese	20 mL
2 tsp	olive oil	10 mL

1. In a small bowl, stir together mozzarella, ricotta, sour cream, milk and Parmesan; set aside.

2. In a pot of boiling water, cook linguine for 8 to 10 minutes or until tender but firm. Rinse under cold running water, drain and stir into cheese mixture.

3. In a nonstick saucepan sprayed with vegetable spray, heat oil over medium-high heat. Add garlic, onions and green peppers; cook for 3 minutes or until softened. Stir in tomato sauce, red kidney beans, white kidney beans and Italian seasoning; reduce heat to low and cook for 5 minutes.

4. *Meanwhile, make the topping:* In a small bowl, combine bread crumbs, Parmesan cheese and olive oil; set aside.

5. Spoon one-half of pasta-cheese mixture into prepared casserole; top with half of bean mixture. Repeat layers. Sprinkle with bread crumb topping. Bake for 25 minutes or until golden and hot.

All-in-One Pasta and Chickpea Ragoût

You only need one pot to prepare this dish. Even the dried pasta is added to the very same pot and cooked until tender in the vegetable-tomato sauce. Spoon into bowls and sprinkle with shredded Fontina or Parmesan cheese, if desired.

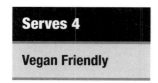

Serves 4

Vegan Friendly

Tips

Keep single servings on hand in the freezer for quick microwave meals.

Add 8 oz (250 g) cubed or sliced smoked sausage such as kielbasa or ham along with chickpeas.

1 tbsp	olive oil	15 mL
1	medium onion, chopped	1
2	cloves garlic, minced	2
1	large green bell pepper, chopped	1
1 tsp	dried oregano	5 mL
½ tsp	dried basil	2 mL
½ tsp	salt	2 mL
¼ tsp	red pepper flakes	1 mL
1	can (28 oz/796 mL) tomatoes, chopped	1
1 cup	vegetable stock	250 mL
1 cup	elbow macaroni	250 mL
2	small zucchini, halved lengthwise and sliced	2
1	can (19 oz/540 mL) chickpeas, rinsed and drained	1

1. In a Dutch oven or large saucepan, heat oil over medium heat. Add onion, garlic, pepper, oregano, basil, salt and red pepper flakes; cook, stirring, for 3 minutes or until vegetables are softened.

2. Add tomatoes and stock; bring to a boil. Reduce heat, cover and simmer, stirring occasionally, for 10 minutes. Stir in pasta; cover and cook for 5 minutes. Stir in zucchini and chickpeas; simmer for 5 to 7 minutes more or until pasta and zucchini are tender.

Roasted Vegetable Lasagna

You can choose seasonal greens for this year-round dish — spinach and dandelion greens in spring, or cabbage, Swiss chard and kale in winter.

Serves 6 to 8

Vegan Friendly

- **Preheat oven to 375°F (190°C)**
- **2 rimmed baking sheets, lightly oiled**
- **11- by 7-inch (2 L) baking pan, lightly oiled**

1	large eggplant, trimmed and cut lengthwise into $1/4$-inch (0.5 cm) slices	1
2	red bell peppers, halved lengthwise	2
5 tbsp	olive oil, divided	75 mL
1 tbsp	balsamic vinegar	15 mL
1	large onion, chopped	1
2 cups	sliced mushrooms	500 mL
2	cloves garlic, minced	2
2 tbsp	chopped fresh mixed herbs, such as oregano, thyme and basil	30 mL
1	can (19 oz/540 mL) crushed tomatoes	1
1	can (14 to 19 oz/398 to 540 mL) lima beans, drained and rinsed	1
3 cups	shredded greens (see above)	750 mL

1. Arrange eggplant slices on one baking sheet and brush with 1 tbsp (15 mL) of the oil. Arrange red pepper halves, cut side down, on the other baking sheet and brush with 1 tbsp (15 mL) of the oil. Bake in preheated oven for 15 minutes or until the tip of a knife easily pierces the eggplant and the skin of the red peppers is dark and blistered. Do not overcook the eggplant. Let cool completely. Slip skin off red peppers and slice into wide strips. In a bowl, toss pepper strips with 1 tbsp (15 mL) of the oil and the vinegar and set aside.

2. In a skillet, heat remaining oil over medium heat. Add onion and mushrooms and cook, stirring frequently, for 6 to 8 minutes or until slightly softened. Add garlic and cook, stirring frequently, for 2 minutes or until onion and garlic are soft. Add herbs and tomatoes. Reduce heat to medium-low and simmer, stirring occasionally, for 10 minutes. Add lima beans and greens and cook for 1 to 5 minutes or until greens are wilted or, in the case of winter greens, tender when pierced with the tip of a knife.

3. Line prepared baking pan with one-third of the eggplant slices. Lay half the red pepper over the eggplant. Spread with one-third of the tomato sauce. Layer another one-third of the eggplant slices and the remaining red pepper slices and spread another one-third of the sauce over. Top with remaining eggplant slices and spread with remaining tomato sauce. Lasagna may be covered and stored in the refrigerator overnight. Bring back to room temperature before baking. Bake in preheated oven for 40 minutes or until sauce is bubbly.

Spicy Rice, Bean and Lentil Casserole

Serves 4 to 6

Vegan Friendly

Tips

This makes an excellent total meal for vegetarians.

Instead of lentils, substitute green or yellow split peas.

Grilled or barbecued corn is excellent in this dish.

Any type of bean can replace the red kidney beans.

This dish is a great source of fiber.

Make Ahead

Prepare up to 2 days in advance and reheat gently.

2 tsp	vegetable oil	10 mL
2 tsp	minced garlic	10 mL
1 cup	chopped onions	250 mL
¾ cup	chopped green bell peppers	175 mL
3¾ cups	vegetable stock	950 mL
¾ cup	brown rice	175 mL
½ cup	green lentils	125 mL
1 tsp	dried basil	5 mL
1 tsp	chili powder	5 mL
1	can (19 oz/540 mL) red kidney beans, rinsed and drained	1
1 cup	canned or frozen corn kernels, drained	250 mL
1 cup	medium salsa	250 mL

1. In a nonstick saucepan, heat oil over medium-high heat. Add garlic, onions and green peppers; cook for 3 minutes. Stir in stock, brown rice, lentils, basil and chili powder; bring to a boil. Reduce heat to medium-low and cook, covered and stirring occasionally, for 30 to 40 minutes or until rice and lentils are tender and liquid is absorbed.

2. Stir in beans, corn and salsa; cover and cook for 5 minutes or until heated through.

Rice and Black Bean Stuffed Peppers

The Greeks stuff just about any vegetable they can get their hands on — from cabbage and vine leaves to zucchinis, tomatoes and eggplants. But peppers are their favorites, especially at harvest time, when they are so affordable. This is an heirloom recipe, that has been fleshed out with the addition of black beans, both for color and taste. These peppers are meant to be eaten at room temperature, when their various flavors really come to the fore. They make a perfect buffet item, especially because they can be (carefully) cut in half to double the number of servings. They also keep well (covered) in the fridge; just let them come back to room temperature before serving.

Serves 6

- **Large roasting pan or baking dish**
- **Preheat oven to 375°F (190°C)**

12	bell peppers, various colors	12
2 lbs	onions, stemmed and peeled	1 kg
1/2 tsp	ground cinnamon	2 mL
1/2 tsp	salt	2 mL
1/4 tsp	freshly ground black pepper	1 mL
1/4 cup	pine nuts	60 mL
1/4 cup	currants	60 mL
1/4 cup	olive oil	60 mL
1 cup	short-grain rice	250 mL
1 cup	diced peeled tomatoes, with juices, or canned tomatoes	250 mL
1 1/2 cups	boiling water, divided	375 mL
1/4 cup	chopped fresh mint (or 1 tbsp/15 mL dried)	60 mL
1/4 cup	chopped fresh drill (or 1 tbsp/15 mL dried)	60 mL
2 cups	cooked black beans or 1 can (19 oz/540 mL) black beans, rinsed and drained	500 mL

1. Slice a 1/2-inch (1 cm) round (including the stem, if any) from the top of each pepper. Set these aside. (They'll serve later as "lids" for the stuffed peppers.) Trim the cavity of the peppers, discarding seed pod and seeds, without puncturing the walls or bottom of the peppers. Set aside.

2. In a bowl, shred the onions through the grater's largest holes (you'll have about 3 cups/750 mL grated onions and juices). Transfer to a large nonstick frying pan. Add cinnamon, salt and pepper; cook, stirring, over high heat for 5 minutes or until most of the juices have evaporated. Add pine nuts, currants and olive oil; cook, stirring, for 3 minutes or until the onions start to catch on bottom of pan.

3. Immediately add rice; cook, stirring, for 2 minutes or until the rice is thoroughly coated with oil. Add tomatoes and $\frac{1}{2}$ cup (125 mL) of the boiling water; cook, stirring, for about 4 minutes or until the tomatoes have broken down and the water is absorbed. Remove from heat. Stir in mint, dill and black beans until well mixed.

4. Stuff a scant $\frac{1}{2}$ cup (125 mL) of the rice-bean stuffing into each pepper. (It should be about two-thirds full to allow for expansion.) Place stuffed peppers into roasting pan, fitting the peppers snugly in a single layer. Place the reserved tops on the peppers to act as lids. Add 1 cup (250 mL) boiling water around the peppers.

5. Cover and bake for 40 minutes, undisturbed. Uncover and bake for 30 to 40 minutes more to char the peppers and reduce the liquid. Remove from oven and cover the peppers. Let them cool down completely (about $1\frac{1}{2}$ hours) before serving.

Assamese Khichri

This is a one-dish vegetarian meal and is served at lunch or dinner with a fried appetizer, such as deep-fried eggplant, and tasty pickle as accompaniments. I find it is delicious with a piece of fried or grilled fish, or fried shrimp. Feel free to substitute any vegetables of your choice.

Serves 6 to 8

Vegan Friendly

3 tbsp	red lentils (masoor dal)	45 mL
3 tbsp	yellow mung beans (yellow mung dal)	45 mL
1 cup	long-grain white rice	250 mL
3 tbsp	ghee or oil, divided	45 mL
2	bay leaves	2
4	whole cloves, crushed	4
2	green cardamom pods, cracked open	2
1	piece cinnamon, 1 inch (2.5 cm) long, crushed	1
1 cup	chopped onions	250 mL
6	small potatoes (any variety), cut in half, or 2 medium potatoes, quartered	6
1/2 cup	chopped green beans (1-inch/2.5 cm pieces)	125 mL
1/2 cup	frozen green peas, thawed	125 mL
1 1/2 tbsp	minced green chiles, preferably serranos	22 mL
1 tbsp	minced peeled gingerroot	15 mL
3	cloves garlic, smashed	3
2 tsp	salt or to taste	10 mL
1/2 tsp	turmeric	2 mL

1. Clean and pick through masoor and mung dals for any small stones and grit. Rinse several times in cold water. Place rice and dals in a large bowl with plenty of cold water and swish vigorously with fingers. Drain. Repeat 4 or 5 times until water is fairly clear. Cover with 3 to 4 inches (7.5 to 10 cm) cold water and set aside to soak for 15 minutes.

2. In a saucepan, heat 1 1/2 tbsp (22 mL) of the ghee over medium heat. Add bay leaves and sauté for 30 seconds. Add cloves, cardamom and cinnamon and sauté for 30 seconds. Add onions and sauté until softened, 5 to 6 minutes. Drain rice mixture and add to saucepan. Add potatoes, green beans, peas, chiles, ginger, garlic, salt and turmeric. Mix well and sauté for 2 minutes.

3. Add 3 1/2 cups (875 mL) fresh water. Cover and bring to a boil over high heat. Reduce heat to as low as possible and cook, covered, without peeking, for 25 minutes.

4. Remove from heat. Drizzle remaining ghee over warm rice. Set lid slightly ajar to allow steam to escape. Let rest for 5 minutes. Gently fluff with a fork and carefully spoon onto platter to serve.

Bengali Khichri

Khichri is the ultimate comfort food for all Indians. It is a combination of rice and lentils cooked together with enough water to make them soft, resembling risotto. Other ingredients and seasonings vary regionally.

Serves 6 to 8

Vegetarian Friendly

1 cup	yellow mung beans (yellow mung dal)	250 mL
¾ cup	long-grain white rice	175 mL
2 tbsp	ghee, divided	30 mL
1 tsp	cumin seeds	5 mL
1 cup	frozen peas, thawed	250 mL
1½ tbsp	minced peeled gingerroot	22 mL
2	bay leaves	2
1½ tsp	salt	7 mL
½ tsp	granulated sugar	2 mL
1 tbsp	minced green chiles, preferably serranos, optional	15 mL

1. Clean and pick through dal for any small stones and grit. Rinse several times in cold water. Drain and spread on dish towel to dry for 30 minutes or for up to 2 hours.

2. Place rice in a bowl with plenty of cold water and swish vigorously with fingers. Drain. Repeat 4 or 5 times until water is fairly clear. Cover with 3 to 4 inches (7.5 to 10 cm) cold water and set aside to soak for at least 15 minutes or for up to 2 hours.

3. Heat a wok over medium heat and add mung beans. Toast, stirring continuously, until beans turn golden, 8 to 10 minutes. Remove from heat.

4. In a saucepan, heat 1 tbsp (15 mL) of the ghee. Add cumin and sauté for 1 minute. Drain rice and add to pan. Add mung beans and sauté for 1 minute. Add 4 cups (1 L) fresh water. Add peas, ginger, bay leaves, salt and sugar. Cover and bring to a boil over high heat. Reduce heat to low and cook, stirring once, until soft and the consistency of risotto, 20 to 25 minutes.

5. Drizzle remaining 1 tbsp (15 mL) of ghee over top. Sprinkle with chiles, if desired, or pass at the table.

Khichri with Tomatoes and Green Peppers

This traditional Indian dish of rice and lentils makes a delicious main course when topped off with a mélange of peppers and tomatoes, so expect requests for seconds. Red lentils work best because they dissolve in the liquid, adding creaminess to the sauce. The pilaf will be liquidy when the rice is cooked, so serve this in soup plates. You don't need to add much — a simple green salad and perhaps some whole-grain bread to soak up the sauce.

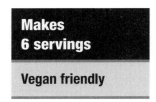

Makes 6 servings

Vegan friendly

Tips

For the best flavor, toast and grind whole cumin seeds rather than buying ground cumin. Simply stir seeds in a dry skillet over medium heat until fragrant, about 3 minutes. Immediately transfer to a spice grinder or mortar and grind.

Substitute 2 cups (500 mL) halved cherry tomatoes for the chopped tomatoes, if you prefer.

2 tbsp	olive oil, divided	30 mL
1	onion, finely chopped	1
2	cloves garlic, minced	2
2 tsp	curry powder	10 mL
1	bay leaf	1
1 cup	brown basmati or brown long-grain rice, rinsed and drained	250 mL
1 cup	dried red lentils	250 mL
4 cups	reduced-sodium vegetable stock	1 L
2	green bell peppers, seeded and diced	2
½ tsp	ground cumin (see Tips, left)	2 mL
½ tsp	salt	2 mL
½ tsp	freshly ground black pepper	2 mL
1	long red or green or Thai chile pepper, optional	1
4	small tomatoes, peeled and chopped (see Tips, left)	4
⅓ cup	ketchup	75 mL
3	hard-cooked eggs, sliced, optional	3

1. In a saucepan, heat 1 tbsp (15 mL) of the oil over medium heat. Add onion and garlic and cook, stirring, until onion softens, about 3 minutes. Stir in curry powder and bay leaf. Add rice and lentils and stir until coated. Add stock and bring to a boil. Reduce heat to low. Cover and simmer until rice is tender, about 50 minutes.

2. Meanwhile, in a skillet, heat remaining 1 tbsp (15 mL) of oil over medium heat. Add bell peppers, cumin, salt, black pepper and chile pepper, if using, and cook, stirring, until peppers are softened, about 5 minutes. Add tomatoes and cook, stirring, for 1 minute. Stir in ketchup. Reduce heat to low and simmer, stirring occasionally, until flavors meld, about 10 minutes.

3. *To serve:* Spread rice mixture evenly over a large deep platter. Arrange pepper mixture over top and garnish with eggs, if using.

Succulent Succotash

Made with freshly picked corn, succotash has become a late summer and autumn tradition. This makes a large batch, but it keeps well.

Serves 8 to 10

Vegan Friendly

Tip

This dish works best made with a robust vegetable stock. If you think your stock may be lacking in flavor, add a bit of vegetable bouillon powder, but be aware that you may have to reduce the quantity of salt in the recipe.

Make ahead

This dish can be partially assembled the night before it is cooked. Complete Step 1 and refrigerate overnight. The next day, continue cooking as directed in Step 2. Alternatively, succotash can be cooked overnight and refrigerated until you're ready to serve.

- **Medium (approx. 4 quart) slow cooker**

1 tbsp	vegetable oil	15 mL
2	onions, finely chopped	2
4	stalks celery, peeled and thinly sliced	4
2	large carrots, cut in quarters lengthwise, then thinly sliced	2
4	cloves garlic, minced	4
2 tsp	paprika	10 mL
2	sprigs fresh rosemary or 1 tbsp (15 mL) dried rosemary leaves	2
1 tsp	each salt and cracked black peppercorns	5 mL
1	can (28 oz/796 mL) tomatoes, including juice, coarsely chopped	1
1½ cups	vegetable stock (see Tip, left)	375 mL
4 cups	frozen lima beans, or 2 cups (500 mL) dried lima beans, cooked and drained (see pages 6 to 10)	1 L
2 cups	corn kernels	500 mL
1 cup	whipping (35%) cream (optional)	250 mL
	Freshly grated Parmesan cheese (optional)	
	Freshly grated nutmeg, to taste	

1. In a skillet, heat oil over medium heat. Add onions, celery and carrots and cook, stirring, until softened, about 7 minutes. Add garlic, paprika, rosemary, salt and peppercorns and cook, stirring, for 1 minute. Stir in tomatoes with juice and stock and bring to a boil. Place beans and corn in stoneware. Add contents of pan and stir well.

2. Cover and cook on Low for 8 hours or on High for 4 hours, until hot and bubbling. Stir in cream and Parmesan, if using, and season with nutmeg.

Mushroom Cholent

Cholent made with brisket, which is prepared on Friday and left to cook overnight, is the traditional midday meal for the Jewish Sabbath. In this version, portobello mushrooms provide heartiness and a mirepoix containing parsnips, as well as the traditional vegetables, adds sweetness and flavor. The mushrooms contribute to a surprisingly rich gravy and the results are very good indeed.

Serves 8

Vegan Friendly

Tip

Although traditional wisdom holds that adding salt to dried beans before they are cooked will make them tough, when food scientist Shirley Corriher actually tested this premise, she found the opposite to be true. Adding salt to beans while they cooked produced a more tender result.

Make ahead

This dish can be assembled before it is cooked. Complete Steps 1 and 2. Cover and refrigerate. When you are ready to cook, continue with Step 3.

- **Large (minimum 4 quart) slow cooker**

1 cup	dried white navy beans	250 mL
1 tbsp	vegetable oil	15 mL
2	onions, finely chopped	2
4	stalks celery, diced	4
2	carrots, peeled and diced	2
2	parsnips, peeled and diced	2
6	cloves garlic, minced	6
1 tbsp	minced gingerroot	15 mL
2 tsp	paprika	10 mL
1 tsp	salt	5 mL
1 tsp	cracked black peppercorns	5 mL
4 cups	vegetable stock	1 L
2	potatoes, peeled and cut into ½-inch (1 cm) cubes	2
12 oz	portobello mushroom caps (about 4 large)	375 g
1 cup	whole or pearl barley, rinsed	250 mL

1. Soak beans according to any method suggested on pages 6 and 7. Drain and rinse and set aside.

2. In a skillet, heat oil over medium heat. Add onions, celery, carrots and parsnips and cook, stirring, until softened, about 7 minutes. Add garlic, gingerroot, paprika, salt and peppercorns and cook, stirring, for 1 minute. Stir in vegetable stock and remove from heat.

3. Pour half the contents of pan into slow cooker stoneware. Set remainder aside. Spread potatoes evenly over mixture. Arrange mushrooms evenly over potatoes, cutting one to fit, if necessary. Spread barley and reserved beans evenly over mushrooms. Add remaining onion mixture to stoneware.

4. Cover and cook on Low for 10 hours, or on High for 5 hours, until beans are tender.

Green Beans Gado Gado

Gado gado, an Indonesian platter of vegetables, is served with a spicy peanut sauce.

Tips

Use soy or rice milk if coconut milk is not available.

In summer, serve the cooked beans over torn lettuce and in winter, use as a vegetable accompaniment to legumes and whole-grain dishes.

- **Heated serving platter**

Gado Gado Sauce

¼ cup	coconut milk (see Tips, left)	60 mL
2 tbsp	peanut or cashew butter	30 mL
1 tbsp	freshly squeezed lemon juice	15 mL
2 tsp	tamari or soy sauce	10 mL
2 tsp	grated fresh gingerroot	10 mL
½	dried cayenne pepper, crushed	½

Green Beans

1 lb	green beans, trimmed and cut in half	500 g
1	small onion, sliced and separated into rings	1
1 tbsp	olive oil	15 mL
1	can (14 oz/398 mL) lima beans, drained and rinsed, or 2 cups (500 mL) cooked lima beans	1
4 oz	bean sprouts	125 g
3 tbsp	chopped peanuts	45 mL

1. *Gado Gado Sauce:* In a small bowl, combine coconut milk, peanut butter, lemon juice, tamari, ginger and cayenne. Stir to mix well.

2. *Green Beans:* In a saucepan, bring 4 cups (1 L) water to a boil over high heat. Drop green beans into boiling water and blanch for 2 to 3 minutes. Using a slotted spoon, transfer green beans to a colander and rinse under cold water. Drain and set aside.

3. In a wok or large saucepan, combine onion rings and oil. Cook gently over medium heat for 7 minutes or until onion is soft. Add Gado Gado Sauce. Reduce heat and simmer for 2 minutes. Stir in green beans, lima beans and bean sprouts. Cook for 1 or 2 minutes or until heated through. Transfer to serving platter or individual plates. Garnish with peanuts and serve immediately.

Variation

Any nuts may be used in place of the peanuts.

Cider Baked Beans

If you often have small quantities of several varieties of dried beans in your pantry, here is a great way to use them up. For a festive presentation, add the bread crumb or caramelized apple topping.

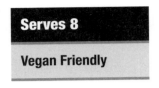

Serves 8

Vegan Friendly

Make Ahead

To manage your time most effectively when making this dish, soak the dried beans overnight. Peel and chop the onions, celery, carrots, parsnips and garlic the night before you plan to cook. Cover and refrigerate overnight. Measure the dried spices and cover. Combine apple cider, water and maple syrup in a 4-cup (1 L) measure. Cover and refrigerate overnight. The next morning, drain and rinse the beans and proceed with the recipe.

• **Medium (approx. 4 quart) slow cooker**

2 cups	assorted dried beans	500 mL
2	onions, finely chopped	2
3	stalks celery, peeled and thinly sliced	3
2	carrots, peeled and thinly sliced	2
2	large parsnips, peeled and thinly sliced	2
2	cloves garlic, minced	2
2 tsp	chili powder	10 mL
1 tsp	salt	5 mL
1 tsp	cracked black peppercorns	5 mL
4	whole cloves	4
1	cinnamon stick piece, about 2 inches (5 cm)	1
1 cup	apple cider or juice	250 mL
1 cup	water	250 mL
½ cup	maple syrup	125 mL
2 tbsp	cornstarch, dissolved in 2 tbsp (30 mL) cold water	30 mL

1. Soak beans according to your preferred method (see pages 6 and 7). Drain and rinse and set aside.

2. In slow cooker stoneware, combine beans, onions, celery, carrots, parsnips, garlic, chili powder, salt, peppercorns, cloves, cinnamon, apple cider, water and maple syrup. Cover and cook on Low for 10 to 12 hours or on High for 5 to 6 hours, until beans are tender.

3. In a bowl, combine dissolved cornstarch with 2 tbsp (30 mL) hot cooking liquid from beans and stir until smooth. Gradually add up to ¼ cup (60 mL) hot bean liquid, stirring until mixture is smooth. Return mixture to stoneware and stir well until sauce thickens.

Variation

Cider Baked Beans with Bread Crumb Topping: Preheat broiler. After beans are cooked, ladle them into individual heatproof tureens or a baking dish. In a bowl, combine 1 cup (250 mL) dry bread crumbs with ¼ cup (60 mL) each melted butter and finely chopped parsley. Sprinkle over beans and place under broiler until topping is lightly browned and beans are bubbling.

Romano Bean Stew

Lovers of hot food will enjoy this combination of spicy sauce, sweetly plump romano beans and fried almonds. It is best served with other spicy dishes, but it works wonderfully to perk up simple meals of rice and plain vegetables.

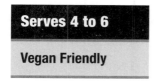

Serves 4 to 6

Vegan Friendly

Tips

For romano beans you can either cook your own or use canned. A 19-ounce (540 mL) can of romano beans, rinsed and drained, will yield exactly 2 cups (500 mL), which you'll need for this recipe.

Romano beans are also known as cranberry or borlotti beans.

2	medium tomatoes	2
1/4 cup	olive oil	60 mL
1/2 tsp	salt	2 mL
1 tsp	whole cumin seeds	5 mL
2	onions, sliced	2
1	fresh jalapeño pepper, diced (with or without seeds, depending on desired hotness)	1
1/2 cup	water	125 mL
1 tbsp	raisins	15 mL
2 cups	cooked romano beans	500 mL
1 tbsp	olive oil	15 mL
1/2 cup	slivered almonds	125 mL

1. Blanch tomatoes in boiling water for 30 seconds. Over a bowl, peel, core and deseed them. Chop tomatoes into chunks and set aside. Strain any accumulated tomato juices from bowl; add the juices to the tomatoes.

2. In a deep frying pan, heat 1/4 cup (60 mL) olive oil over high heat for 1 minute. Add salt and cumin seeds and stir-fry for 1 minute. Add onions and stir-fry for 2 minutes or until softened. Add jalapeño pepper (and seeds, if desired). Stir-fry for 1 to 2 minutes or until ingredients are well coated and starting to char.

3. Add reserved tomato and juices. Stir-fry for 2 to 3 minutes, until tomatoes are breaking up. Add water and let it come to a boil. Stir in raisins, then fold in beans. Reduce heat to medium-low and simmer for 5 minutes, stirring occasionally to prevent scorching. Transfer to a serving bowl.

4. In a frying pan, heat 1 tbsp (15 mL) oil over high heat for 30 seconds. Add slivered almonds and fry for 1 to 2 minutes, stirring and turning constantly, until browned. Take off heat and immediately transfer to a cool dish. Scatter the almonds on top of the beans. This dish will be at its best if allowed to rest for 1 or 2 hours, then served at room temperature.

Red Beans and Greens

Few meals could be more healthful than this delicious combination of hot leafy greens over flavorful beans. Collard greens are particularly delicious, but other dark leafy greens such as kale work well, too. The smoked paprika makes the dish more robust but it isn't essential.

Serves 6 to 8

Vegan Friendly

Tip

If you're cooking for a smaller group, make the full quantity of beans, spoon off what is needed, and serve with the appropriate quantity of cooked greens. Refrigerate or freeze the leftover beans for another meal.

Make Ahead

This dish can be partially prepared the night before it is cooked. Complete Steps 1 and 2. Cover and refrigerate overnight. The next day continue cooking as directed.

- **Medium (approx. 4 quart) slow cooker**

2 cups	dried kidney beans	500 mL
1 tbsp	vegetable oil	15 mL
2	large onions, finely chopped	2
2	stalks celery, finely chopped	2
4	cloves garlic, minced	4
1 tsp	dried oregano leaves	5 mL
1 tsp	salt	5 mL
1/2 tsp	cracked black peppercorns	2 mL
1/2 tsp	dried thyme leaves	2 mL
1/4 tsp	ground allspice or 6 whole allspice, tied in a piece of cheesecloth	1 mL
2	bay leaves	2
4 cups	vegetable stock	1 L
1 tsp	smoked paprika (optional)	5 mL

Greens

2 lbs	greens, thoroughly washed, stems removed and chopped	1 kg
	Butter or butter substitute	
1 tbsp	balsamic vinegar	15 mL
	Salt and freshly ground black pepper	

1. Soak beans according to your preferred method (see pages 6 and 7). Drain and rinse and set aside.

2. In a skillet, heat oil over medium heat. Add onions and celery and cook, stirring, until softened, about 5 minutes. Add garlic, oregano, salt, peppercorns, thyme, allspice and bay leaves and cook, stirring, for 1 minute. Transfer to slow cooker stoneware. Add beans and vegetable stock.

3. Cover and cook on Low for 8 hours or on High for 4 hours. Stir in smoked paprika, if using.

4. *Greens:* Steam greens until tender, about 10 minutes for collards. Toss with butter or butter substitute and balsamic vinegar. Season with salt and pepper to taste. Add to beans and stir to combine. Serve immediately.

Vegetable Tamale Pie

You would never know by the richness and the flavor that this recipe is both vegan and gluten-free!

Tip

For flavor notes that range from savory to sweet, use a combination of green, yellow, red and/or orange bell peppers in this recipe, instead of just one color.

- **8-inch (20 cm) square baking dish**

½ cup	polenta (yellow cornmeal)	125 mL
¼ cup	shredded vegan Cheddar cheese alternative	60 mL
1½ tsp	vegetable oil	7 mL
3	cloves garlic, minced	3
1	onion, finely chopped	1
1	small zucchini, diced	1
½	red, yellow or orange bell pepper, finely chopped	½
1 tbsp	chili powder	15 mL
1 tsp	ground cumin	5 mL
1 tsp	dried oregano	5 mL
1	can (14 to 19 oz/398 to 540 mL) pinto beans, drained and rinsed	1
1	can (14½ oz/411 mL) tomato purée (or 1¾ cups/425 mL crushed tomatoes)	1
½ cup	frozen corn kernels	125 mL
2 tsp	brown rice flour	10 mL
¼ cup	cold water	60 mL
½ tsp	each salt and freshly ground black pepper	2 mL

1. In a medium saucepan, bring 2 cups (500 mL) water to a boil over high heat. Stir in polenta, reduce heat and simmer, stirring often, for 30 minutes or until thick. Add cheese replacement and stir until melted. Remove from heat and set aside. Preheat oven to 375°F (190°C).

2. In a large skillet, heat oil over medium-high heat. Sauté garlic and onion for 5 to 7 minutes or until tender. Add zucchini, red pepper, chili powder, cumin and oregano; sauté for 5 minutes. Stir in beans, tomato purée and corn.

3. In a small bowl, whisk together rice flour and cold water to form a slurry. Stir into vegetable mixture and cook, stirring, for 3 minutes or until mixture thickens slightly. Season with salt and pepper. Spread in baking dish. Spread polenta mixture over top. Bake for 40 minutes or until bubbling. Let cool for 5 minutes before serving.

Leek-Potato-Lentil Pie

The subtly flavored filling of this pie highlights the sweet, earthy tastes of its main ingredients.

Tip

Be sure to wash leek thoroughly, splitting down the middle and paying special care to the grit that hides where the green and white parts meet.

- **Preheat oven to 400°F (200°C)**
- **4 ramekins, 1½-cup (375 mL) capacity, measuring 1 to 2 inches (2.5 to 5 cm) deep and 5 inches (12.5 cm) wide**

¼ cup	olive oil	60 mL
¼ tsp	salt	1 mL
¼ tsp	black pepper	1 mL
8 oz	boiled potatoes (about 2), cubed	250 g
2	leeks, green and white parts alike, finely chopped	2
½ cup	tomato sauce	125 mL
1½ cups	tomato juice	375 mL
2 cups	cooked lentils	500 mL
1 cup	thinly shredded spinach, packed	250 mL
¼ cup	finely chopped fresh parsley	60 mL
4	sheets Olive Oil Crust (page 245)	4
1	egg	1
1 tbsp	milk	15 mL

1. In a large, deep frying pan, heat olive oil over high heat. Add salt and pepper and stir. Add potatoes and leeks. Actively stir-fry for 5 minutes or until leeks have cooked down to ¼ of their original volume.

2. Add tomato sauce and tomato juice; stir to bring back to a boil. Reduce heat to medium. Add lentils and cook, stirring, for 5 minutes or until everything is piping hot and well mixed. Add shredded spinach, turn a few times and transfer mixture to a bowl. Add chopped parsley and mix in. Let mixture cool for about 20 minutes, uncovered and unrefrigerated.

3. Put one-quarter of the mixture (about 1¼ cups/ 300 mL) into each ramekin. Cover the filling with a sheet of crust, pinching the excess pastry over the edges of rims. Whisk together the egg and milk and brush over the crusts. Bake for 20 to 22 minutes or until golden brown and crusty.

Olive Oil Crust

This is an all-purpose crust for savory pies and serves as a serious competitor to store-bought phyllo. It is easy to work with: trimmings can be re-rolled with no loss, and it lives happily in the fridge for up to 5 days. It can also be frozen, but must be fully defrosted, and the oil that will have seeped out must be worked back into the dough.

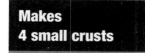

**Makes
4 small crusts**

1¾ cups	all-purpose flour	425 mL
1½ tsp	salt	7 mL
1½ tsp	baking powder	7 mL
½ cup	olive oil	125 mL
½ cup	milk	125 mL
1	whole egg, beaten	1
	Additional flour (as needed)	

1. In a bowl, sift together flour, salt and baking powder. In a separate bowl, whisk together olive oil, milk and beaten egg. Add the liquid ingredients all at once to the dry ingredients. Using fingers or an electric mixer with dough hook, blend the liquids into the flour. (If you use a mixer, scrape down the sides of the bowl several times.) This shouldn't take long; the dough will have absorbed the liquids and have the texture of an earlobe. If dough does not have the correct texture, work in another 2 tbsp (30 mL) flour.

2. Transfer the dough to a storage bowl, cover and refrigerate for at least ½ hour. When ready to use, knead any oil that may have seeped out back into the dough.

3. To roll crusts for making pies, divide the dough into 4 equal pieces. On a floured work surface, take one piece of dough and flatten it into a round with your hand. Turn it over and flour the other side. Using a floured rolling pin, roll dough into a round sheet about 8 or 9 inches (20 or 23 cm) in diameter and about ⅛ inch (3 mm) thick. It will shrink a little on its own but can be stretched by hand later. Transfer onto a piece of waxed paper. Repeat procedure for 3 remaining pieces of dough and stack them, separated by waxed paper, to ensure that they peel off easily when ready to use. The stack can then be covered and refrigerated.

Vegetarian Shepherd's Pie with Peppered Potato Topping

Tips

This shepherd's pie rivals the beef version — creamy, thick and rich tasting. Beans provide the meat-like texture.

For a different twist, try sweet potatoes.

Try other cheeses such as mozzarella or Swiss.

Make Ahead

Prepare up to 1 day in advance. Reheat gently.

Freeze for up to 3 weeks.

- **Preheat oven to 350°F (180°C)**
- **13- by 9-inch (3 L) baking dish**

2 tsp	vegetable oil	10 mL
2 tsp	minced garlic	10 mL
1 cup	chopped onions	250 mL
¾ cup	finely chopped carrots	175 mL
1½ cups	prepared tomato pasta sauce	375 mL
1 cup	canned red kidney beans, rinsed and drained	250 mL
1 cup	canned chickpeas, rinsed and drained	250 mL
½ cup	vegetable stock or water	125 mL
1½ tsp	dried basil	7 mL
2	bay leaves	2
4 cups	diced potatoes	1 L
½ cup	2% milk	125 mL
⅓ cup	light sour cream	75 mL
¼ tsp	freshly ground black pepper	1 mL
¾ cup	shredded Cheddar cheese	175 mL
3 tbsp	grated Parmesan cheese	45 mL

1. In a saucepan, heat oil over medium-high heat. Add garlic, onions and carrots; cook 4 minutes or until onions are softened. Stir in tomato sauce, kidney beans, chickpeas, stock, basil and bay leaves. Reduce heat to medium-low and cook, covered, for 15 minutes or until vegetables are tender. Remove bay leaves. Transfer sauce to a food processor; pulse on and off just until chunky. Spread over bottom of baking dish.

2. Place potatoes in a saucepan and add cold water to cover; bring to a boil. Reduce heat and simmer for 10 to 12 minutes or until tender. Drain; mash with milk, sour cream and pepper. Spoon on top of sauce in baking dish. Sprinkle with Cheddar and Parmesan cheese. Bake, uncovered, for 20 minutes or until hot.

Lentil Shepherd's Pie

Here's a flavorful rendition of an old favorite, in which lentils are substituted for the traditional meat. Serve with a tossed salad for a nutritious and satisfying meal.

Serves 4

Vegetarian Friendly

Tips

Use shredded Cheddar cheese instead of the Italian 4-cheese mixture, if you prefer.

Substitute ½ cup (125 mL) loosely packed parsley leaves for the green onions, if you prefer.

Be careful not to overprocess the potato mixture or the topping will be mushy. Small lumps of potato should remain.

- **Preheat oven to 350°F (180°C)**
- **Food processor**
- **8-cup (2 L) baking or casserole dish, lightly greased**

Topping

2 cups	diced cooked potatoes	500 mL
½ cup	milk	125 mL
1 cup	shredded Italian 4-cheese mix	250 mL
½ cup	dry bread crumbs	125 mL
4	green onions (white part only), coarsely chopped	4
1 tbsp	butter, softened	15 mL
½ tsp	salt	2 mL
	Freshly ground black pepper	

Filling

1 tbsp	vegetable oil	15 mL
2 cups	diced onion	500 mL
1 cup	diced celery	250 mL
1	can (28 oz/796 mL) tomatoes, drained and coarsely chopped	1
1	can (19 oz/540 mL) lentils, drained and rinsed	1
2 tbsp	prepared basil pesto	30 mL
2 tbsp	shredded Italian 4-cheese mix	30 mL

1. *Topping:* In a food processor fitted with metal blade, combine potatoes and milk. Pulse several times to combine. Add cheese, bread crumbs, onions, butter, salt, and black pepper to taste. Process until blended but potatoes are still a bit lumpy. Set aside.

2. *Filling:* In a skillet, heat oil over medium heat. Add onion and celery and cook, stirring, until celery is softened, about 8 minutes. Add tomatoes and lentils. Bring to a boil. Stir in pesto and pour into prepared baking dish.

3. Spread reserved potato mixture evenly over lentil mixture. Sprinkle with shredded cheese. Bake in preheated oven until top is browned and mixture is bubbling, about 25 minutes.

Zesty Black Bean Pie

If your taste buds have grown weary of the old standards, try this savory pie with a cracker crumb crust. Just add a simple green salad for a nutritious and tasty meal.

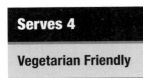

Serves 4

Vegetarian Friendly

Tips

Use a mild or hot tomato salsa, depending upon your preference.

If you are using a blender to make the cracker crumbs, add the crackers in batches and process, scraping down the sides after each addition.

- **Preheat oven to 350°F (180°C)**
- **9-inch (23 cm) pie plate**
- **Food processor or blender**

Crust

30	cheese-flavored crackers, such as Ritz (about half an 8 oz/250 g box)	30
¼ cup	butter, melted	60 mL

Filling

1 tbsp	vegetable oil	15 mL
1 cup	diced onion	250 mL
1 tsp	minced garlic	5 mL
1 tsp	ground cumin	5 mL
1	can (19 oz/540 mL) black beans, drained and rinsed	1
1	can (12 oz/341 mL) corn kernels, drained	1
1 cup	tomato salsa	250 mL
4 oz	cream cheese, cut into ½-inch (1 cm) cubes and softened	125 g

1. *Crust:* In a food processor or blender (see Tips, left), pulse crackers until they resemble coarse crumbs.

2. In a bowl, combine cracker crumbs and butter. Press into pie plate. Bake in preheated oven until golden, about 8 minutes.

3. *Filling:* Meanwhile, in a skillet, heat oil over medium heat. Add onion and cook, stirring, until softened, about 3 minutes. Add garlic and cumin and cook, stirring, for 1 minute.

4. Stir in beans, corn and salsa. Bring to a boil. Add cream cheese, and cook, stirring, until cheese is melted and mixture holds together, about 2 minutes. Remove from heat.

5. Spread mixture evenly over cooked crust. Bake in preheated oven for 10 minutes to combine flavors.

Variations

Add 1 jalapeño pepper, finely chopped, along with the garlic. Add 1 or 2 finely chopped roasted red peppers along with the corn.

Black Bean, Corn and Leek Frittata

Tips

Here's a great variation on the traditional omelet — but with less fat and cholesterol.

Replace beans and vegetables with other varieties of your choice.

Cilantro can be replaced with dill, parsley and basil.

Make Ahead

Combine entire mixture early in the day. Cook just before serving.

1½ tsp	vegetable oil	7 mL
2 tsp	minced garlic	10 mL
¾ cup	chopped leeks	175 mL
½ cup	chopped red bell peppers	125 mL
½ cup	canned or frozen corn kernels, drained	125 mL
½ cup	canned black beans, rinsed and drained	125 mL
⅓ cup	chopped fresh cilantro	75 mL
2	eggs	2
3	egg whites	3
⅓ cup	2% milk	75 mL
¼ tsp	salt	1 mL
¼ tsp	freshly ground black pepper	1 mL
2 tbsp	grated Parmesan cheese	30 mL

1. In a nonstick saucepan sprayed with vegetable spray, heat oil over medium-high heat. Add garlic, leeks and red peppers; cook 4 minutes or until softened. Remove from heat; stir in corn, black beans and cilantro.

2. In a bowl, whisk together whole eggs, egg whites, milk, salt and pepper. Stir in cooled vegetable mixture.

3. Spray a 12-inch (30 cm) nonstick frying pan with vegetable spray. Heat over medium-low heat. Pour in frittata mixture. Cook for 5 minutes, gently lifting sides of frittata to let uncooked egg mixture flow under frittata. Sprinkle with Parmesan cheese. Cover and cook another 3 minutes or until frittata is set. Slip frittata onto a serving platter. Cut into wedges and serve immediately.

Creamy Chipotle Black Bean Burrito Bake

Authentic Mexican flavors abound in this vegetarian recipe, with smoky chipotle peppers in adobo sauce, black beans, corn and creamy Monterey Jack cheese. Serve garnished with avocado slices and chopped fresh cilantro.

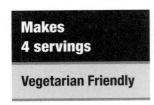

**Makes
4 servings**

Vegetarian Friendly

Tips

You can adjust the heat in the recipe by choosing mild, medium or hot salsa. Turn it up a little bit more by adding another chipotle pepper or two.

Look for canned chipotle peppers in adobo sauce in the international foods section of your supermarket. They're a great addition to soups, stews, sauces and dressings — anywhere you want to add heat and smoky flavor.

- **Preheat oven to 350°F (180°C)**
- **11- by 7-inch (28 by 18 cm) glass baking dish, greased**

1/2 cup	reduced-fat sour cream	125 mL
1	chipotle pepper in adobo sauce, finely chopped	1
1	can (14 to 19 oz/398 to 540 mL) black beans, drained and rinsed	1
1 cup	frozen corn kernels, thawed	250 mL
4	8- to 10-inch (20 to 25 cm) reduced-fat flour tortillas	4
1 cup	salsa	250 mL
1/2 cup	shredded part-skim Monterey Jack cheese	125 mL

1. In a medium bowl, combine sour cream and chipotle pepper. Stir in beans and corn.
2. Spoon 1/2 cup (125 mL) of the bean mixture down the center of each tortilla. Roll up and place seam side down in prepared baking dish. Spread salsa evenly over tortillas. Sprinkle with cheese.
3. Cover and bake in preheated oven for 20 minutes or until bubbling.

Southwest Butternut Squash Tortilla Bake

This easy casserole, filled with traditional flavors of the Southwest, is a wonderful way to showcase butternut squash.

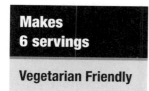

**Makes
6 servings**

Vegetarian Friendly

Tips

For more heat, use 2 jalapeños and leave in the seeds. But be careful — the ribs and seeds really add to the heat!

Butternut squash is easier to dice if you microwave it on High for about 2 minutes before peeling.

If you want to use canned corn, use a 14 or 15 oz (398 or 425 mL) can and drain before using.

- **Preheat oven to 400°F (200°C)**
- **8-cup (2 L) round casserole dish**

2 tbsp	olive oil, divided	30 mL
1	onion, thinly sliced	1
2	cloves garlic, minced	2
1	jalapeño pepper, seeded and minced	1
1 tsp	paprika	5 mL
1 tsp	ground cumin	5 mL
1 tsp	dried oregano	5 mL
1	can (16 oz/454 mL) crushed tomatoes	1
1 lb	butternut squash, peeled, seeded and diced	500 g
1 cup	vegetable broth	250 mL
1	can (14 to 19 oz/398 to 540 mL) black beans, drained and rinsed	1
1½ cups	corn kernels (thawed if frozen)	375 mL
¼ tsp	salt	1 mL
¼ tsp	freshly ground black pepper	1 mL
8	6-inch (15 cm) corn tortillas, cut into ¾-inch (2 cm) strips	8
½ cup	shredded reduced-fat sharp (old) Cheddar cheese	125 mL

1. In a large nonstick skillet, heat half the oil over medium heat. Sauté onion for 5 to 7 minutes or until softened. Add garlic and jalapeño; sauté for 1 minute. Add paprika, cumin and oregano; sauté for 1 minute. Add tomatoes, squash and broth; bring to a simmer. Reduce heat to low, cover and simmer for about 10 minutes or until squash is just tender. Stir in beans, corn, salt and pepper.

2. Spoon squash mixture into casserole dish. Layer tortilla strips over top. Brush with the remaining oil.

3. Bake in preheated oven for 25 to 30 minutes or until topping is golden brown and filling is bubbling. Sprinkle with cheese and bake for 3 minutes or until cheese is melted.

Enchiladas in Salsa Verde

Serve this tasty Mexican dish with a simple avocado and onion salad.

Tips

Salsa verde is available in the Mexican foods section of many supermarkets or in specialty food stores.

Corn tortillas have a more authentic Mexican flavor than those made with flour.

Garnish this dish to suit your taste. Finely chopped red or green onion, finely chopped cilantro leaves, shredded lettuce and/ or sour cream all make a nice finish.

- **Preheat oven to 350°F (180°C)**
- **13- by 9-inch (33 by 23 cm) baking dish**

1 tbsp	vegetable oil	15 mL
1 cup	diced onion	250 mL
1 tbsp	minced garlic	15 mL
1 tsp	ground cumin	5 mL
2 cups	diced cooked potatoes	500 mL
1	package (10 oz/300 g) frozen chopped spinach, including liquid, thawed, or 1 bag (10 oz/300 g) spinach, stems removed, coarsely chopped	1
1	can (14 oz/398 mL) vegetarian refried beans	1
3 cups	shredded Monterey Jack cheese or Mexican cheese mix, divided	750 mL
3 cups	salsa verde, divided (see Tips, left)	750 mL
16	6-inch (15 cm) tortillas, preferably corn (see Tips, left)	16

1. In a skillet, heat oil over medium heat. Add onion and cook, stirring, until softened, about 3 minutes. Add garlic and cumin and cook, stirring, for 1 minute. Add potatoes and spinach and cook, stirring, until spinach is incorporated, about 3 minutes. Stir in refried beans and bring to a boil. Add 1¾ cups (425 mL) of the cheese and cook, stirring, until cheese melts, about 2 minutes. Remove from heat.

2. Pour 1 cup (250 mL) salsa verde into a bowl. One at a time, dip tortillas into sauce, turning to ensure all parts are moistened. Lay 1 tortilla on a plate and spread with ¼ cup (60 mL) of the bean mixture. Roll up and place, seam side down, in baking dish. Repeat with remaining tortillas and filling.

3. Pour remaining salsa verde over tortillas and sprinkle with remaining cheese. Cover and bake in preheated oven until hot and bubbling, about 30 minutes. Let casserole rest for 5 minutes. Add garnishes (see Tips, left) and serve.

Variation

If you are a heat seeker, add 1 finely chopped jalapeño pepper along with the garlic.

Southwest Bread Pudding

Serves 6

Vegetarian Friendly

- **Preheat oven to 350°F (180°C)**
- **12-cup (3 L) casserole dish**

	Olive oil spray	
10	slices good-quality white bread	10
2	jars (each 16 oz/454 mL) salsa verde (green salsa)	2
1	can (14 to 19 oz/398 to 540 mL) pinto beans, drained and rinsed	1
1 cup	sour cream	250 mL
1½ cups	shredded Monterey Jack cheese	375 mL

1. Spray a baking sheet with oil. Place bread on pan in a single layer and spray with more oil. Bake for about 10 minutes, until slightly toasted and warm; cut into 1-inch (2.5 cm) cubes.

2. Place one-quarter of the salsa in the bottom of casserole dish and top with one-third of the bread cubes, arranged in an even layer. Layer with half the beans, another quarter of the salsa, half the sour cream, and one-third of the cheese. Repeat layers, then finish with the remaining bread, remaining salsa, and remaining cheese.

3. Bake in preheated oven for about 20 minutes, until browned and bubbling.

Variation

Mexican Torta: Follow preceding recipe, but replace the bread with 10 corn tortillas, cut into wedges, and replace the pinto beans with navy beans.

Peas and Greens

This delicious combination of black-eyed peas and greens is a great dish for busy weeknights. It also makes a wonderful side dish for roasted meat, particularly lamb.

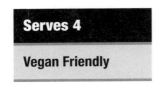

Serves 4

Vegan Friendly

Tips

To prepare fennel, before removing the core, chop off the top shoots and discard. If the outer sections of the bulb seem old and dry, peel them with a vegetable peeler before using.

You can use any kind of paprika in this recipe: regular; hot, which produces a nicely peppery version; or smoked, which adds a delicious note of smokiness. If you have regular paprika and would like a bit a heat, dissolve ¼ tsp (1 mL) cayenne pepper in the lemon juice along with the paprika.

Toasting fennel seeds intensifies their flavor. To toast fennel seeds, stir them in a dry skillet over medium heat until fragrant, about 3 minutes. Transfer to a mortar or spice grinder and grind.

- **Medium to large (3½ to 5 quart) slow cooker**

1 tbsp	vegetable oil	15 mL
2	onions, finely chopped	2
1	bulb fennel, cored and thinly sliced on the vertical	1
4	cloves garlic, minced	4
½ tsp	salt (or to taste)	2 mL
½ tsp	cracked black peppercorns	2 mL
¼ tsp	fennel seeds, toasted and ground (see Tips, left)	1 mL
1	can (14 oz/398 mL) diced tomatoes, with juice	1
2 cups	cooked black-eyed peas, drained and rinsed	500 mL
1 tsp	paprika (see Tips, left) dissolved in 2 tbsp (30 mL) freshly squeezed lemon juice	5 mL
4 cups	chopped spinach or Swiss chard (about 1 bunch), stems removed	1 L

1. In a skillet, heat oil over medium heat for 30 seconds. Add onions and fennel; cook, stirring, until fennel is softened, about 5 minutes. Add garlic, salt, peppercorns and fennel seeds; cook, stirring, for 1 minute. Add tomatoes with juice and bring to a boil. Transfer to slow cooker stoneware.

2. Stir in peas. Cover and cook on Low for 8 hours or on High for 4 hours, until peas are tender. Stir in paprika solution. Add spinach, stirring until submerged. Cover and cook on High for 20 minutes, until spinach is tender.

Make Ahead

Complete Step 1. Cover and refrigerate for up to 2 days. When you're ready to cook, continue with the recipe.

Potato and Adzuki Latkes

A fast and nutritious meal that is both satisfying and great tasting, this dish can be adapted to almost any vegetable that is in your refrigerator. The egg holds the ingredients together and the flour absorbs the liquid from the freshly grated vegetables to keep the pancakes from falling apart.

Serves 4

Vegetarian Friendly

- **Preheat oven to 325°F (160°C)**
- **Baking sheet, lined with paper towels**

2	medium potatoes, shredded and drained	2
1 cup	cooked adzuki beans	250 mL
1	carrot, shredded	1
1/2	onion, chopped or shredded	1/2
1/2 cup	shredded Swiss or Cheddar cheese	125 mL
1	clove garlic, minced	1
1 tbsp	chopped fresh savory	15 mL
1 tbsp	chopped fresh oregano	15 mL
1/2 tsp	salt	2 mL
1	large egg, beaten	1
1/4 cup	unbleached all-purpose or whole wheat flour (approx.)	60 mL
2 to 4 tbsp	olive oil	30 to 60 mL
1 cup	drained yogurt or Yogurt Cheese, (page 98), optional	250 mL

1. In a large bowl, combine potatoes, beans, carrot, onion, cheese, garlic, savory, oregano and salt, mixing well. Stir in egg. Sprinkle in flour, 1 tbsp (15 mL) at a time, stirring until the mixture holds together well.

2. In a large skillet, heat 1 tbsp (15 mL) of the oil over medium heat. Drop 1/4 cup (60 mL) of the potato mixture into the skillet and flatten lightly with a fork (keep latke compact and at least 1/2 inch/1 cm thick). Repeat to make 1 or 2 more latkes. Cook for 4 minutes on one side. Flip and cook for 3 to 4 minutes on the other side or until browned. Using a slotted lifter, transfer to prepared baking sheet and keep warm in preheated oven. Repeat with remaining vegetable mixture, adding more oil as necessary. Serve hot with a dollop of yogurt, if using.

Variation

Use any cooked legume (lima, red kidney or pinto beans) or lentils (red or green) in place of the adzuki beans.

Moroccan Chickpea Tagine

This is a very nice slow-cooked stew, but to save time, it may be cooked on the stovetop (see Tips, below).

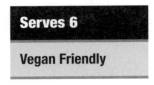
Tips

To cook Moroccan Chickpea Tagine on the stovetop: In a Dutch oven or large saucepan, heat 1 tbsp (15 mL) olive oil over high heat. Reduce heat to medium. Add onion and cook, stirring frequently, for 6 to 8 minutes or until soft. Add all other ingredients. Reduce heat to low, cover and cook, stirring once or twice, for 45 minutes or until sweet potato is tender.

Use 1¼ cups (300 mL) vegetable stock if using canned chickpeas and their liquid.

- **Preheat oven to 350°F (180°C)**
- **Tagine or Dutch oven**

4 cups	cooked chickpeas, rinsed and drained, or 2 cans (14 to 19 oz/398 to 540 mL) chickpeas with liquid (see Tips, left)	1 L
2 cups	vegetable stock or water	500 mL
	Juice of 1 lemon	
2 cups	diced sweet potato, sweet or pie pumpkin or butternut squash	500 mL
½ cup	quinoa, rinsed	125 mL
1	onion, chopped	1
¼ cup	chopped dried apricots	60 mL
¼ cup	chopped raisins	60 mL
4	sun-dried tomato halves, thinly sliced	4
2	slices (⅛ inch/3 mm) fresh gingerroot, finely chopped	2
½ tsp	ground cumin	2 mL
½ tsp	ground coriander	2 mL
¼ tsp	ground cinnamon	1 mL
¼ tsp	hot pepper flakes	1 mL
	Sea salt and freshly ground pepper	

1. In the base of tagine, combine chickpeas, stock, lemon juice, sweet potato, quinoa, onion, apricots, raisins, sun-dried tomatoes, ginger, cumin, coriander, cinnamon and hot pepper flakes.

2. Bake in preheated oven for 1½ hours or until sweet potato is tender when pierced with the tip of a knife. Season to taste with salt and pepper.

Garlic Greens with Chickpeas and Cumin

This makes an excellent main dish, or serve smaller portions as a warm salad course or vegetable side dish. The best thing about it is that it takes less than half an hour from start to finish.

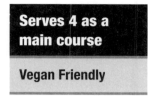

Serves 4 as a main course

Vegan Friendly

Tip

If cumin seeds are not available, use 2 tsp (10 mL) ground cumin and skip the toasting and grinding in Step 1.

1 tbsp	cumin seeds (see Tip, left)	15 mL
1 tsp	hot pepper flakes	5 mL
½ tsp	ground cinnamon	2 mL

Garlic Greens

3 tbsp	olive oil	45 mL
2	onions, coarsely chopped	2
4	cloves garlic, chopped	4
8	dried apricot halves, thinly sliced	8
1	can (14 to 19 oz/398 to 540 mL) chickpeas with liquid	1
	Juice of 1 lemon	
4 cups	packed fresh spinach, trimmed (about 10 oz/300 g)	1 L
	Sea salt and freshly ground pepper	

1. In a small skillet, toast cumin seeds over medium heat until aromatic, 1 to 2 minutes. Remove from heat and let cool. Using a mortar and pestle or spice grinder, pulverize or grind the toasted seeds. In a bowl, combine with hot pepper flakes and cinnamon. Set aside.

2. *Garlic Greens:* In a deep skillet or saucepan, heat oil over medium heat. Add onions and cook, stirring frequently, for 6 to 8 minutes or until soft.

3. Stir in cumin mixture, garlic and apricots and cook, stirring occasionally, for 2 minutes. Add chickpeas with liquid and lemon juice. Bring to a boil and add spinach. Cover, reduce heat and simmer, stirring once, for 5 minutes. Season to taste with salt and pepper.

Lentil Sloppy Joes

Here's a kids' favorite that grown-ups enjoy, too. It makes a great dinner for those busy nights when everyone is coming and going at different times. Leave the slow cooker on Low or Warm, the buns on the counter and the fixins' of salad in the fridge and let everyone help themselves.

Tip

Use 1 can (14 to 19 oz/398 to 540 mL) green or brown lentils, drained and rinsed, or cook 1 cup (250 mL) dried lentils (see page 10 or Variation, page 277).

Make Ahead

Complete Step 1. Cover and refrigerate for up to 2 days. When you're ready to cook, complete the recipe.

- **Small to medium (1½ to 4 quart) slow cooker**

1 tbsp	oil	15 mL
1	onion, finely chopped	1
4	stalks celery, diced	4
4	cloves garlic, minced	4
½ tsp	dried oregano	2 mL
½ tsp	salt	2 mL
	Freshly ground black pepper	
½ cup	tomato ketchup	125 mL
¼ cup	water	60 mL
1 tbsp	balsamic vinegar	15 mL
1 tbsp	brown sugar	15 mL
1 tbsp	Dijon mustard	15 mL
2 cups	cooked brown or green lentils, drained and rinsed (see Tip, left)	500 mL
	Hot pepper sauce, optional	
	Toasted hamburger buns	

1. In a skillet, heat oil over medium heat. Add onion and celery and cook, stirring, until softened, about 5 minutes. Add garlic, oregano, salt, and pepper, to taste, and cook, stirring, for 1 minute. Stir in ketchup, water, balsamic vinegar, brown sugar and mustard. Transfer to slow cooker stoneware. Add lentils and stir well.

2. Cover and cook on Low for 6 hours or on High for 3 hours, until hot and bubbly. Add hot pepper sauce, to taste, if using. Ladle over hot toasted buns and serve immediately.

Poached Eggs on Spicy Lentils

This delicious combination is a great cold-weather dish. Add the chiles if you prefer a little spice and accompany with warm Indian bread, such as naan, and hot rice. The Egg and Lentil Curry (see Variation, below) is a great dish for a buffet table or as part of an Indian-themed meal.

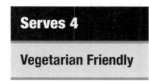

Serves 4

Vegetarian Friendly

Tips

To poach eggs: In a deep skillet, bring about 2 inches (5 cm) lightly salted water to a boil over medium heat. Reduce heat to low. Break eggs into a measuring cup and, holding the cup close to the surface of the water, slip the eggs into the pan. Cook until whites are set and centers are still soft, 3 to 4 minutes. Remove with a slotted spoon.

If you are halving this recipe, be sure to use a small ($1\frac{1}{2}$ to $3\frac{1}{2}$ quart) slow cooker.

Make Ahead

Complete Step 1. Cover and refrigerate for up to 2 days. When you're ready to cook, complete the recipe.

- **Medium (approx. 4 quart) slow cooker**

1 tbsp	oil	15 mL
2	onions, finely chopped	2
1 tbsp	minced garlic	15 mL
1 tbsp	minced gingerroot	15 mL
1 tsp	ground coriander	5 mL
1 tsp	ground cumin	5 mL
1 tsp	cracked black peppercorns	5 mL
1 cup	red lentils, rinsed	250 mL
1	can (28 oz/796 mL) tomatoes with juice, coarsely chopped	1
2 cups	vegetable broth	500 mL
1 cup	coconut milk	250 mL
	Salt	
1	long green chile pepper or 2 Thai bird's-eye chiles, finely chopped, optional	1
4	eggs	4
	Finely chopped fresh parsley, optional	

1. In a large skillet, heat oil over medium heat. Add onions and cook, stirring, until softened, about 3 minutes. Add garlic, ginger, coriander, cumin and peppercorns and cook, stirring, for 1 minute. Add lentils, tomatoes with juice and vegetable broth and bring to a boil. Transfer to slow cooker stoneware.

2. Cover and cook on Low for 6 hours or on High for 3 hours, until lentils are tender and mixture is bubbly. Stir in coconut milk, salt, to taste, and chile pepper, if using. Cover and cook for 20 to 30 minutes, until heated through.

3. When ready to serve, ladle into soup bowls and top each serving with a poached egg (see Tips, left). Garnish with parsley, if using.

Variation

Egg and Lentil Curry: Substitute 4 to 6 hard-cooked eggs for the poached. Peel them and cut into halves. Ladle the curry into a serving dish, arrange the eggs on top and garnish.

Cumin-Laced Lentils with Sun-Dried Tomatoes and Roasted Peppers

The slightly Middle Eastern flavors that underscore this dish are luscious. It is very forgiving. If you don't have sun-dried tomatoes, substitute tomato paste. As for harissa, substitute cayenne (see Tips, below).

Serves 6

Vegan Friendly

Tips

Use some red lentils in this recipe because they dissolve into the liquid, producing a lusciously creamy result, but if you don't have any, use brown or green lentils for the total quantity.

If you don't have sun-dried tomatoes, substitute 1 tbsp (15 mL) tomato paste.

If you don't have harissa, dissolve $\frac{1}{2}$ tsp (2 mL) cayenne pepper in 1 tbsp (15 mL) freshly squeezed lemon juice and stir in along with the red peppers.

Make Ahead

Complete Step 1. Cover and refrigerate for up to 2 days. When you're ready to cook, complete the recipe.

• **Medium (approx. 4 quart) slow cooker**

1 tbsp	olive oil	15 mL
1	onion, finely chopped	1
2	stalks celery, diced	2
4	cloves garlic, minced	4
1 tbsp	ground cumin (see Tip, page 261)	15 mL
1 tbsp	ground coriander	15 mL
1 tsp	salt	5 mL
1 tsp	cracked black peppercorns	5 mL
1 cup	brown or green lentils, rinsed	250 mL
$\frac{1}{2}$ cup	red lentils, rinsed (see Tips, left)	125 mL
1	can (14 oz/398 mL) diced tomatoes, with juice	1
2	finely chopped sun-dried tomatoes (see Tips, left)	2
2 cups	vegetable broth	500 mL
2	roasted red peppers, thinly sliced	2
1 to 2 tsp	harissa (see Tips, left)	5 to 10 mL
	Finely chopped cilantro	

1. In a skillet, heat oil over medium heat. Add onion and celery and cook, stirring, until softened, about 5 minutes. Add garlic, cumin, coriander, salt and peppercorns and cook, stirring, for 1 minute. Add brown and red lentils and toss until well coated with mixture. Add tomatoes with juice and sun-dried tomatoes. Transfer to slow cooker stoneware.

2. Stir in vegetable broth. Cover and cook on Low for 6 hours or on High for 3 hours, until lentils are tender. Add roasted peppers and harissa and stir well. Cover and cook on High for 15 minutes to meld flavors. Garnish with cilantro.

Indian-Spiced Lentils with Peppery Apricots

Although the flavors are exotic, this delicious mélange qualifies as comfort food. Savory lentils seasoned with spices that are traditionally associated with the East are punctuated by sweet, chewy apricots sprinkled with piquant cayenne. It's a marriage made in heaven.

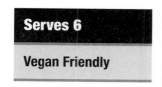

Serves 6

Vegan Friendly

Tip

For best results, toast and grind the cumin and coriander seeds yourself. *To toast seeds:* Place in a dry skillet over medium heat and cook, stirring, until fragrant, about 3 minutes. Immediately transfer to a spice grinder or mortar and grind finely.

Make Ahead

Complete Step 1. Cover and refrigerate for up to 2 days. When you're ready to cook, complete the recipe.

- **Medium (approx. 4 quart) slow cooker**

1 tbsp	oil	15 mL
2	onions, finely chopped	2
4	stalks celery, diced	4
4	cloves garlic, minced	4
1 tbsp	minced gingerroot	15 mL
2 tsp	ground cumin (see Tip, left)	10 mL
2 tsp	ground coriander	10 mL
1 tsp	ground turmeric	5 mL
1	piece (2 inches/5 cm) cinnamon stick	1
1½ cups	brown or green lentils, rinsed	375 mL
4 cups	vegetable broth	1 L
1	sweet potato, peeled and diced	1
½ tsp	cayenne pepper	2 mL
1 cup	chopped dried apricots	250 mL
	Finely chopped fresh parsley	

1. In a skillet, heat oil over medium heat. Add onions and celery and cook, stirring, until softened, about 5 minutes. Add garlic, ginger, cumin, coriander, turmeric and cinnamon stick and cook, stirring, for 1 minute. Transfer to slow cooker stoneware. Stir in lentils and vegetable broth.

2. Add sweet potato and stir well. Cover and cook on Low for 6 to 8 hours or on High for 3 to 4 hours, until lentils are tender.

3. In a small bowl, sprinkle cayenne evenly over apricots. Add to stoneware and stir well. Cover and cook on High for 15 minutes to meld flavors. Discard cinnamon stick. Garnish with parsley.

Eggplant Lentil Ragoût

This is a delicious combination of flavors and textures. Just add a green salad for a satisfying meal.

Tips

To sweat eggplant:
Place cubed eggplant
in a colander, sprinkle
liberally with salt, toss
well and set aside for
30 minutes to 1 hour.
If time is short, blanch
the pieces for a minute
or two in heavily salted
water. In either case,
rinse thoroughly in
fresh cold water and,
using your hands,
squeeze out excess
moisture. Pat dry with
paper towels and it's
ready for cooking.

For the best flavor,
toast and grind cumin
seeds yourself. *To toast
seeds:* Place in a dry
skillet over medium
heat and cook,
stirring, until fragrant,
about 3 minutes.
Immediately transfer
to a spice grinder
or mortar and
grind finely.

Make Ahead

Complete Steps 1
and 2. Cover and
refrigerate for up
to 2 days. When
you're ready to cook,
complete the recipe.

- **Medium (approx. 4 quart) slow cooker**

1	medium eggplant (about 1 lb/500 g) peeled, cubed (2 inch/5 cm) and sweated (see Tips, left)	1
2 tbsp	olive oil (approx.)	30 mL
2	onions, finely chopped	2
4	cloves garlic, minced	4
1 tbsp	ground cumin (see Tips, left)	15 mL
1 tsp	finely grated lemon zest	5 mL
1 tsp	salt	5 mL
1/2 tsp	cracked black peppercorns	2 mL
1 cup	brown or green lentils, rinsed	250 mL
3 cups	vegetable broth	750 mL
1 tbsp	freshly squeezed lemon juice	15 mL
1/2 cup	finely chopped dill	125 mL

1. In a skillet, heat oil over medium-high heat. Add eggplant, in batches, and cook until browned, adding more oil as necessary. Transfer to slow cooker stoneware.

2. Add onions to pan, adding more oil, if necessary, and cook, stirring, until softened, about 3 minutes. Add garlic, cumin, lemon zest, salt and peppercorns and cook, stirring, for 1 minute. Add lentils and toss until coated. Transfer to slow cooker stoneware. Stir in broth.

3. Cover and cook on Low for 6 to 8 hours or on High for 3 to 4 hours, until lentils are tender. Stir in lemon juice and dill.

Sides and Small Plates

Pea Tops with Pancetta and Tofu 264

Soy-Braised Tofu, Cabbage and Ginger
   with Cellophane Noodles 265

Butter Beans and Grilled Red Pepper . . . 266

White Beans with Tomato 267

Greek Beans with Onions 268

Red Beans and Red Rice 269

Pumpkin and Black Beans 270

Lentils Cooked with Wine and Tomato . . 271

Spiced Rice and Lentil Pilaf 272

Lentils-Rice-Spinach 273

Frijoles Borrachos Mexicanos 274

Tomatoes Stuffed with Corn,
   Black Beans and Pine Nuts 275

Basic Pinto Beans 275

Quick Refried Beans 276

Stove-Top Refried Beans 276

Basic Beans in the Slow Cooker 277

Pea Tops with Pancetta and Tofu

Pea tops are the shoots of snow pea plants. They're now available almost year-round in Asian markets. They are tasty in salads and have a subtle, nutty flavor when cooked. However, they are quite perishable and won't last much longer than a couple of days in your refrigerator.

Serves 4

1	3-inch (7.5 cm) square medium tofu	1
2 tbsp	vegetable oil, divided	30 mL
	Salt and pepper to taste	
1 tsp	sesame oil	5 mL
2	slices pancetta or prosciutto, finely chopped	2
2 tsp	minced garlic	10 mL
8 oz	pea tops or arugula	250 g
2 tbsp	chicken stock or vegetable stock	30 mL

1. Slice tofu into pieces $\frac{1}{2}$ inch (1 cm) thick by $1\frac{1}{2}$ inches (3.5 cm) square.

2. In a nonstick skillet, heat 1 tbsp (15 mL) oil over medium-high heat for 30 seconds. Add tofu and season lightly with salt, pepper and sesame oil; fry 1 minute per side or until golden. Remove from skillet; arrange on a platter and keep warm.

3. Add remaining oil to skillet and heat for 30 seconds. Add pancetta and garlic; fry briefly for 20 to 30 seconds or until fragrant. Add pea tops and stock; stir-fry until pea tops are just wilted. Arrange evenly over tofu and serve.

Soy-Braised Tofu, Cabbage and Ginger with Cellophane Noodles

Braising is a key component of Chinese cooking — it adds rich flavor to otherwise bland ingredients such as tofu. Baking also firms the tofu and allows the flavorings to penetrate. For added flavor, roast the cabbage along with the tofu. Bean thread noodles are very slippery and best eaten with chopsticks.

Serves 4

- **Preheat oven to 375°F (190°C)**
- **Greased baking sheet**

4 oz	bean thread noodles or 8 oz (250 g) dried angel hair pasta	125 g
4 oz	medium-firm tofu, cut into ½-inch (1 cm) cubes	125 g
1 tbsp	vegetable oil, plus oil for coating noodles	15 mL
2 tbsp	soy sauce	30 mL
2 tbsp	minced gingerroot	30 mL
1 tbsp	minced garlic	15 mL
4 cups	vegetable stock or apple juice	1 L
2 cups	shredded green cabbage	500 mL
1 tbsp	chopped cilantro	15 mL
2 tbsp	tomato ketchup	30 mL
1 tbsp	horseradish	15 mL
1 tbsp	cornstarch dissolved in 2 tbsp (30 mL) water	15 mL
	Salt and pepper to taste	

1. In a heatproof bowl or pot, cover noodles with boiling water and soak for 3 minutes. Drain. (If using pasta, prepare according to package directions and coat with a little oil.) Set aside.

2. In a large bowl, combine tofu, oil, soy sauce, ginger and garlic. Place on a baking sheet and roast for 15 minutes or until firm and browned. Remove from oven and allow to cool slightly.

3. Meanwhile, in a saucepan over medium-high heat, combine stock, cabbage, tofu, cilantro, ketchup and horseradish. Bring to a boil. Reduce heat and simmer for 5 minutes. Add dissolved cornstarch and cook until mixture begins to thicken. Add noodles and stir until heated through. Season with salt and pepper; serve immediately.

Butter Beans and Grilled Red Pepper

This recipe combines the soft sweetness of beans with the pungency of grilled red peppers and chunks of tomato. Butter beans are known as dried lima beans in the American South. Just about any large bean, or assortment of beans, may be substituted for butter beans in this recipe.

Serves 6 to 8

3	red bell peppers, grilled, seeded and cut into strips	3
1	large white onion, peeled, halved and thinly sliced	1
1	clove garlic, minced	1
3	cans (each 19 oz/540 mL) butter beans, rinsed and drained	3
2 cups	canned Italian plum tomatoes, drained, seeded and chopped	500 mL
1/2 cup	chopped flat-leaf parsley	125 mL
3 tbsp	extra virgin olive oil	45 mL
1/4 cup	fresh lemon juice	60 mL
1 tsp	finely grated lemon zest	5 mL
	Salt and freshly ground black pepper, to taste	

1. In a large bowl, combine red peppers, onion, garlic, beans, tomatoes and parsley. Toss to combine well.

2. In a small bowl, whisk together olive oil, lemon juice, lemon zest, salt and pepper. Pour over bean mixture; stir to combine. Cover bowl with plastic wrap; let stand for 30 minutes at room temperature. Serve.

White Beans with Tomato

Turn leftovers into a fabulous soup the day after enjoying these flavorful Tuscan-style baked beans scented with fresh rosemary and enriched with Pecorino Romano.

Serves 4 to 6

- **Preheat oven to 375°F (190°C)**
- **8-cup (2 L) casserole with lid**

¼ cup	olive oil	60 mL
¼ cup	chopped flat-leaf parsley	60 mL
8	fresh sage leaves	8
2	branches rosemary	2
4	cloves garlic, finely chopped	4
1 cup	canned Italian plum tomatoes, chopped, with juices	250 mL
	Salt and freshly ground black pepper	
2 cups	dried cannellini (white kidney beans) or navy beans, soaked overnight in water to cover	500 mL
1 cup	grated Pecorino Romano cheese, divided	250 mL

1. In a large skillet, heat olive oil over medium-low heat. Add parsley, sage, rosemary and garlic; cook, stirring occasionally, for 6 minutes or until the garlic is softened and the herbs are fragrant. Stir in tomatoes with juice and a pinch each of salt and pepper; cook for 3 minutes or until slightly thickened.

2. In casserole dish, stir together tomato mixture, drained beans and half of the Pecorino Romano. Add enough cold water to cover beans; stir well. Cover casserole and bake for 2½ hours or until beans are tender, testing for doneness every 30 minutes. (Cooking time will depend on freshness of the beans.)

3. Remove and discard rosemary branches, which should be bare. Sprinkle remaining cheese over the surface. Cook, uncovered, for 10 minutes longer or until cheese is golden. Serve from casserole.

Yahni

Greek Beans with Onions

The affinity of beans with onions is no culinary secret, but this heirloom recipe stretches the notion to its limits. A mixture of approximately equal amounts of onion and beans, it is further onion-enhanced with a garnish of raw onion at the end. It results in a sweet, satisfyingly flavored bean dish that can be used on the side of any Mediterranean main course.

Serves 6

Tip

If using canned kidney beans, a 19-oz (540 mL) can of beans, rinsed and drained, will yield the 2 cups (500 mL) required for this recipe.

2	medium tomatoes	2
1/4 cup	olive oil	60 mL
1/4 tsp	salt	1 mL
1/4 tsp	black pepper	1 mL
2 cups	thinly sliced onions	500 mL
1	stick celery, finely diced	1
4	cloves garlic, thinly sliced	4
1 cup	water	250 mL
1/4 cup	chopped fresh parsley, packed down	60 mL
1 tbsp	red wine vinegar	15 mL
1 tsp	sugar	5 mL
2 cups	cooked white kidney beans	500 mL
	Extra virgin olive oil, to taste	
1/4 cup	finely diced red onions	60 mL

1. Blanch tomatoes in boiling water for 30 seconds. Over a bowl, peel, core and deseed them. Chop tomatoes into chunks and set aside. Strain any accumulated tomato juices from bowl; add the juices to the tomatoes.

2. In a large frying pan, heat oil over high heat for 30 seconds. Add salt and pepper and stir. Add onions and celery and stir-fry for 5 minutes or until wilted. Add garlic and stir-fry for 1 minute or until garlic is well coated with oil and everything is shiny.

3. Add tomato and its juices. Stir-fry for 2 minutes, mixing well. Add water, parsley, vinegar and sugar; bring back to a boil. Reduce heat to medium-low and cook for 5 to 6 minutes. Stir occasionally, mashing the tomato until it has broken down and the sauce is pink.

4. Fold beans into the sauce. Cook, stirring occasionally (and gently), for 5 to 6 minutes or until most of the liquid has been absorbed and everything is well integrated.

5. Transfer to a serving dish. Drizzle with extra virgin olive oil and top with red onions. Let rest, covered and unrefrigerated, for 1 to 2 hours to develop flavor. Serve at room temperature.

Red Beans and Red Rice

Here's a fresh twist on the classic Southern dish of red beans and rice. Bulked up with muscular red rice, this is very hearty — with the addition of salad, it's a meal in itself. The green peas add a burst of color, making this a visually attractive dish that looks good on a buffet. It is particularly tasty as an accompaniment to roast chicken or pork, pork chops or a platter of roasted vegetables.

Makes 8 servings

Vegan friendly

Tips

If you're using chicken stock rather than water to cook the rice, you may not need the added salt.

Red rice is very colorful in this dish, but brown rice or a mixture of brown rice and wild rice would work well, too. The cooking time is the same.

You can cook your own dried beans or use 1 can (14 to 19 oz/398 to 540 mL) no-salt-added red kidney or small red beans, drained and rinsed.

1 tbsp	olive oil	15 mL
1	onion, finely chopped	1
1	green bell pepper, seeded and diced	1
4	stalks celery, diced	4
4	cloves garlic, minced	4
1 tsp	dried thyme leaves	5 mL
½ tsp	salt (see Tips, left)	2 mL
½ tsp	cracked black peppercorns	2 mL
¼ tsp	cayenne pepper	1 mL
1 cup	Wehani or Camargue red rice, rinsed and drained (see Tips, left)	250 mL
2 cups	water or reduced-sodium chicken stock	500 mL
2 cups	cooked red beans (see Tips, left)	500 mL
2 cups	cooked green peas	500 mL

1. In a Dutch oven, heat oil over medium heat for 30 seconds. Add onion, bell pepper, celery and garlic and cook, stirring, until pepper is softened, about 5 minutes. Add thyme, salt, peppercorns and cayenne and cook, stirring, for 1 minute.

2. Add rice and toss to coat. Add water and bring to a boil. Reduce heat to low. Cover and simmer until rice is tender and most of the water is absorbed, about 1 hour. Stir in beans and peas and cook, covered, until heated through, about 10 minutes.

Variation

Red Rice, Sausage and Beans: To turn this into a heartier dish, perfect for a pot luck or buffet, add 4 oz (125 g) diced kielbasa along with the peas.

Pumpkin and Black Beans

Orange and black for Halloween, this dish is frighteningly nutritious.

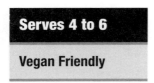

Serves 4 to 6

Vegan Friendly

1	onion, chopped	1
2 tbsp	olive oil	30 mL
2	cloves garlic, minced	2
1	red bell pepper, chopped	1
1 cup	vegetable stock	250 mL
2 cups	cubed peeled pumpkin	500 mL
1½ cups	cooked or canned black beans, rinsed and drained	375 mL
2 tbsp	chopped fresh savory or oregano	30 mL
1 tbsp	minced fresh gingerroot	15 mL
1 tbsp	freshly squeezed lemon juice	15 mL
1 tbsp	tamari or soy sauce	15 mL

1. In a large skillet, combine onion and oil. Sauté over medium heat for 5 minutes. Add garlic and bell pepper and sauté for another 3 minutes.

2. Stir in stock. Increase heat to high and bring to a boil. Stir in pumpkin, black beans, savory, ginger, lemon juice and tamari. Cover, reduce heat to medium-low and cook gently for 8 to 10 minutes or until pumpkin is tender-crisp. Serve immediately.

Variations

Substitute sweet potatoes or squash for the pumpkin, if desired.

Use any cooked legume, such as chickpeas, soybeans, lentils or black-eyed peas, in place of the black beans.

Lenticchie in Umido

Lentils Cooked with Wine and Tomato

Serves 4 to 6

Vegan Friendly

Tip

The best lentils for this dish are the little dark green ones called cavellucchi in Italy and Puy in France. They remain firm during cooking — unlike the conventional orange or pale green lentils, which become a little too mushy.

2 tbsp	olive oil	30 mL
2	cloves garlic, finely chopped	2
1	onion, finely chopped	1
1	carrot, finely chopped	1
1½ cups	lentils (see Tip, left) soaked in cold water overnight	375 mL
1 cup	dry red wine	250 mL
1 cup	passata (puréed, sieved tomatoes) or canned ground plum tomatoes	250 mL
1 cup	chicken stock or vegetable stock	250 mL
½ tsp	salt	2 mL
¼ tsp	freshly ground black pepper	1 mL
1 lb	spinach	500 g

1. In a large skillet, heat olive oil over medium-high heat. Add garlic, onion and carrot; cook, stirring occasionally, for 7 minutes or until vegetables are softened. Stir in drained lentils; cook 2 minutes longer.

2. Pour in wine. Bring to a boil; boil for 2 minutes. Reduce heat to medium-low. Stir in passata, stock, salt and pepper. Cover and cook, stirring occasionally, for 20 minutes or until lentils are tender. Meanwhile, prepare spinach.

3. Trim and wash spinach. Put the spinach in a large saucepan with just the water that clings to the leaves after washing. Cook, covered, over high heat until steam begins to escape from beneath lid. Remove lid, toss spinach and cook 1 minute or until tender. Remove from heat. Drain, pressing spinach against sides of colander to squeeze out as much water as possible. Chop spinach roughly. Set aside.

4. When lentils are tender, stir in spinach. Adjust seasoning as necessary and serve.

Spiced Rice and Lentil Pilaf

Readily available spices transform a simple rice and lentil dish into something quite exotic.

Serves 6

Tip

You can turn this pilaf into a main course by stirring in cubes of leftover cooked poultry or meat (or cooked shrimp) about 10 minutes before the rice is ready.

Make Ahead

The pilaf can be refrigerated, covered, for up to 3 days. Reheat in the microwave on High for 6 to 8 minutes or in a 350°F (180°C) oven for 20 to 30 minutes or until piping hot.

1 tbsp	canola oil or vegetable oil	15 mL
1	onion, chopped	1
2	cloves garlic, minced	2
1 tsp	minced gingerroot	5 mL
1 tsp	turmeric	5 mL
1 tsp	ground coriander	5 mL
1 tsp	ground cumin	5 mL
¼ tsp	salt	1 mL
¼ tsp	black pepper	1 mL
Pinch	cayenne pepper (or more to taste)	Pinch
1 cup	green lentils, rinsed and drained	250 mL
4 cups	beef stock	1 L
1 cup	long-grain rice	250 mL
2	tomatoes, chopped	2
¼ cup	chopped fresh mint	60 mL
¼ cup	chopped fresh cilantro or parsley	60 mL

1. In a large skillet, heat oil over medium-high heat. Add onion, garlic and ginger; cook, stirring, for 3 to 5 minutes or until onion is soft but not brown. Add turmeric, coriander, cumin, salt, pepper and cayenne; cook, stirring, for 1 minute.

2. Add lentils; stir to coat with spice mixture. Stir in stock and bring to a boil over high heat. Reduce heat to medium-low; simmer, covered, for 15 minutes.

3. Add rice. Simmer, covered, for 20 minutes or until rice and lentils are tender. Stir in tomatoes, mint and cilantro. If desired, season to taste with additional salt and pepper. Transfer to a warm shallow serving dish; serve at once.

Lentils-Rice-Spinach

This is a variation of spanako-rizo (spinach-rice), a rustic winter staple of the eastern Mediterranean, where spinach is one of the leafy vegetables that keep growing in the cold months. The lentils are an addition, but they are in keeping with the traditions of this kind of cuisine. They also bolster this dish into main-course status.

Serves 4 to 6

Tip

The Lentils-Rice-Spinach can be served immediately, or it can wait for up to 2 hours, covered and unrefrigerated.

¼ cup	olive oil	60 mL
¼ tsp	salt	1 mL
¼ tsp	black pepper	1 mL
2 cups	diced onions	500 mL
1	medium tomato, cubed	1
4 cups	chopped fresh spinach leaves, packed down	1 L
1½ cups	cooked rice (from ½ cup/125 mL raw rice)	375 mL
2 cups	cooked green lentils	500 mL
1	lemon, cut into wedges	1

1. In a pot or large skillet, heat oil over high heat for 30 seconds. Add salt and pepper and stir for 30 seconds. Add onions and stir-fry for 2 minutes or until softened. Add cubed tomato and stir-fry for 1 minute.

2. Add all the spinach at once; cook, turning over several times, for 1 minute or until the spinach has been reduced to one-third of its volume.

3. Reduce heat to medium-low and add rice and lentils. Stir-cook for 3 to 4 minutes or until well mixed and everything is piping hot. Remove from heat, cover and let rest for 5 to 6 minutes as it develops flavor. Serve with lemon wedges on the side.

Frijoles Borrachos Mexicanos

Borrachos *means "drunken" in Spanish and, in this recipe, refers to the fact that both tequila and beer lend their special qualities to the humble pinto bean. Very good with warmed tortillas or as a side dish with Mexican-style grilled fish.* Pinto *is Spanish for "painted" — an apt description for these beans, which feature streaks of reddish-brown. Along with pink beans, these are the beans most commonly used in the making of refried beans.*

Serves 8

Tip

Look for cans of chipotle chile peppers (smoked jalapeños) in the international section of large supermarkets or in Mexican or Latin American markets.

1 lb	dried pinto beans	500 g
1½ cups	Mexican beer	375 mL
5 cups	water	1.25 L
2	chipotle chile peppers, seeded and finely chopped	2
4	cloves garlic, minced	4
1 tsp	cumin seeds, toasted	5 mL
2 tbsp	vegetable oil	30 mL
1	onion, chopped	1
2	cloves garlic, minced	2
4	tomatoes (fresh or canned), chopped	4
2	fresh jalapeños, seeded and chopped	2
	Salt and freshly ground black pepper, to taste	
½ cup	tequila	125 mL
1 cup	chopped fresh cilantro	250 mL

1. In a colander, rinse pinto beans, discarding any stones. Transfer beans to a large pot. Add beer, water, chipotles, garlic and cumin seeds; bring to a boil. Reduce heat and simmer gently, covered, for 1 to 1½ hours or until tender.

2. Meanwhile, heat oil in a skillet over medium heat. Add onion and garlic; cook for 5 minutes or until softened. Add tomatoes, jalapeños, salt and pepper. Simmer, stirring occasionally, for 5 minutes or until thickened. Remove from heat.

3. When beans are done, stir in tomato mixture and tequila; simmer for 5 to 10 minutes. Remove from heat and stir in cilantro. Serve immediately.

Tomatoes Stuffed with Corn, Black Beans and Pine Nuts

Tips

These tomatoes are visually stunning. Serve as an appetizer or a side.

If black beans are unavailable, use chickpeas or white navy beans.

The filling is great as a salad by itself.

4	medium tomatoes	4
1/2 cup	canned corn kernels, drained	125 mL
1/2 cup	canned black beans, rinsed and drained	125 mL
1/4 cup	each chopped cilantro, green onions and red pepper	60 mL
2 tbsp	light mayonnaise	30 mL
2 tbsp	toasted pine nuts	30 mL
1 tbsp	grated Parmesan cheese	15 mL
2 tsp	freshly squeezed lemon juice	10 mL
1 tsp	Dijon mustard	5 mL

1. Slice tops off tomatoes and reserve. Scoop out and discard seeds and core.
2. In a small bowl, mix together corn, black beans, cilantro, green onions, red pepper, mayonnaise, pine nuts, Parmesan, lemon juice and Dijon.
3. Divide mixture evenly between tomato shells, about 1/3 cup (75 mL) per tomato. Cover with reserved tomato tops and serve.

Basic Pinto Beans

This is a simple recipe for basic mashed pinto beans.

Tips

Test beans by smashing one bean between thumb and index finger.

Store beans in an airtight container and refrigerate for up to 2 days or freeze for up to 4 months.

3 cups	dried pinto beans	750 mL
1 tbsp	garlic powder	15 mL
1 tbsp	onion powder	15 mL

1. Place beans in a large pot. Add enough water to cover by 4 inches (10 cm) and bring to a boil over medium-high heat. Reduce heat and boil gently until soft (see Tips, left), $2\frac{1}{2}$ to 3 hours. Let cool completely to room temperature, about 2 to 3 hours.

Variation

Substitute black beans or kidney beans for the pinto beans.

Quick Refried Beans

Here is a quick way to get an authentic-tasting batch of refried beans in a hurry.

**Makes about
2 cups (500 mL)**

2	cans (each 14 to 19 oz/398 to 540 mL) pinto beans, slightly drained, reserving liquid (see Tip, left)	2
1½ tbsp	lard	22 mL
	Salt	

Tip

Dehydrated refried beans are quick to prepare and have a great flavor. You can find them in the Mexican food section at your supermarket. Add ½ cup (125 mL) less water than directed when rehydrating them, for a firmer consistency.

1. In a large skillet, bring beans to a boil over medium-high heat and boil for 2 minutes. Reduce heat to medium-low. Using a potato masher, gently mash beans. Beans should be like a thick paste, not runny. If too thick, add reserved liquid, 1 tsp (5 mL) at a time, until just thick, but not stiff.

2. Increase heat to medium. Scoop beans to one side of skillet and add lard. Let lard start melting and slowly stir beans and lard until well blended and bubbling. Season with salt to taste.

Variation

Substitute vegetable or canola oil for the lard for a vegetarian option.

Stove-Top Refried Beans

These beans can be whipped up in minutes. A truly authentic Mexican flavor is best achieved by refrying these beans in lard. They are delicious.

**Makes 2 cups
(500 mL)**

2 cups	cooked pinto beans, drained, reserving liquid (Basic Pinto Beans, page 275)	500 mL
2 tbsp	lard	30 mL
	Salt	

Tip

Substitute 2 tbsp (30 mL) vegetable or canola oil for the lard.

1. In a large skillet, heat beans and ¼ cup (60 mL) reserved liquid over medium-high heat. Bring to a boil and boil for 2 minutes. Reduce heat to medium-low. Using a potato masher, gently mash beans. Beans should be like a thick paste, not runny. If too thick, add more reserved liquid, 1 tsp (5 mL) at a time, until bean mixture is thick, but not stiff. Repeat until all beans are mashed.

2. In another large skillet, melt lard over medium-high heat. Add mashed beans and stir until well blended and bubbling, 4 to 6 minutes. Season with salt to taste.

Basic Beans in the Slow Cooker

The slow cooker excels at transforming legumes into potentially sublime fare. This recipe is also extraordinarily convenient. Put presoaked beans into the slow cooker before you go to bed, and in the morning they are ready for whatever recipe you intend to make.

Makes approximately 2 cups (500 mL)
Vegan Friendly

Tips

This recipe may be doubled or tripled to suit the quantity of beans required for a recipe.

Soybeans and chickpeas take longer than other legumes to cook. They will likely take the full 12 hours on Low (about 6 hours on High).

Once cooked, legumes should be covered and stored in the refrigerator, where they will keep for up to 5 days. Cooked legumes can also be frozen, with liquid to cover, in an airtight container. They will keep frozen for up to 6 months.

- **Small to medium (2 to 3½ quart) slow cooker**

1 cup	dried beans (see Tips, left)	250 mL
3 cups	water	750 mL
	Garlic, optional	
	Bay leaves, optional	
	Bouquet garni, optional	

Long soak: In a bowl, combine beans and water. Soak for at least 6 hours or overnight. Drain and rinse thoroughly with cold water. Beans are now ready for cooking.

Quick soak: In a pot, combine beans and water. Cover and bring to a boil. Boil for 3 minutes. Turn off heat and soak for 1 hour. Drain and rinse thoroughly under cold water. Beans are now ready to cook.

Cooking: In slow cooker stoneware, combine 1 cup (250 mL) presoaked beans and 3 cups (750 mL) fresh cold water. If desired, season with garlic, bay leaves or a bouquet garni made from your favorite herbs tied together in cheesecloth. Cover and cook on Low for 10 to 12 hours or overnight, or on High for 5 to 6 hours, until beans are tender. If not using immediately, cover and refrigerate. In either case, drain and rinse before using.

Variation

These instructions also work for dried lentils, with the following changes: Do not presoak them, and reduce the cooking time to about 6 hours on Low.

Contributing Authors

Julia Aitken is the author of the *125 Best Entertaining Recipes*. Recipes from that book are found on pages 37, 72, 75 and 272.

Byron Ayanoglu is the author of *125 Best Vegetarian Recipes*. Recipes from that book are found on pages 225, 226, 241, 244, 245, 268 and 273. Byron co-authored *Simply Mediterranean Cooking* with **Algis Kemezys**, and recipes from that book are found on pages 38, 77, 196, 204, 208 and 232. He is also the co-author, with **Jennifer Mackenzie**, of *The Complete Curry Cookbook*. Recipes from that book are found on pages 150, 151, 157, 158, 159, 160, 161, 162, 164 and 168.

Johanna Burkhard is the author of *500 Best Comfort Food Recipes*, and recipes from that book are found on pages 55, 62, 76, 125, 183, 188, 190 and 229.

Andrew Chase is the author of *The Asian Bistro Cookbook*. Recipes from that book are found on pages 156 and 180.

Cinda Chavich is the author of *The Wild West Cookbook*. Recipes from that book are found on pages 20, 23, 27, 52, 57, 82, 83, 110, 126, 129, 141, 179, 184 and 185. Cinda also wrote *200 Best Pressure Cooker Recipes*, and material from that book appears on pages 7, 8, 9 and 10.

Kelley Cleary Coffeen is the author of *300 Best Taco Recipes*. Recipes from that book appear on pages 102, 105, 106, 107, 108, 109, 275 and 276.

Tiffany Collins wrote *300 Best Casserole Recipes*. Recipes from that book appear on pages 24, 112, 174, 177, 203, 206, 212, 243, 250 and 251.

Pat Crocker is the author of *The Healing Herbs Cookbook*. Recipes from that book are found on pages 91, 114, 116 and 147. She is also the author of *The Vegetarian Cook's Bible*; recipes from that book appear on pages 45, 89, 93, 97, 98, 146, 219, 239, 255, and 270. Pat also wrote *The Vegan Cook's Bible*. Recipes from that book appear on pages 33, 34, 35, 65, 71, 88, 90, 230, 256 and 257.

Meredith Deeds and **Carla Snyder** wrote *300 Sensational Soups*. Recipes from that book appear on pages 49, 51, 53, 56, 58, 59, 60, 63, 66 and 70. They are also the authors of *Everyday to Entertaining: 200 Sensational Recipes That Transform from Casual to Elegant*. Recipes from that book appear on pages 16, 17, 28, 29, 92, and 93.

Judith Finlayson is the author of *The Convenience Cook*. Recipes from that book appear on pages 18, 21, 31, 104, 131, 133, 139, 143, 175, 247, 248 and 252. She also wrote *The Complete Whole Grains Cookbook*, and recipes from that book appear on pages 48, 87, 191, 236 and 269. Recipes from her slow cooker books, *Sensational Slow Cooker Gourmet*, *Slow Cooker Comfort Food*, *The Vegetarian Slow Cooker* and *125 Best Vegetarian Slow Cooker Recipes* appear on pages 26, 36, 64, 68, 124, 128, 130, 132, 134, 136, 138, 140, 142, 144, 145, 172, 176, 186, 187, 192, 194, 198, 199, 200, 202, 218, 220, 222, 223, 224, 236, 237, 238, 240, 242, 254, 258, 259, 260, 261, 262 and 277. Judith co-authored *650 Best Food Processor Recipes* with **George Geary**; recipes from that book appear on pages 19, 22, 29, 30, 32, 42, 50, 115 and 210.

Bill Jones and **Stephen Wong** are co-authors of *100 Best Asian Noodle Recipes* and *100 Best Chinese Recipes*. Recipes from those books are found on pages 41, 43, 182, 214, 264 and 265.

Tracy Kett compiled and edited *The Organic Gourmet*. Recipes from that book are found on pages 54 and 69.

Alison Lewis is the author of *400 Best Sandwich Recipes*. Recipes from that book are found on pages 31, 100, 101, 103, 111, 119, 121 and 122.

Jane Rodmell is the author of *All the Best Recipes*. Recipes from that book are found on pages 25, 74, 78, 84, 86, 97, 127, 189 and 213.

Andre Schloss, with **Ken Bookman**, wrote *2500 Recipes: Everyday to Extraordinary*. Recipes from that book appear on pages 84, 94, 95, 96, 153, 193, 205 and 253.

Kathleen Sloan-McIntosh is the author of *125 Best Italian Recipes*. Recipes from that book are found on pages 18, 44, 46, 61, 67, 178, 267 and 271. She also wrote *125 Best Grilling Recipes*, and recipes from that book appear on pages 266 and 274.

Krystal Taylor, a dietitian, contributed Teriyaki Rice Noodles with Veggies and Beans, which appears on page 217. It is taken from *Dietitians of Canada, Simply Great Food: 250 Quick, Easy & Delicious Recipes*, edited by Patricia Chuey, MSc, RD, Eileen Campbell and Mary Sue Waisman, MSc, RD.

Suneeta Vaswani is the author of *The Complete Book of Indian Cooking*. Recipes from that book appear on pages 152, 154, 165, 166, 167, 169, 170, 171, 234 and 235.

Index

A

alcoholic beverages. *See* beer;
    spirits; wine
All-in-One Pasta and Chickpea
    Ragoût, 229
Amaranth Chili, 146
anchovies
    Mediterranean Pork and Beans,
        186
    Saucy Halibut on a Bed of
        Lentils, 210
Andhra Yellow Lentils with
    Tomatoes, 170
appetizers, 15–38
Asian Tofu Dressing, 96
Assamese Khichri, 234
avocado
    Beyond Bean Dip, 23
    Black Bean and Corn Salsa Mini
        Tostadas with Chipotle Sour
        Cream, 28
    Black Bean Nachos, 20
    Easy Tostadas, 111
    Hominy and Red Bean Chili (tip),
        142

B

bacon. *See also* pancetta
    Beer-Braised Chili, 132
    Cabbage, Bean and Bacon
        Chowder, 52
    Caribbean Black Bean Soup, 58
    Green Lentil Soup, 70
    Home-Style Pork and Beans, 187
    Maple Baked Pork and Beans
        with Caramelized Apples, 185
    Molasses Baked Beans, 188
    Quick Cassoulet, 193
barley
    Baked Beans 'n' Barley, 192
    Best-Ever Cholent, 176
    Mushroom Cholent, 238
    Southwestern Bean and Barley
        Salad with Roasted Peppers,
        87
Basic Beans in the Slow Cooker,
    277
Basic Pinto Beans, 275
basil. *See also* herbs
    Basil and White Bean Spread, 18
    Saucy Halibut on a Bed of
        Lentils, 210
    Thai Dry Vegetable Curry, 156
    Thai Red Curry Tofu with Sweet
        Mango and Basil, 151
beans. *See also specific types of
    beans (below)*
    cooking, 8–10
    Assamese Khichri, 234
    Basic Beans in the Slow Cooker,
        277
    Beans, Beef and Biscuits, 174

Bean Salad with Mustard-Dill
    Dressing, 76
Best-Ever Cholent, 176
Cantonese Noodles, 219
Cider Baked Beans, 240
Corn and Three-Bean Salad, 79
Firehouse Chili Soup, 53
Grande Beef Nachos, 22
Green Beans Gado Gado, 239
Italian Bean Pasta Salad, 81
Lamb Soup with Red Wine,
    Romano Beans and Chèvre, 54
Lamb with Flageolet Gratin,
    200
Make-Ahead Southwestern Pork
    Stew, 183
Minestrone Genovese, 48
Parsi Chicken Stew with Lentils
    and Vegetables, 154
Potato and Adzuki Latkes, 255
Red Chili con Carne Soft Tacos,
    107
Romano Bean Stew, 241
Salmon over White-and-Black
    Bean Salsa, 211
Teriyaki Rice Noodles with
    Veggies and Beans, 217
Tex-Mex Chili, 127
Three-Bean Tacos, 106
20-Minute Chili, 125
Two-Bean Turkey Chili, 140
Very Veggie Chili, 143
beans, black
    Bean Burgers with Dill Sauce,
        120
    Black Bean, Butternut Squash
        and Poblano Chile Soup, 59
    Black Bean, Corn and Leek
        Frittata, 249
    Black Bean and Bulgur Salad, 84
    Black Bean and Corn Salsa Mini
        Tostadas with Chipotle Sour
        Cream, 28
    Black Bean and Rice Salad, 83
    Black Bean and Roasted Corn
        Salsa, 29
    Black Bean and Sausage Gumbo,
        57
    Black Bean Burgers, 121
    Black Bean Chili, 147
    Black Bean Chili with Hominy
        and Sweet Corn, 145
    Black Bean Chipotle Dip, 30
    Black Bean Nachos, 20
    Black Bean Quesadillas, 101
    Caribbean Black Bean Soup, 58
    Chicken and Black Bean Chili,
        139
    Chicken Baked with Black Beans
        and Lime, 205
    Chunky Black Bean Chili, 124
    Creamy Chipotle Black Bean
        Burrito Bake, 250
    Easy Tostadas, 111

Pork and Beef Chili with Ancho
    Sauce, 126
Pork and Black Bean Stew with
    Sweet Potatoes, 184
Pumpkin and Black Beans, 270
Rice and Black Bean Stuffed
    Peppers, 232
Roasted Eggplant and Artichoke
    Dip, 35
Sausage and Black Bean Chili,
    131
Slow Cooker Black Bean and
    Salsa Dip, 26
Southwest Butternut Squash
    Tortilla Bake, 251
Southwestern Shepherd's Pie, 174
Spicy Black Bean Gazpacho, 55
Tomatoes Stuffed with Corn,
    Black Beans and Pine Nuts, 275
Wild West Bean Caviar with
    Roasted Tomatoes, 27
Zesty Black Bean Pie, 248
beans, kidney. *See also* beans, red;
    beans, white
    Butternut Chili, 134
    Chicken Enchilada Casserole
        with Teriyaki Sauce, 112
    Chili con Carne Pronto, 133
    Greek Chili with Black Olives
        and Feta Cheese, 135
    Potluck Bean and Pasta Salad, 82
    Three-Cheese Creamy Pasta
        Bean Bake, 228
beans, lima. *See also* beans
    Brunswick-Style Chicken Pot Pie,
        206
    Butter Beans and Grilled Red
        Pepper, 266
    Corn and Rice Chowder with
        Parsley Persillade, 45
    Cracked Wheat and Lima Bean
        Wrap, 114
    Grilled Corn and Lima Bean
        Salad, 78
    Lemon-Laced Butterbean Dip, 19
    Roasted Vegetable Lasagna, 230
    Succotash Sausage Soup, 56
    Succulent Succotash, 237
beans, mung (yellow). *See also*
    beans
    Bengali Khichri, 235
    Cajun Blackened Potato and
        Mung Bean Salad, 89
    Punjabi Creamy Yellow Mung
        Beans, 165
    Rajasthani Mixed Dal, 167
beans, pinto. *See also* beans; beans,
    refried
    Basic Pinto Beans, 275
    Cheesy Beans and Hot Dogs, 203
    Chicken, Pinto Beans and Green
        Chile Soup, 60
    Frijoles Borrachos Mexicanos, 274
    Frybread Tostadas, 110

beans, pinto (*continued*)
Lime-Spiked Turkey Chili with Pinto Beans, 138
Not-Too-Corny Turkey Chili with Sausage, 136
Prairie Fire Beans, 179
Quick Refried Beans, 276
Red Chili with Anchos, 128
Southwest Bread Pudding, 253
Stove-Top Refried Beans, 276
Vegetable Tamale Pie, 243
Wagon Boss Chili, 129
beans, red. *See also* beans, kidney
Baked Orzo and Beans, 226
Bean and Sweet Potato Chili on Garlic Polenta, 147
Caribbean Red Bean, Spinach and Potato Curry, 162
Chicken Tortillas, 109
Easy Chili con Carne, 130
Easy Vegetable Chili, 144
Hominy and Red Bean Chili, 142
Red Beans and Greens, 242
Red Beans and Red Rice, 269
Red Beans and Rice Soft Tacos with Cajun Sauce, 108
Southwestern Bean and Barley Salad with Roasted Peppers, 87
Spicy Bean Dip, 25
Spicy Rice, Bean and Lentil Casserole, 231
Tex-Mex Rotini Salad, 80
Tortilla Bean Salad with Creamy Salsa Dressing, 85
Vegetarian Chili, 141
Vegetarian Shepherd's Pie with Peppered Potato Topping, 246
beans, refried
Baked Shrimp Enchiladas, 212
Beyond Bean Dip, 23
Easy Chicken Tacos, 104
Easy Tostadas, 111
Enchiladas in Salsa Verde, 252
Kim's Mexican Casserole, 177
Oaxaca Chicken Tacos, 105
Oven-Fried Beef and Bean Chimichangas, 103
Refried Nachos, 21
Sirloin and Chorizo Frijole Tacos, 102
Taco Burgers, 119
Warm Mexican Layered Dip, 24
beans, white, 16. *See also* beans; beans, kidney
Baked Beans 'n' Barley, 192
Basil and White Bean Spread, 18
Braised Lamb with Beans and Dates, 204
Cabbage, Bean and Bacon Chowder, 52
Cheater's Cassoulet, 194
Greek Bean and Tomato Salad, 77
Greek Beans with Onions, 268
Home-Style Pork and Beans, 187
Linguine with Tuna, White Beans and Dill, 209

Maple Baked Pork and Beans with Caramelized Apples, 185
Mediterranean Pork and Beans, 186
Southwest Bread Pudding (variation), 253
Molasses Baked Beans, 188
Mushroom Cholent, 238
Navy Bean and Ham Soup, 51
Pasta e Fagioli, 42
Penne with Creamy White Bean Sauce, 227
Pork 'n' Beans, The Best, 189
Pyaza Paneer and Navy Bean Curry, 160
Quick Cassoulet, 193
Red Pepper Hummus (tip), 31
Ribollita, 46
Stuffed Veal Rolls with White Beans, 178
Tuscan Shrimp and Beans, 213
Tuscan White Bean and Tomato Salad, 74
Wheat Berry Minestrone, 50
White Bean Salad with Lemon-Dill Vinaigrette, 75
White Bean Salsa, 16
White Bean Soup with Swiss Chard, 44
White Beans with Tomato, 267
White Bean with Mint, 18
Wild Mushroom and Navy Bean Soup, 49
beef. *See also* beef, ground
Best-Ever Cholent, 176
Caribbean Curried Beef and Chickpeas, 150
Chunky Black Bean Chili, 124
Easy Tostadas (variation), 111
Make-Ahead Southwestern Pork Stew (tip), 183
Pork and Beef Chili with Ancho Sauce, 126
Sirloin and Chorizo Frijole Tacos, 102
Tex-Mex Chili, 127
Wagon Boss Chili, 129
beef, ground
Beans, Beef and Biscuits, 174
Butternut Chili, 134
Chili con Carne Pronto, 133
Easy Chili con Carne, 130
Firehouse Chili Soup, 53
Grande Beef Nachos, 22
Greek Chili with Black Olives and Feta Cheese, 135
Kim's Mexican Casserole, 177
Oven-Fried Beef and Bean Chimichangas, 103
Red Chili con Carne Soft Tacos, 107
Southwestern Shepherd's Pie, 174
Taco Burgers, 119
20-Minute Chili, 125
Warm Mexican Layered Dip, 24
beer
Beer-Braised Chili, 132
Chunky Black Bean Chili, 124

Frijoles Borrachos Mexicanos, 274
Tex-Mex Chili, 127
Bengali Khichri, 235
Bengali Red Lentils, 169
Best-Ever Cholent, 176
The Best Pork 'n' Beans, 189
Beyond Bean Dip, 23
biscuit dough
Beans, Beef and Biscuits, 174
Brunswick-Style Chicken Pot Pie, 206
Bok Choy, Noodle and Tofu Soup, 40
breads (as ingredient). *See also* burgers; pita breads; tortillas
Crostini, 17
Cuban-Style Tofu Sandwich, 100
Lentil Sloppy Joes, 258
Ribollita, 46
Southwest Bread Pudding, 253
White Bean Soup with Swiss Chard, 44
broccoli
Curry-Fried Tofu Soup with Vegetables and Udon Noodles, 41
Penne with Creamy White Bean Sauce (tip), 227
Steamed Shrimp-Stuffed Tofu with Broccoli, 214
Teriyaki Rice Noodles with Veggies and Beans, 217
Brunswick-Style Chicken Pot Pie, 206
burgers, 117–23
Butter Beans and Grilled Red Pepper, 266
Butternut Chili, 134

C

cabbage
Bok Choy, Noodle and Tofu Soup (tip), 40
Cabbage, Bean and Bacon Chowder, 52
Minestrone Genovese, 48
Soy-Braised Tofu, Cabbage and Ginger with Cellophane Noodles, 265
Cajun Blackened Potato and Mung Bean Salad, 89
Cajun Black Spice, 98
Cajun Potato and Red Lentil Salad, 91
Cajun Sauce, 108
Cajun-Style Tofu with Tomatoes and Okra, 220
Cantonese Noodles, 219
Caribbean Black Bean Soup, 58
Caribbean Chickpea Curry with Potatoes, 161
Caribbean Curried Beef and Chickpeas, 150
Caribbean Red Bean, Spinach and Potato Curry, 162

carrots. See also vegetables
  Chickpea-Herb Burgers, 116
  Roasted Vegetable Hummus, 34
  Tomato Dal with Spinach, 172
cassoulet, 5, 193–94
celery, 175. See also vegetables
celery root
  Best-Ever Cholent, 176
  Hominy and Red Bean Chili, 142
celery seed, 133
Cheater's Cassoulet, 194
cheese. See also specific types of
    cheese (below)
  Baked Orzo and Beans, 226
  Baked Shrimp Enchiladas, 212
  Black Bean Quesadillas, 101
  Easy Chicken Tacos, 104
  Enchiladas in Salsa Verde, 252
  Grande Beef Nachos, 22
  Lamb Soup with Red Wine,
    Romano Beans and Chèvre, 54
  Lentil Shepherd's Pie, 247
  Manicotti Stuffed with
    Chickpeas and Cheese, 206
  Mexican Casserole, Kim's, 177
  Moussaka with Tofu Topping, 222
  Oaxaca Chicken Tacos, 105
  Paneer with Chickpeas in
    Creamy Tomato Curry, 157
  Potato and Adzuki Latkes, 255
  Pyaza Paneer and Navy Bean
    Curry, 160
  Refried Nachos, 21
  Ribollita, 46
  Spicy Bean Dip (variation), 25
  Three-Bean Tacos, 106
  Three-Cheese Creamy Pasta
    Bean Bake, 228
  Vegetarian Shepherd's Pie with
    Peppered Potato Topping, 246
  Warm Mexican Layered Dip, 24
  White Bean Soup with Swiss
    Chard, 44
  White Beans with Tomato, 267
cheese, Cheddar
  Beyond Bean Dip, 23
  Cheesy Beans and Hot Dogs, 203
  Chicken Enchilada Casserole
    with Teriyaki Sauce, 112
  Frybread Tostadas, 110
  Oven-Fried Beef and Bean
    Chimichangas, 103
  Prairie Fire Beans, 179
  Red Chili con Carne Soft Tacos,
    107
cheese, cream
  Black Bean and Roasted Corn
    Salsa, 29
  Black Bean Chipotle Dip, 30
  Slow Cooker Black Bean and
    Salsa Dip, 26
  Zesty Black Bean Pie, 248
cheese, feta
  Black-Eyed Pea Salad with
    Tomato and Feta, 86
  Greek Bean and Tomato Salad, 77
  Greek Chili with Black Olives
    and Feta Cheese, 135

Grilled Corn and Lima Bean
  Salad, 78
Italian Bean Pasta Salad, 81
Lentil Salad with Dried
  Cranberries and Pistachios, 93
Lentil Salad with Feta Cheese, 92
cheese, Jack
  Black Bean Nachos, 20
  Chicken Baked with Black Beans
    and Lime, 205
  Creamy Chipotle Black Bean
    Burrito Bake, 250
  Easy Tostadas, 111
  Sirloin and Chorizo Frijole Tacos,
    102
  Southwest Bread Pudding, 253
  Taco Burgers, 119
chicken. See also turkey
  Black Bean Quesadillas
    (variation), 101
  Bok Choy, Noodle and Tofu Soup
    (tip), 40
  Brunswick-Style Chicken Pot Pie,
    206
  Chicken, Pinto Beans and Green
    Chile Soup, 60
  Chicken and Black Bean Chili,
    139
  Chicken Baked with Black Beans
    and Lime, 205
  Chicken Curry Baked with
    Lentils, 153
  Chicken Enchilada Casserole
    with Teriyaki Sauce, 112
  Chicken Tortillas, 109
  Easy Chicken Tacos, 104
  Easy Tostadas (variation), 111
  Oaxaca Chicken Tacos, 105
  Oven-Fried Beef and Bean
    Chimichangas (variation), 103
  Parsi Chicken Stew with Lentils
    and Vegetables, 154
chickpeas, 9
  All-in-One Pasta and Chickpea
    Ragoût, 229
  Amaranth Chili, 146
  Bean Salad with Mustard-Dill
    Dressing, 76
  Black Bean Chili, 147
  Caribbean Chickpea Curry with
    Potatoes, 161
  Caribbean Curried Beef and
    Chickpeas, 150
  Chickpea and Roasted Pepper
    Salad, 84
  Chickpea-Herb Burgers, 116
  Chickpea Soup with Chorizo and
    Garlic, 63
  Chickpea Tofu Burgers with
    Cilantro Mayonnaise, 118
  Chickpea Tofu Stew, 225
  Coconut Curried Chickpea Soup,
    66
  Corn and Three-Bean Salad, 79
  Cracked Wheat and Lima Bean
    Wrap (variation), 114
  Curried Couscous with Tomatoes
    and Chickpeas, 163

Falafel Burgers with Creamy
  Sesame Sauce, 117
Falafel in Pita, 115
Garlic Greens with Chickpeas
  and Cumin, 257
Harira, 64
Hearty Potato and Leek Soup, 65
Hominy and Red Bean Chili
  (variation), 142
Hummus and Sautéed Vegetable
  Wraps, 113
Hummus from Scratch, 32
Italian Bean Pasta Salad, 81
Manicotti Stuffed with
  Chickpeas and Cheese, 206
Moroccan Chickpea Tagine, 256
Moroccan Spiced Lentil Soup,
  72
Moussaka with Tofu Topping, 222
Paneer with Chickpeas in
  Creamy Tomato Curry, 157
Pappardelle and Chickpea Soup,
  61
Potato and Chickpea Stew with
  Spicy Sausage, 196
Potluck Bean and Pasta Salad, 82
Quick Chickpea and Pasta Soup,
  62
Red Hot Hummus, 33
Red Pepper Hummus, 31
Roasted Vegetable Hummus, 34
Roasted Vegetable Salad, 88
Smoked Oyster Hummus, 31
Spicy Lamb with Chickpeas, 202
Tortilla Bean Salad with Creamy
  Salsa Dressing, 85
Vegetarian Chili, 141
Vegetarian Shepherd's Pie with
  Peppered Potato Topping, 246
chiles, green. See peppers, green
  chile
chilies, 123–48
cholent, 176, 238
Cider Baked Beans, 240
cilantro
  Baked Shrimp Enchiladas, 212
  Bengali Red Lentils (variation),
    169
  Butternut Chili, 134
  Chickpea Tofu Burgers with
    Cilantro Mayonnaise, 118
  Chunky Black Bean Chili, 124
  Cilantro-Yogurt Sauce, 122
  Curried Couscous with Tomatoes
    and Chickpeas, 163
  Easy Vegetable Chili, 144
  Frijoles Borrachos Mexicanos,
    274
  Lamb with Lentils, 152
  Not-Too-Corny Turkey Chili with
    Sausage, 136
  Pork and Black Bean Stew with
    Sweet Potatoes, 184
  Pyaza Paneer and Navy Bean
    Curry, 160
  Rajasthani Mixed Dal, 167
  Red Lentil Curry with Coconut
    and Cilantro, 168

coconut milk
  Coconut Curried Chickpea Soup, 66
  Curried Squash and Red Lentil Soup with Coconut, 68
  Green Beans Gado Gado, 239
  Poached Eggs on Spicy Lentils, 259
  Red Lentil Curry with Coconut and Cilantro, 168
  Thai Red Curry Tofu with Sweet Mango and Basil, 151
  Tofu and Snow Peas in Tamarind Ginger Curry, 158
  Tofu with Lime, Lemongrass and Coconut Curry, 164
corn and hominy. See also vegetables
  Baked Shrimp Enchiladas, 212
  Black Bean, Corn and Leek Frittata, 249
  Black Bean and Corn Salsa Mini Tostadas with Chipotle Sour Cream, 28
  Black Bean and Roasted Corn Salsa, 29
  Black Bean Chili with Hominy and Sweet Corn, 145
  Brunswick-Style Chicken Pot Pie, 206
  Cajun Blackened Potato and Mung Bean Salad, 89
  Cajun-Style Tofu with Tomatoes and Okra, 220
  Corn and Rice Chowder with Parsley Persillade, 45
  Corn and Three-Bean Salad, 79
  Creamy Chipotle Black Bean Burrito Bake, 250
  Easy Chicken Tacos, 104
  Grilled Corn and Lima Bean Salad, 78
  Hominy and Red Bean Chili, 142
  Make-Ahead Southwestern Pork Stew, 183
  Not-Too-Corny Turkey Chili with Sausage, 136
  Southwest Butternut Squash Tortilla Bake, 251
  Southwestern Bean and Barley Salad with Roasted Peppers, 87
  Southwestern Shepherd's Pie, 174
  Spicy Rice, Bean and Lentil Casserole, 231
  Succotash Sausage Soup, 56
  Succulent Succotash, 237
  Tex-Mex Rotini Salad, 80
  Tomatoes Stuffed with Corn, Black Beans and Pine Nuts, 275
  Zesty Black Bean Pie, 248
cornmeal
  Bean and Sweet Potato Chili on Garlic Polenta, 147
  Vegetable Tamale Pie, 243
couscous
  Amaranth Chili (variation), 146
  Curried Couscous with Tomatoes and Chickpeas, 163
  Teriyaki Rice Noodles with Veggies and Beans (variation), 217
Crostini, 17
Cuban-Style Tofu Sandwich, 100
cucumber
  Black Bean and Bulgur Salad, 84
  Cilantro-Yogurt Sauce, 122
  Grilled Mediterranean Vegetable and Lentil Salad, 90
  Tabbouleh with Lentils, 95
Cumin-Laced Lentils with Sun-Dried Tomatoes and Roasted Peppers, 260
Curried Squash and Red Lentil Soup with Coconut, 68
curries and dal, 149–72
Curry-Fried Tofu Soup with Vegetables and Udon Noodles, 41

D

dal. See lentils
Dijon Vinaigrette, 96
dill
  Bean Burgers with Dill Sauce, 120
  Bean Salad with Mustard-Dill Dressing, 76
  Eggplant Lentil Ragoût, 262
  Linguine with Tuna, White Beans and Dill, 209
  Penne with Creamy White Bean Sauce, 227
  White Bean Salad with Lemon-Dill Vinaigrette, 75
dressings (salad), 95–98

E

Easy Chicken Tacos, 104
Easy Chili con Carne, 130
Easy Tostadas, 111
Easy Vegetable Chili, 144
eggplant
  Braised Stuffed Bean Curd (variation), 180
  Eggplant Lentil Ragoût, 262
  Greek Chili with Black Olives and Feta Cheese, 135
  Grilled Mediterranean Vegetable and Lentil Salad, 90
  Hummus from Scratch (variation), 32
  Moussaka with Tofu Topping, 222
  Parsi Chicken Stew with Lentils and Vegetables, 154
  Roasted Eggplant and Artichoke Dip, 35
  Roasted Vegetable Lasagna, 230
  Tofu Ratatouille, 218
  Tofu with Lime, Lemongrass and Coconut Curry, 164

eggs
  Black Bean, Corn and Leek Frittata, 249
  Cajun Potato and Red Lentil Salad, 91
  Poached Eggs on Spicy Lentils, 259
Enchiladas in Salsa Verde, 252

F

Falafel Burgers with Creamy Sesame Sauce, 117
Falafel in Pita, 115
fennel (bulb)
  Bistro Lentils with Smoked Sausage, 190
  Lamb Soup with Red Wine, Romano Beans and Chèvre, 54
  Lamb with Flageolet Gratin, 200
  Peas and Greens, 254
  Sausage-Spiked Peas 'n' Rice, 191
Firehouse Chili Soup, 53
fish. See also anchovies; seafood
  Asian Tofu Dressing (variation), 96
  Linguine with Tuna, White Beans and Dill, 209
  Salmon over White-and-Black Bean Salsa, 211
  Saucy Halibut on a Bed of Lentils, 210
Frijoles Borrachos Mexicanos, 274
fruit. See also fruit, dried; lime
  Black Bean and Bulgur Salad, 84
  Caribbean Black Bean Soup, 58
  Maple Baked Pork and Beans with Caramelized Apples, 185
  Quince-Laced Lamb Shanks with Yellow Split Peas, 198
  Roasted Vegetable Salad, 88
  Thai Red Curry Tofu with Sweet Mango and Basil, 151
fruit, dried
  Braised Lamb with Beans and Dates, 204
  Garlic Greens with Chickpeas and Cumin, 257
  Indian-Spiced Lentils with Peppery Apricots, 261
  Lentil Salad with Dried Cranberries and Pistachios, 93
  Moroccan Chickpea Tagine, 256
  Potato and Chickpea Stew with Spicy Sausage, 196
  Rice and Black Bean Stuffed Peppers, 232
  Rice and Red Lentil Pilaf with Fried Zucchini, 208
Frybread Tostadas, 110

G

garlic. See also vegetables
  Cajun-Style Tofu with Tomatoes and Okra, 220
  Chickpea Tofu Stew, 225

Garlic Greens with Chickpeas and Cumin, 257
Lentil Sloppy Joes, 258
Lentils with Spicy Sausage, 38
Lime-Spiked Turkey Chili with Pinto Beans, 138
Mediterranean-Style Braised Tofu, 224
Peas and Greens, 254
Pork and Black Bean Stew with Sweet Potatoes, 184
Quince-Laced Lamb Shanks with Yellow Split Peas, 198
Roasted Eggplant and Artichoke Dip, 35
Roasted Garlic and Lentil Soup, 71
Santorini-Style Fava Spread, 36
Smoked Oyster Hummus, 31
Tomato Dal with Spinach, 172
Two-Bean Turkey Chili, 140
White Bean with Mint, 18
ginger
Braised Roasted Pork with Tofu and Green Onions, 182
Braised Stuffed Bean Curd, 180
Moroccan Chickpea Tagine, 256
Parsi Chicken Stew with Lentils and Vegetables, 154
Soy-Braised Tofu, 224
Soy-Braised Tofu, Cabbage and Ginger with Cellophane Noodles, 265
Spicy Lamb with Chickpeas, 202
Tofu and Snow Peas in Tamarind Ginger Curry, 158
grains. See also barley; rice
Black Bean and Bulgur Salad, 84
Chickpea-Herb Burgers (variation), 116
Cracked Wheat and Lima Bean Wrap, 114
Curried Couscous with Tomatoes and Chickpeas (tip), 163
Moroccan Chickpea Tagine, 256
Tabbouleh with Lentils, 95
Wheat Berry Minestrone, 50
Greek Bean and Tomato Salad, 77
Greek Beans with Onions, 268
Greek Chili with Black Olives and Feta Cheese, 135
greens. See also greens, salad; spinach
Peas and Greens, 254
Quick Chickpea and Pasta Soup (variation), 62
Red Beans and Greens, 242
Roasted Vegetable Lasagna, 230
Wheat Berry Minestrone, 50
White Bean Soup with Swiss Chard, 44
greens, salad. See also lettuce
Grilled Corn and Lima Bean Salad, 78
Pea Tops with Pancetta and Tofu, 264
Roasted Vegetable Salad, 88
Three-Bean Tacos, 106

H
ham and ham hocks
All-in-One Pasta and Chickpea Ragoût (tip), 229
Navy Bean and Ham Soup, 51
Prairie Fire Beans, 179
Harira, 64
herbs (fresh). See also specific herbs
Chickpea-Herb Burgers, 116
Saucy Halibut on a Bed of Lentils, 210
Spiced Rice and Lentil Pilaf, 272
White Beans with Tomato, 267
White Bean with Mint, 18
Hoisin Stir-Fried Vegetables and Tofu over Rice Noodles, 216
Home-Style Pork and Beans, 187
hummus, 5, 31–34
Hummus and Sautéed Vegetable Wraps, 113
Hummus from Scratch, 32

I
Indian-Spiced Lentils with Peppery Apricots, 261
isoflavones, 13–14
Italian Bean Pasta Salad, 81

K
khichri, 234–36
Kim's Mexican Casserole, 177

L
lamb
Braised Lamb with Beans and Dates, 204
Cheater's Cassoulet, 194
Chicken Curry Baked with Lentils (variation), 153
Greek Chili with Black Olives and Feta Cheese, 135
Lamb Soup with Red Wine, Romano Beans and Chèvre, 54
Lamb with Flageolet Gratin, 200
Lamb with Lentils, 152
Parsi Chicken Stew with Lentils and Vegetables (variation), 154
Quince-Laced Lamb Shanks with Yellow Split Peas, 198
Spicy Lamb with Chickpeas, 202
leeks. See also vegetables
Bean and Sweet Potato Chili on Garlic Polenta, 147
Black Bean, Corn and Leek Frittata, 249
Corn and Rice Chowder with Parsley Persillade, 45
Hearty Potato and Leek Soup, 65
Leek-Potato-Lentil Pie, 244
Ribollita, 46
Succotash Sausage Soup, 56
legumes, 5. See also beans; lentils; peas
buying and storing, 6

cooking, 8–10
gas problem, 7
health benefits, 11–14
long-soak method, 6–7
in microwave, 7, 8
in pressure cooker, 7, 8–10
quick-soak method, 7
Lemon-Laced Butterbean Dip, 19
lentils, 5, 92. See also lentils, green or brown; lentils, red
cooking, 9, 10
Amaranth Chili, 146
Andhra Yellow Lentils with Tomatoes, 170
Basic Beans in the Slow Cooker (variation), 277
Bistro Lentils with Smoked Sausage, 190
Cajun Blackened Potato and Mung Bean Salad (variation), 89
Chicken Curry Baked with Lentils, 153
Cracked Wheat and Lima Bean Wrap (variation), 114
Grilled Mediterranean Vegetable and Lentil Salad, 90
Leek-Potato-Lentil Pie, 244
Lentil and Pancetta Antipasto, 37
Lentil Burgers with Yogurt Sauce, 122
Lentil Salad with Dried Cranberries and Pistachios, 93
Lentil Salad with Feta Cheese, 92
Lentil Shepherd's Pie, 247
Lentil Soup with Rice, 67
Lentils with Spicy Sausage, 38
Parsi Chicken Stew with Lentils and Vegetables, 154
Potato and Adzuki Latkes (variation), 255
Rajasthani Mixed Dal, 167
Roasted Garlic and Lentil Soup, 71
lentils, green or brown
Brown Lentils with Peanuts, 171
Country-Style Salted Pork with Lentils, 199
Cumin-Laced Lentils with Sun-Dried Tomatoes and Roasted Peppers, 260
Eggplant Lentil Ragoût, 262
Green Lentil Soup, 70
Indian-Spiced Lentils with Peppery Apricots, 261
Lamb with Lentils, 152
Lentils Cooked with Wine and Tomato, 271
Lentil Sloppy Joes, 258
Lentils-Rice-Spinach, 273
Marinated Lentil Salad, 94
Saucy Halibut on a Bed of Lentils, 210
Spiced Rice and Lentil Pilaf, 272
Spicy Rice, Bean and Lentil Casserole, 231
Tabbouleh with Lentils, 95

lentils, red
  Assamese Khichri, 234
  Bengali Red Lentils, 169
  Cajun Potato and Red Lentil
    Salad, 91
  Curried Squash and Red Lentil
    Soup with Coconut, 68
  Harira, 64
  Khichri with Tomatoes and
    Green Peppers, 236
  Moroccan Spiced Lentil Soup, 72
  Poached Eggs on Spicy Lentils,
    259
  Potato and Chickpea Stew with
    Spicy Sausage, 196
  Red Lentil Curry with Coconut
    and Cilantro, 168
  Rice and Red Lentil Pilaf with
    Fried Zucchini, 208
  Savory Red Lentil Soup, 69
lettuce. See also greens, salad
  Cracked Wheat and Lima Bean
    Wrap, 114
  Red Beans and Rice Soft Tacos
    with Cajun Sauce, 108
  Red Chili con Carne Soft Tacos,
    107
  Sirloin and Chorizo Frijole Tacos,
    102
  Taco Burgers, 119
  Tortilla Bean Salad with Creamy
    Salsa Dressing, 85
lime
  Chicken Baked with Black Beans
    and Lime, 205
  Lime-Spiked Turkey Chili with
    Pinto Beans, 138
  Spicy Lamb with Chickpeas, 202
  Tofu with Lime, Lemongrass and
    Coconut Curry, 164
  Two-Bean Turkey Chili, 140
  Linguine with Tuna, White Beans
    and Dill, 209

M

Make-Ahead Southwestern Pork
  Stew, 183
Manicotti Stuffed with Chickpeas
  and Cheese, 206
maple syrup
  Baked Beans 'n' Barley, 192
  Cider Baked Beans, 240
  Home-Style Pork and Beans, 187
  Maple Baked Pork and Beans
    with Caramelized Apples, 185
  Soy-Braised Tofu, 224
Marinated Lentil Salad, 94
Mediterranean Pork and Beans, 186
Mediterranean-Style Braised Tofu,
  224
milk and soy/rice milk
  Cantonese Noodles (variation),
    219
  Cheesy Beans and Hot Dogs, 203
  Corn and Rice Chowder with
    Parsley Persillade, 45
Minestrone Genovese, 48

molasses
  The Best Pork 'n' Beans, 189
  Molasses Baked Beans, 188
  Quince-Laced Lamb Shanks with
    Yellow Split Peas, 198
Moroccan Chickpea Tagine, 256
Moroccan Spiced Lentil Soup, 72
Moussaka with Tofu Topping, 222
mushrooms
  Black Bean Quesadillas, 101
  Braised Roasted Pork with Tofu
    and Green Onions, 182
  Braised Stuffed Bean Curd, 180
  Cantonese Noodles, 219
  Greek Chili with Black Olives
    and Feta Cheese, 135
  Hoisin Stir-Fried Vegetables and
    Tofu over Rice Noodles, 216
  Minestrone Genovese, 48
  Mushroom Cholent, 238
  Roasted Vegetable Lasagna, 230
  Saffron Curry Mushrooms and
    Tofu, 159
  Stuffed Veal Rolls with White
    Beans, 178
  Tofu Ratatouille, 218
  White Bean Soup with Swiss
    Chard, 44
  Wild Mushroom and Navy Bean
    Soup, 49

N

nachos, 20–22
noodles. See also pasta
  Bok Choy, Noodle and Tofu
    Soup, 40
  Cantonese Noodles, 219
  Curry-Fried Tofu Soup with
    Vegetables and Udon Noodles,
    41
  Hoisin Stir-Fried Vegetables and
    Tofu over Rice Noodles, 216
  Soy-Braised Tofu, Cabbage
    and Ginger with Cellophane
    Noodles, 265
  Teriyaki Rice Noodles with
    Veggies and Beans, 217
nuts
  Brown Lentils with Peanuts, 171
  Lentil Salad with Dried
    Cranberries and Pistachios, 93
  Rice and Black Bean Stuffed
    Peppers, 232
  Romano Bean Stew, 241

O

Oaxaca Chicken Tacos, 105
olive oil
  garlic-infused, 19
  Olive Oil Crust, 245
olives
  Cracked Wheat and Lima Bean
    Wrap, 114
  Greek Chili with Black Olives
    and Feta Cheese, 135
  Marinated Lentil Salad, 94

Mediterranean Pork and Beans,
  186
Potluck Bean and Pasta Salad, 82
onions. See also garlic; leeks;
  vegetables
  Greek Beans with Onions, 268
  Lamb with Lentils, 152
  Rice and Black Bean Stuffed
    Peppers, 232

P

pancetta. See also bacon
  Baked Beans 'n' Barley, 192
  Lentil and Pancetta Antipasto,
    37
  Lentil Soup with Rice, 67
  Pasta e Fagioli, 42
  Pea Tops with Pancetta and Tofu,
    264
  Stuffed Veal Rolls with White
    Beans, 178
Pappardelle and Chickpea Soup, 61
Parsi Chicken Stew with Lentils
  and Vegetables, 154
parsley. See also herbs
  Butter Beans and Grilled Red
    Pepper, 266
  Lentil Shepherd's Pie (tip), 247
  Mediterranean Pork and Beans,
    186
  Pork and Black Bean Stew with
    Sweet Potatoes, 184
parsnips
  Cider Baked Beans, 240
  Lamb Soup with Red Wine,
    Romano Beans and Chèvre, 54
  Mushroom Cholent, 238
  Spicy Lamb with Chickpeas, 202
pasta. See also couscous; noodles
  All-in-One Pasta and Chickpea
    Ragoût, 229
  Baked Orzo and Beans, 226
  Corn and Three-Bean Salad, 79
  Italian Bean Pasta Salad, 81
  Linguine with Tuna, White
    Beans and Dill, 209
  Manicotti Stuffed with
    Chickpeas and Cheese, 206
  Pappardelle and Chickpea Soup,
    61
  Pasta e Fagioli, 42
  Penne with Creamy White Bean
    Sauce, 227
  Potluck Bean and Pasta Salad, 82
  Quick Chickpea and Pasta Soup,
    62
  Tex-Mex Rotini Salad, 80
  Three-Cheese Creamy Pasta
    Bean Bake, 228
peas, 9, 10. See also chickpeas;
  peas, green
  Beer-Braised Chili, 132
  Black-Eyed Pea Salad with
    Tomato and Feta, 86
  Grilled Mediterranean Vegetable
    and Lentil Salad, 90
  Peas and Greens, 254

Quince-Laced Lamb Shanks with
  Yellow Split Peas, 198
Rajasthani Mixed Dal, 167
Santorini-Style Fava Spread, 36
Sausage-Spiked Peas 'n' Rice, 191
Spicy Rice, Bean and Lentil
  Casserole (tip), 231
Split Yellow Peas with Zucchini,
  166
Tomato Dal with Spinach, 172
Wild West Bean Caviar with
  Roasted Tomatoes, 27
peas, green
Assamese Khichri, 234
Bengali Khichri, 235
Bok Choy, Noodle and Tofu
  Soup, 40
Hummus and Sautéed Vegetable
  Wraps, 113
Mixed Vegetable Herb Broth with
  Soft Tofu, 43
Pea Tops with Pancetta and Tofu,
  264
Penne with Creamy White Bean
  Sauce, 227
Red Beans and Red Rice, 269
Tofu and Snow Peas in Tamarind
  Ginger Curry, 158
Penne with Creamy White Bean
  Sauce, 227
peppers, bell. See also peppers,
  roasted red; vegetables
Bok Choy, Noodle and Tofu
  Soup, 40
Butter Beans and Grilled Red
  Pepper, 266
Corn and Three-Bean Salad, 79
Hummus and Sautéed Vegetable
  Wraps, 113
Khichri with Tomatoes and
  Green Peppers, 236
Make-Ahead Southwestern Pork
  Stew, 183
Potluck Bean and Pasta Salad, 82
Rice and Black Bean Stuffed
  Peppers, 232
Roasted Vegetable Lasagna, 230
peppers, chipotle
Beer-Braised Chili, 132
Black Bean and Corn Salsa Mini
  Tostadas with Chipotle Sour
  Cream, 28
Black Bean and Roasted Corn
  Salsa, 29
Black Bean Chipotle Dip, 30
Creamy Chipotle Black Bean
  Burrito Bake, 250
Hominy and Red Bean Chili,
  142
peppers, green chile (mild)
Andhra Yellow Lentils with
  Tomatoes, 170
Assamese Khichri, 234
Baked Shrimp Enchiladas, 212
Bengali Red Lentils, 169
Lamb with Lentils, 152
Lime-Spiked Turkey Chili with
  Pinto Beans, 138

Oven-Fried Beef and Bean
  Chimichangas, 103
Rajasthani Mixed Dal, 167
Refried Nachos, 21
Split Yellow Peas with Zucchini,
  166
peppers, hot. See also peppers,
  chipotle; peppers, jalapeño
Black Bean, Butternut Squash
  and Poblano Chile Soup, 59
Black Bean Chili, 147
Black Bean Nachos, 20
Butternut Chili, 134
Cajun Black Spice, 98
Caribbean Chickpea Curry with
  Potatoes, 161
Caribbean Curried Beef and
  Chickpeas, 150
Caribbean Red Bean, Spinach
  and Potato Curry, 162
Chicken, Pinto Beans and Green
  Chile Soup, 60
Chili con Carne Pronto
  (variation), 133
Chunky Black Bean Chili, 124
Curried Squash and Red Lentil
  Soup with Coconut, 68
Easy Chicken Tacos (variation),
  104
Easy Vegetable Chili, 144
Frijoles Borrachos Mexicanos,
  274
Not-Too-Corny Turkey Chili with
  Sausage, 136
Parsi Chicken Stew with Lentils
  and Vegetables, 154
Pico de Gallo, 29
Poached Eggs on Spicy Lentils,
  259
Pork and Beef Chili with Ancho
  Sauce, 126
Punjabi Creamy Yellow Mung
  Beans, 165
Red Chili with Anchos, 128
Red Lentil Curry with Coconut
  and Cilantro (variation), 168
Tex-Mex Chili, 127
Tofu in Indian-Spiced Tomato
  Sauce, 223
peppers, jalapeño
Beyond Bean Dip, 23
Black Bean and Rice Salad, 83
Black Bean Chili with Hominy
  and Sweet Corn, 145
Cabbage, Bean and Bacon
  Chowder, 52
Enchiladas in Salsa Verde
  (variation), 252
Oaxaca Chicken Tacos, 105
Romano Bean Stew, 241
Sausage and Black Bean Chili,
  131
Southwest Butternut Squash
  Tortilla Bake, 251
Spicy Bean Dip, 25
Three-Bean Tacos, 106
Wild West Bean Caviar with
  Roasted Tomatoes, 27

Zesty Black Bean Pie (variation),
  248
peppers, roasted red, 26
Chickpea and Roasted Pepper
  Salad, 84
Cumin-Laced Lentils with Sun-
  Dried Tomatoes and Roasted
  Peppers, 260
Easy Chicken Tacos, 104
Falafel in Pita (variation), 115
Red Pepper Hummus, 31
Smoked Oyster Hummus, 31
Southwestern Bean and Barley
  Salad with Roasted Peppers, 87
Zesty Black Bean Pie (variation),
  248
Pico de Gallo, 29
pita breads
Falafel in Pita, 115
Pita Chips, 17
Refried Nachos (variation), 21
pork
Beer-Braised Chili, 132
The Best Pork 'n' Beans, 189
Braised Roasted Pork with Tofu
  and Green Onions, 182
Braised Stuffed Bean Curd, 180
Cheater's Cassoulet, 194
Chicken Tortillas (tip), 109
Country-Style Salted Pork with
  Lentils, 199
Home-Style Pork and Beans, 187
Make-Ahead Southwestern Pork
  Stew, 183
Mediterranean Pork and Beans,
  186
Pork and Beef Chili with Ancho
  Sauce, 126
Pork and Black Bean Stew with
  Sweet Potatoes, 184
Red Chili with Anchos, 128
potatoes. See also vegetables
Amaranth Chili, 146
Assamese Khichri, 234
Best-Ever Cholent, 176
Cabbage, Bean and Bacon
  Chowder, 52
Cajun Blackened Potato and
  Mung Bean Salad, 89
Cajun Potato and Red Lentil
  Salad, 91
Caribbean Chickpea Curry with
  Potatoes, 161
Caribbean Red Bean, Spinach
  and Potato Curry, 162
Coconut Curried Chickpea Soup,
  66
Enchiladas in Salsa Verde, 252
Hearty Potato and Leek Soup,
  65
Leek-Potato-Lentil Pie, 244
Lentil Shepherd's Pie, 247
Potato and Adzuki Latkes, 255
Potato and Chickpea Stew with
  Spicy Sausage, 196
Pyaza Paneer and Navy Bean
  Curry, 160
Southwestern Shepherd's Pie, 174

potatoes (*continued*)
 Vegetarian Shepherd's Pie with
  Peppered Potato Topping, 246
Potluck Bean and Pasta Salad, 82
Prairie Fire Beans, 179
Pumpkin and Black Beans, 270
Punjabi Creamy Yellow Mung
 Beans, 165
Pyaza Paneer and Navy Bean
 Curry, 160

Q

Quick Cassoulet, 193
Quick Chickpea and Pasta Soup, 62
Quick Refried Beans, 276
Quince-Laced Lamb Shanks with
 Yellow Split Peas, 198

R

Rajasthani Mixed Dal, 167
Red Chili con Carne Soft Tacos, 107
Red Chili with Anchos, 128
Red Hot Hummus, 33
Red Pepper Hummus, 31
Red Wine Vinaigrette, 97
Refried Nachos, 21
Ribollita, 46
rice. *See also* grains
 Assamese Khichri, 234
 Bengali Khichri, 235
 Black Bean and Rice Salad, 83
 Chicken Curry Baked with
  Lentils (variation), 153
 Corn and Rice Chowder with
  Parsley Persillade, 45
 Khichri with Tomatoes and
  Green Peppers, 236
 Lentil Soup with Rice, 67
 Lentils-Rice-Spinach, 273
 Minestrone Genovese, 48
 Red Beans and Red Rice, 269
 Red Beans and Rice Soft Tacos
  with Cajun Sauce, 108
 Rice and Black Bean Stuffed
  Peppers, 232
 Rice and Red Lentil Pilaf with
  Fried Zucchini, 208
 Roasted Garlic and Lentil Soup,
  71
 Sausage-Spiked Peas 'n' Rice, 191
 Spiced Rice and Lentil Pilaf, 272
 Spicy Rice, Bean and Lentil
  Casserole, 231

S

Saffron Curry Mushrooms and
 Tofu, 159
salads, 74–95
Salmon over White-and-Black Bean
 Salsa, 211
salsa, 16, 20
salsa (as ingredient)
 Black Bean and Corn Salsa Mini
  Tostadas with Chipotle Sour
  Cream, 28

Chicken Enchilada Casserole
 with Teriyaki Sauce, 112
Creamy Chipotle Black Bean
 Burrito Bake, 250
Enchiladas in Salsa Verde, 252
Refried Nachos, 21
Slow Cooker Black Bean and
 Salsa Dip, 26
Southwest Bread Pudding, 253
Spicy Rice, Bean and Lentil
 Casserole, 231
Taco Burgers, 119
Warm Mexican Layered Dip, 24
Zesty Black Bean Pie, 248
sandwiches and wraps, 100–116
Santorini-Style Fava Spread, 36
sausage, 131
 All-in-One Pasta and Chickpea
  Ragoût (tip), 229
 Bistro Lentils with Smoked
  Sausage, 190
 Black Bean and Bulgur Salad, 84
 Black Bean and Sausage Gumbo,
  57
 Cheater's Cassoulet, 194
 Cheesy Beans and Hot Dogs, 203
 Chicken and Black Bean Chili
  (variation), 139
 Chicken Baked with Black Beans
  and Lime, 205
 Chickpea Soup with Chorizo and
  Garlic, 63
 Firehouse Chili Soup (variation),
  53
 Grande Beef Nachos (variation),
  22
 Lentils with Spicy Sausage, 38
 Not-Too-Corny Turkey Chili with
  Sausage, 136
 Pork and Beef Chili with Ancho
  Sauce, 126
 Potato and Chickpea Stew with
  Spicy Sausage, 196
 Quick Cassoulet, 193
 Red Beans and Red Rice
  (variation), 269
 Sausage and Black Bean Chili,
  131
 Sausage-Spiked Peas 'n' Rice, 191
 Sirloin and Chorizo Frijole Tacos,
  102
 Stuffed Veal Rolls with White
  Beans, 178
 Succotash Sausage Soup, 56
seafood. *See also* fish
 Baked Shrimp Enchiladas, 212
 Bok Choy, Noodle and Tofu Soup
  (tip), 40
 Easy Tostadas (variation), 111
 Smoked Oyster Hummus, 31
 Steamed Shrimp-Stuffed Tofu
  with Broccoli, 214
 Tuscan Shrimp and Beans, 213
Sesame Tofu Vinaigrette, 95
snow peas. *See* peas, green
soups, 39–72
sour cream
 Beyond Bean Dip, 23

Black Bean and Corn Salsa Mini
 Tostadas with Chipotle Sour
 Cream, 28
Cracked Wheat and Lima Bean
 Wrap (variation), 114
Creamy Chipotle Black Bean
 Burrito Bake, 250
Southwest Bread Pudding, 253
Three-Cheese Creamy Pasta
 Bean Bake, 228
Warm Mexican Layered Dip, 24
Southwest Bread Pudding, 253
Southwest Butternut Squash
 Tortilla Bake, 251
Southwestern Bean and Barley
 Salad with Roasted Peppers, 87
Southwestern Shepherd's Pie, 174
Soy-Braised Tofu, 224
Soy-Braised Tofu, Cabbage and
 Ginger with Cellophane
 Noodles, 265
Spiced Rice and Lentil Pilaf, 272
Spicy Bean Dip, 25
Spicy Black Bean Gazpacho, 55
Spicy Lamb with Chickpeas, 202
Spicy Rice, Bean and Lentil
 Casserole, 231
spinach. *See also* greens
 Cantonese Noodles, 219
 Caribbean Red Bean, Spinach
  and Potato Curry, 162
 Coconut Curried Chickpea Soup,
  66
 Enchiladas in Salsa Verde, 252
 Garlic Greens with Chickpeas
  and Cumin, 257
 Leek-Potato-Lentil Pie, 244
 Lentils Cooked with Wine and
  Tomato, 271
 Lentils-Rice-Spinach, 273
 Punjabi Creamy Yellow Mung
  Beans, 165
 Tomato Dal with Spinach, 172
spirits. *See also* beer; wine
 Frijoles Borrachos Mexicanos,
  274
 Maple Baked Pork and Beans
  with Caramelized Apples, 185
squash. *See also* zucchini
 Black Bean, Butternut Squash
  and Poblano Chile Soup, 59
 Butternut Chili, 134
 Curried Squash and Red Lentil
  Soup with Coconut, 68
 Hominy and Red Bean Chili, 142
 Moroccan Chickpea Tagine, 256
 Parsi Chicken Stew with Lentils
  and Vegetables, 154
 Pumpkin and Black Beans, 270
 Southwest Butternut Squash
  Tortilla Bake, 251
 Very Veggie Chili (variation), 143
Steamed Shrimp-Stuffed Tofu with
 Broccoli, 214
Stove-Top Refried Beans, 276
Stuffed Veal Rolls with White
 Beans, 178
Succotash Sausage Soup, 56

Succulent Succotash, 237
sweet potatoes
Bean and Sweet Potato Chili on
Garlic Polenta, 147
Indian-Spiced Lentils with
Peppery Apricots, 261
Moroccan Chickpea Tagine, 256
Pork and Black Bean Stew with
Sweet Potatoes, 184
Pumpkin and Black Beans
(variation), 270
Vegetarian Shepherd's Pie with
Peppered Potato Topping (tip),
246

T

Tabbouleh with Lentils, 95
Taco Burgers, 119
taco shells
Easy Chicken Tacos, 104
Refried Nachos (variation), 21
tamarind
Brown Lentils with Peanuts, 171
Tofu and Snow Peas in Tamarind
Ginger Curry, 158
Teriyaki Rice Noodles with Veggies
and Beans, 217
Tex-Mex Chili, 127
Tex-Mex Rotini Salad, 80
Thai Dry Vegetable Curry, 156
Thai Red Curry Tofu with Sweet
Mango and Basil, 151
tofu, 5, 10, 13–14. See also specific
types (below)
tofu, firm or medium
Bok Choy, Noodle and Tofu
Soup, 40
Braised Stuffed Bean Curd, 180
Cajun-Style Tofu with Tomatoes
and Okra, 220
Cantonese Noodles, 219
Chickpea Tofu Burgers with
Cilantro Mayonnaise, 118
Chickpea Tofu Stew, 225
Cuban-Style Tofu Sandwich, 100
Curry-Fried Tofu Soup with
Vegetables and Udon Noodles,
41
Hoisin Stir-Fried Vegetables and
Tofu over Rice Noodles, 216
Make-Ahead Southwestern Pork
Stew (tip), 183
Mediterranean-Style Braised
Tofu, 224
Moussaka with Tofu Topping,
222
Pea Tops with Pancetta and Tofu,
264
Pyaza Paneer and Navy Bean
Curry (variation), 160
Saffron Curry Mushrooms and
Tofu, 159
Soy-Braised Tofu, 224
Soy-Braised Tofu, Cabbage
and Ginger with Cellophane
Noodles, 265
Thai Dry Vegetable Curry, 156

Thai Red Curry Tofu with Sweet
Mango and Basil, 151
Tofu and Snow Peas in Tamarind
Ginger Curry, 158
Tofu in Indian-Spiced Tomato
Sauce, 223
Tofu Ratatouille, 218
Tofu with Lime, Lemongrass and
Coconut Curry, 164
tofu, soft or silken
Asian Tofu Dressing, 96
Braised Roasted Pork with Tofu
and Green Onions, 182
Mixed Vegetable Herb Broth with
Soft Tofu, 43
Sesame Tofu Vinaigrette, 95
Steamed Shrimp-Stuffed Tofu
with Broccoli, 214
Tofu Mayonnaise, 97
tomatoes. See also tomatoes, sun-
dried; tomato sauces; vegetables
All-in-One Pasta and Chickpea
Ragoût, 229
Amaranth Chili, 146
Andhra Yellow Lentils with
Tomatoes, 170
Bean and Sweet Potato Chili on
Garlic Polenta, 147
Bengali Red Lentils (variation),
169
Black Bean Chili, 147
Black Bean Chili with Hominy
and Sweet Corn, 145
Black Bean Nachos, 20
Black-Eyed Pea Salad with
Tomato and Feta, 86
Butter Beans and Grilled Red
Pepper, 266
Butternut Chili, 134
Cajun-Style Tofu with Tomatoes
and Okra, 220
Chickpea Tofu Stew, 225
Chunky Black Bean Chili, 124
Cracked Wheat and Lima Bean
Wrap, 114
Curried Couscous with Tomatoes
and Chickpeas, 163
Curried Squash and Red Lentil
Soup with Coconut, 68
Easy Chili con Carne, 130
Greek Bean and Tomato Salad,
77
Greek Chili with Black Olives
and Feta Cheese, 135
Harira, 64
Hominy and Red Bean Chili, 142
Italian Bean Pasta Salad, 81
Khichri with Tomatoes and
Green Peppers, 236
Lamb Soup with Red Wine,
Romano Beans and Chèvre, 54
Lamb with Lentils, 152
Lentil Salad with Feta Cheese, 92
Lentils Cooked with Wine and
Tomato, 271
Lentil Shepherd's Pie, 247
Make-Ahead Southwestern Pork
Stew, 183

Moroccan Spiced Lentil Soup, 72
Not-Too-Corny Turkey Chili with
Sausage, 136
Paneer with Chickpeas in
Creamy Tomato Curry, 157
Parsi Chicken Stew with Lentils
and Vegetables, 154
Pasta e Fagioli, 42
Pico de Gallo, 29
Poached Eggs on Spicy Lentils,
259
Pork and Beef Chili with Ancho
Sauce, 126
Rajasthani Mixed Dal, 167
Red Chili with Anchos, 128
Roasted Garlic and Lentil Soup,
71
Salmon over White-and-Black
Bean Salsa, 211
Savory Red Lentil Soup, 69
Spicy Black Bean Gazpacho, 55
Spicy Lamb with Chickpeas, 202
Succulent Succotash, 237
Tex-Mex Rotini Salad, 80
Tofu in Indian-Spiced Tomato
Sauce, 223
Tofu Ratatouille, 218
Tomato Dal with Spinach, 172
Tomatoes Stuffed with Corn,
Black Beans and Pine Nuts,
275
Tuscan Shrimp and Beans, 213
Tuscan White Bean and Tomato
Salad, 74
Two-Bean Turkey Chili, 140
Wagon Boss Chili, 129
White Bean Salad with Lemon-
Dill Vinaigrette, 75
White Beans with Tomato, 267
Wild West Bean Caviar with
Roasted Tomatoes, 27
tomatoes, sun-dried
Cumin-Laced Lentils with Sun-
Dried Tomatoes and Roasted
Peppers, 260
Moroccan Chickpea Tagine, 256
Red Hot Hummus, 33
Santorini-Style Fava Spread, 36
Southwestern Bean and Barley
Salad with Roasted Peppers, 87
tomato sauces (as ingredient). See
also salsa
Baked Beans 'n' Barley, 192
Baked Shrimp Enchiladas, 212
Beans, Beef and Biscuits, 174
Cheater's Cassoulet, 194
Chicken and Black Bean Chili,
139
Chicken Tortillas, 109
Chili con Carne Pronto, 133
Home-Style Pork and Beans, 187
Leek-Potato-Lentil Pie, 244
Lime-Spiked Turkey Chili with
Pinto Beans, 138
Molasses Baked Beans, 188
Moussaka with Tofu Topping,
222
Pork 'n' Beans, The Best, 189

tomato sauces (as ingredient)
(*continued*)
  Sausage and Black Bean Chili,
    131
  Three-Cheese Creamy Pasta
    Bean Bake, 228
  20-Minute Chili, 125
  Vegetarian Shepherd's Pie with
    Peppered Potato Topping, 246
  Very Veggie Chili, 143
tortilla chips
  Black Bean Nachos, 20
  Grande Beef Nachos, 22
  Tortilla Bean Salad with Creamy
    Salsa Dressing, 85
tortillas
  Baked Shrimp Enchiladas, 212
  Black Bean Quesadillas, 101
  Caribbean Chickpea Curry with
    Potatoes (variation), 161
  Chicken Enchilada Casserole
    with Teriyaki Sauce, 112
  Chicken Tortillas, 109
  Cracked Wheat and Lima Bean
    Wrap, 114
  Creamy Chipotle Black Bean
    Burrito Bake, 250
  Easy Tostadas, 111
  Enchiladas in Salsa Verde, 252
  Hummus and Sautéed Vegetable
    Wraps, 113
  Kim's Mexican Casserole, 177
  Oaxaca Chicken Tacos, 105
  Oven-Fried Beef and Bean
    Chimichangas, 103
  Red Beans and Rice Soft Tacos
    with Cajun Sauce, 108
  Red Chili con Carne Soft Tacos,
    107
  Sirloin and Chorizo Frijole Tacos,
    102
  Southwest Bread Pudding
    (variation), 253
  Southwest Butternut Squash
    Tortilla Bake, 251
  Three-Bean Tacos, 106
turkey. *See also* chicken
  Firehouse Chili Soup (variation),
    53

  Lime-Spiked Turkey Chili with
    Pinto Beans, 138
  Not-Too-Corny Turkey Chili with
    Sausage, 136
  20-Minute Chili, 125
  Two-Bean Turkey Chili, 140
  Warm Mexican Layered Dip, 24
Tuscan Shrimp and Beans, 213
Tuscan White Bean and Tomato
    Salad, 74
20-Minute Chili, 125

V

veal
  Chicken Tortillas (tip), 109
  Stuffed Veal Rolls with White
    Beans, 178
vegetables (mixed). *See also specific
    vegetables*
  Bistro Lentils with Smoked
    Sausage, 190
  Cabbage, Bean and Bacon
    Chowder, 52
  Cajun-Style Tofu with Tomatoes
    and Okra, 220
  Cider Baked Beans, 240
  Curry-Fried Tofu Soup with
    Vegetables and Udon Noodles,
    41
  Easy Vegetable Chili, 144
  Grilled Mediterranean Vegetable
    and Lentil Salad, 90
  Hoisin Stir-Fried Vegetables and
    Tofu over Rice Noodles, 216
  Minestrone Genovese, 48
  Mixed Vegetable Herb Broth with
    Soft Tofu, 43
  Mushroom Cholent, 238
  Roasted Vegetable Hummus, 34
  Roasted Vegetable Salad, 88
  Thai Dry Vegetable Curry, 156
  Tofu Ratatouille, 218
  Vegetable Tamale Pie, 243
  Vegetarian Chili, 141
  Vegetarian Shepherd's Pie with
    Peppered Potato Topping, 246
  Very Veggie Chili, 143
  Wheat Berry Minestrone, 50

W

Wagon Boss Chili, 129
Warm Mexican Layered Dip, 24
Wild Mushroom and Navy Bean
    Soup, 49
Wild West Bean Caviar with
    Roasted Tomatoes, 27
wine
  Cheater's Cassoulet, 194
  Country-Style Salted Pork with
    Lentils, 199
  Lamb Soup with Red Wine,
    Romano Beans and Chèvre,
    54
  Lentils Cooked with Wine and
    Tomato, 271
  Mediterranean Pork and Beans,
    186
  Pork and Black Bean Stew with
    Sweet Potatoes, 184

Y

yogurt
  Cajun Sauce, 108
  Chicken Curry Baked with
    Lentils, 153
  Cilantro-Yogurt Sauce, 122
  Cracked Wheat and Lima Bean
    Wrap, 114
  Yogurt Cheese, 98

Z

Zesty Black Bean Pie, 248
zucchini. *See also* vegetables
  All-in-One Pasta and Chickpea
    Ragoût, 229
  Chickpea Soup with Chorizo and
    Garlic, 63
  Coconut Curried Chickpea Soup,
    66
  Greek Chili with Black Olives
    and Feta Cheese, 135
  Rice and Red Lentil Pilaf with
    Fried Zucchini, 208
  Split Yellow Peas with Zucchini,
    166

Library and Archives Canada Cataloguing in Publication

250 best beans, lentils & tofu recipes : healthy, wholesome foods.

Includes index.
ISBN 978-0-7788-0416-1

1. Cooking (Beans). 2. Cooking (Lentils). 3. Cooking (Tofu). 4. Cookbooks.
I. Title: Two hundred fifty best beans, lentils & tofu recipes.

TX803.B4T86 2012   641.6'565   C2012-902817-7